AF602087

Transforming Rural Areas through
Veterinary Science

The Editors

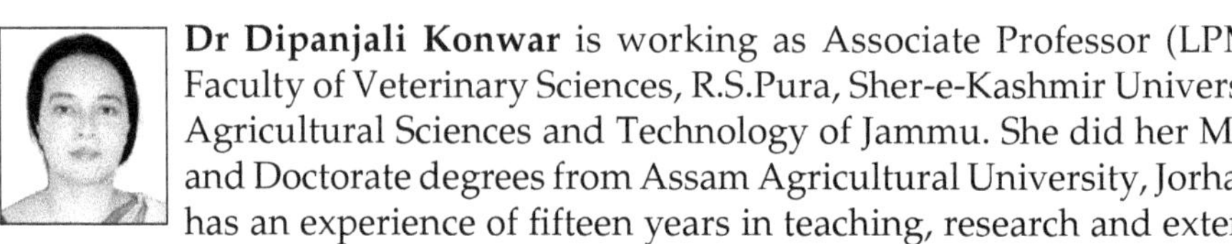

Dr Dipanjali Konwar is working as Associate Professor (LPM), in Faculty of Veterinary Sciences, R.S.Pura, Sher-e-Kashmir University of Agricultural Sciences and Technology of Jammu. She did her Masters and Doctorate degrees from Assam Agricultural University, Jorhat. She has an experience of fifteen years in teaching, research and extension. Presently she is working on managemental practices for enhancing productivity in livestock. She has been more than fifty publications to her credit, which includes research papers, technical bulletins, extension folders, & practical manuals.

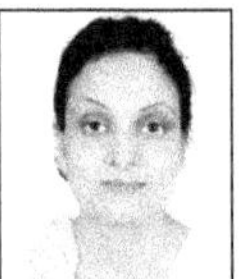

Dr Shilpa Sood is working as Associate Professor (Veterinary Pathology), in Faculty of Veterinary Sciences, R.S. Pura, Sher-e-Kashmir University of Agricultural Sciences and Technology of Jammu. She did her Master's from Hisar Agriculture University and Doctorate degree from Tennessee, USA. She has an experience of fifteen years in teaching, research and extension. Presently she is working on disease diagnostics of Livestock and Poultry. She has been more than fifty publications to her credit, which includes research papers, technical bulletins, extension folders, & practical manuals.

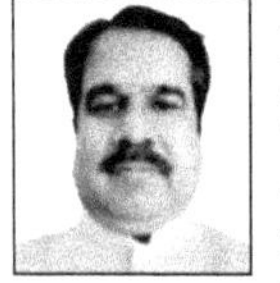

Dr Shahid Ahamad presently working as Chief Scientist/Associate Director Research at Directorate of Research in Sher-e-Kashmir University of Agricultural Sciences & Technology of Jammu (Chatha) J.&K. Earlier he served as Jr. Scientist (Plant Pathology), Sr. Scientist/ Programme Coordinator in KVKs and Dy. Director Research. He is also working as Nodal Officer, PME Cell. His research interests are plant diseases management, maize pathology, organic crop production and research management. He has been published more than two hundred publications in national and international reputed journals/magazines/News papers etc. including ten books in different aspects of agriculture/ plant pathology. He is having twenty years of experience in research, extension and teaching activities in the field of plant pathology in general and agriculture in particular.

Transforming Rural Areas through
Veterinary Science

– Editors –

Dipanjali Konwar
Shilpa Sood
Shahid Ahamad

2019
Daya Publishing House®
A Division of
Astral International Pvt. Ltd.
New Delhi – 110 002

ISBN: 9789389569186 (Int. Edition)

Published by : Daya Publishing House®
A Division of
Astral International Pvt. Ltd.
– ISO 9001:2015 Certified Company –
4736/23, Ansari Road, Darya Ganj
New Delhi-110 002
Ph. 011-43549197, 23278134
E-mail: info@astralint.com
Website: www.astralint.com

Preface

A recent survey by the Economist revealed that the world population has increased by 90 per cent in the past 40 years while food production has increased only by 25 per cent per head. With an additional 1.5 billion mouths to feed by 2020, farmers worldwide have to produce 39 per cent more. The new millennium promises excitement and hope for the future by new advancement in agriculture research. Doubling farmers' income by 2022 is the mission of Government of India. Hence Indian agriculture awaits for transformation through innovative technological interventions.

There has been a long felt need for a book exclusively on the "Socio-Economic Transformation in Rural Areas through Innovative Veterinary Technologies and Animal Husbandry Practices". An effort has been made to collect information on various aspects of veterinary sciences *viz.* Transformation of rural areas through modern dairy farming, strategies to raise income by small ruminants rearing in the hilly areas, transforming rural livelihoods through scientific dairying and dairy entrepreneurship, commercial broiler chicken farming ,giant freshwater prawn farming, utilization of animal by-products, mitigation of climatic stress and technologies to reduce greenhouse gas emissions from livestock, conservation of animal genetic resources, livestock sector contribution and challenges in Indian agricultural system, major constraints and strategies for milk production in hilly and kandi areas of Jammu, Common diseases of Cattle, Recent trends for teat and udder surgery in ruminants, edible vaccines, Constraints and Strategies for Chevon Production, Pig Farming as an Emerging Enterprise, Constraints and Strategies for Mutton & Wool Production in Hilly and Kandi areas of Jammu & Kashmir, etc. Chapters in this book have been contributed by noted Veterinary Scientists.

We are grateful and indebted to all the learned galaxy of contributors who have spent their considerable time in contributing the chapters on various important aspects of animal science and solicit their cooperation in future also.

A deep sense of respect and gratitude to Prof. Pradeep K. Sharma, Hon'ble Vice Chancellor, SKUAST-JAMMU, Dr.J.P.Sharma, Director Research, Dr. Deepak Kher, Director, Planning & Monitoring, Dr.R.K.Arora, ADE & I/c KVKs for their technical guidance and help in bringing out this book. We feel that this book shall find use with the researchers, policy makers and useful for veterinary, fisheries and agriculture students and other stake-holders in Indian agriculture.

Last but not the least, we must acknowledge and oblige the M/S Astral Publishing House, New Delhi who has been always considerate and positive to our contentions and efforts. Services of M/S Astral Publishers to the academic world are pure, socialistic and commendable. We look forward that this book will be made available to teachers, scientists, students and other stake holders at reasonable and economic price.

Dr. Dipanjali Konwar

Dr. Shilpa Sood

Dr. Shahid Ahamad

List of Contributors

Dr. Suraj A. Amrutkar Assistant Professor, Poultry Science, Division of ILFC, F.V.Sc. & A.H., SKUAST-J, R.S.Pura, Jammu	Dr. M. Rashid Associate Professor, Division of VPHE, , F.V.Sc. & A.H., SKUAST-J, R.S.Pura, Jammu
Dr. Pranav Kumar Assistant Professor, Division of VAHEE, , F.V.Sc. & A.H., SKUAST-J, R.S.Pura, Jammu	Dr. Amit Mandal College of Fisheries, GADVASU, Ludhiana
Dr. Amandeep Singh Division VAHEE, , F.V.Sc. & A.H., SKUAST-J, R.S.Pura, Jammu	Dr. Prem Kumar Scientist, KVK, Jammu SKUAST-J, R.S.Pura
Dr. Akhil Gupta Scientist, FSRC, SKUAST-J, Chatha	Dr. Sahar Masud Assoc. Professor, FSRC, SKUAST-J, Chatha
Dr. Raj Kumar Scientist, FSRC, SKUAST-J, Chatha	Dr. Anil k. Taku Professor & Head, Division VMC, , F.V.Sc. & A.H., SKUAST-J, R.S.Pura, Jammu
Dr. Nawab Nashiruddullah Professor & Head, Division VPP, FVSc& AH, SKUAST-J, R.S.Pura	Dr. JafrinAra Ahmed Associate Professor, Division VP& B, , F.V.Sc. & A.H., SKUAST-J, R.S.Pura, Jammu

Dr. Asma Khan Professor & Head, Division LPM, , F.V.Sc. & A.H., SKUAST-J, R.S.Pura, Jammu	Dr. Dhirendra Kumar Assistant Professor, Division AGB, FVSc& AH, SKUAST-J, R.S.Pura
Dr. Surinder K. Gupta Professor & University Librarian, Division Veterinary Medicine, F.V.Sc. & A.H., SKUAST-J, R.S.Pura, Jammu	Dr. Nazam Khan Assistant Professor, Animal Nutrition, Division ILFC, F.V.Sc. & A.H., SKUAST-J, R.S.Pura, Jammu
Dr. Dipanjali Konwar Associate Professor, Division LPM, , F.V.Sc. & A.H., SKUAST-J, R.S.Pura, Jammu	Dr. Vikas Mahajan Assistant Professor, Animal Genetics, Division ILFC, , F.V.Sc. & A.H., SKUAST-J, R.S.Pura, Jammu
Dr. Biswajit Brahma Associate Professor, Division LPM, FVSc& AH, SKUAST-J, R.S.Pura	Dr. A. K. Pandey Assistant Professor, Division VGO, F.V.Sc. & A.H., SKUAST-J, R.S.Pura, Jammu
Dr. S. A. Khandi Assistant Professor, Division VAHEE, F.V.Sc. & A.H., SKUAST-J, R.S.Pura, Jammu	Dr. Rajesh Katoch Professor & Head, Division VPA, F.V.Sc. & A.H., SKUAST-J, R.S.Pura, Jammu
Dr. AnishYadav Professor & ICAR National Fellow, Division of VPA, F.V.Sc. & A.H., SKUAST-J, R.S.Pura, Jammu	Dr. Rajesh Godara Assistant Professor, Division VPA, , F.V.Sc. & A.H., SKUAST-J, R.S.Pura, Jammu
Dr. Sanjay Agarwal Assistant Professor, Division VGO,F.V.Sc. & A.H., SKUAST-J, R.S.Pura, Jammu	Dr. Utsav Sharma Professor & Head, Division VGO, F.V.Sc. & A.H., SKUAST-J, R.S.Pura, Jammu
Dr. Rakjshan Jeelani F.V.Sc. & A.H., Division of LPM SKUAST-J, R.S.Pura, Jammu	Dr. Mir Mudasir F.V.Sc. & A.H., Division VGO SKUAST-J, R.S.Pura, Jammu
Dr. Md. Moin Ansari Assoc. Prof. F.V.Sc. & A.H., SKUAST-K, Suhama, Srinagar, Kashmir, J.&K.	Dr. Rajan Sharma F.V.Sc. & A.H., SKUAST-J, R.S.Pura, Jammu
Dr. Shafiya Imtiaz Rafiqui F.V.Sc. & A.H., Division of VPA SKUAST-J, R.S.Pura, Jammu	Dr. Pallavi Khajuria F.V.Sc. & A.H., SKUAST-J, R.S.Pura, Jammu
Dr. Shiv Kumar Sharma Scientist Krishi Vigyan Kendra, Kashipu	Dr. Shahid Ahamad Chief Scientist/Associate Director Research Directorate of Research, SKUAST-Jammu

Contents

Transforming Rural Areas through Veterinary Science *Pages* **1–14**
Editor: Dipanjali Konwar, Shilpa Sood & Shahid Ahamad
Published by: **ASTRAL INTERNATIONAL PVT. LTD., NEW DELHI**

1 Socio-Economic Transformation of Rural Areas through Modern Dairy Farming

Dr. M. Rashid & Dr. Asma Khan

Introduction

Farming with innovative technology is a major key in transformation. The forces of transformation are many and widespread such as increased quality, safety and traceability demands of processors and consumers of food products, implementation of information and process control technologies that facilitate biological manufacturing of crop and livestock products, adoption of technologies and business practices that exploit economies of size, opting leasing and other outsourcing strategies to promote growth and control expansion of resource, strategic alliance and cooperative business models to facilitate more effective and efficient vertical coordination in the production/distribution linkages. Both the livestock and grain sectors are changing from small scale business to larger businesses.

This chapter describes the fundamental drivers of structural change in dairy farming by describing innovative farming operations developing in India that appear to be leading and shaping the industry, which can also paves the way in Jammu & Kashmir state for enhance productivity.

The first driver of management system is **Heading** which includes, housing, health and hygiene. For efficient management of cattle housing should be well planned and adequate. Improper planning in the management of animal housing may result in additional labour charges and thus reduce the profit of the farmer. During construction of a house for dairy cattle, care should be taken to provide comfortable accommodation for individual cattle. Full importance should also be given to the proper sanitation, durability and ventilation, arrangement for the production of clean milk under convenient and economic conditions.

So while discussing the housing for dairy cattle, the first question arises is that why do we house dairy cattle?

There are probability three main reasons namely:

1. To protect the dairy cows from extremes of environment. The talk of extremes of weather conditions is true in our country. This stress from environment should be avoided so that animals may remain healthy, comfortable and produce full and reproduce to their maximum capacity.
2. To control and thereby maximize nutrient intake and production.
3. To Protect pastures from the effect of large number of cows regularly wailing over wetland, an event which would seriously damage the sward and depress grassland production in the following year.

User Friendly

Housing system must be designed to be convenient and user friendly for both cows and herdsman. If the system is difficult to manage, the herdsman have less time to look after the cows and to carry out the basic, but important daily task which differentiate a good herdsman from a bad one. In addition if the stockman has spent a frustrating day repairing and outdated piece of equipment which should have been replaced long ago. It's not unnatural that, by the milking time temper will be frayed and patience in handling cows will be seriously reduced. So, housing brings man and cows into a very close association and this can be beneficial like any other close relationship.

Location of Dairy Building

The points which should be before the erection of dairy building are as follows:

1. Topography and drainage
2. Soil Type
3. Exposure to sun and protection from winds.
4. Accessibility
5. Durability and attractiveness
6. Water supply
7. Surroundings
8. Labor
9. Marketing
10. Electricity
11. Facilities and food.

Types of Housing Systems

There are three types of animal houses. These are:

1. Conventional Housing System
   a. Tail to tail type of housing system
   b. Face to face type of housing system
2. Loose Housing System
3. Semi-loose Housing system.

Table 1. Comparative Housing Requirement of Different Animals

	Poultry	*Pigs*	*Ruminants*	*Horses*
Shelter	Yes	Yes	Yes	Yes
Controlled Temp.	Yes	Yes	No	No
Controlled Light	Yes	No	No	No
Wind Proof	Yes	Yes	Yes	Yes
Draught Proof	Yes	Yes	Yes	Yes
Only in Environment controlled House	Yes	No	No	No
Rain Proof	Yes	Yes	Yes	Yes
Free from Condensation	Yes	Yes	Yes	Yes

New Techniques in Cattle Housing

A) Cubical Design

The design of a resting area which is essentially the cubical is very important to the well being of a cow. Inadequate bed length and hard beds are the main reasons why some cows refuse to use cubical.

1. The design of the cubical should be based on the cow weight, chest girth and diagonal body length.

Cow Body Weight (kg)	375	425	475	525	575	625	675	725	775	825
Clear Cubical Length (m)	2	2.04	2.08	2.12	2.16	2.20	2.24	2.28	2.30	2.33
Clear Cubical Length (m)	1.10	1.10	1.0	1.20	1.20	1.20	1.20	1.20	1.20	1.20

2. The cow's body weight should be based on the average body weights of the largest cow.
3. Forward space should be provided for rising movement. The Dutch, "comfort type" allows a cow good head space when its moves forward to rise on its hind legs (Fig.1)
4. There should not be side restriction in the pelvic region which will help in reducing the risk of injury when the cow is lying down or rising.

5. The concrete floor of the cubicles should be well bedded. By doing so the animal will feel comfortable and use cubicle for more time. It's better to use soft carpet type bedding material as compared to straw or saw dust which has to be dragged at each time. This practice should be encouraged as health benefits of having all cows tying in clean, dry cubicles are considerable.

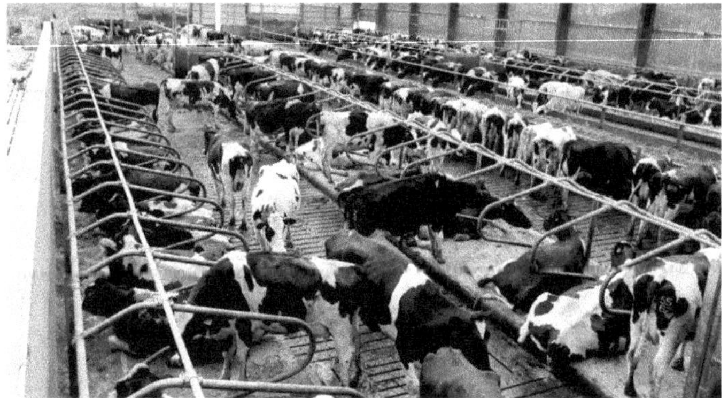

Fig. 1. Cubicle Design

B) Feed Barrier Design

Another zone of great social interaction is the feed area. Performance specifications for feed barriers have been outlined. The points to be taken care of are:

- ☆ The most important factor is to obtain initial dimensions correctly, so that the animals do not compete aggressively for feed.
- ☆ Poorly designed barriers can cause injuries, particularly to the nape and brisket. They can also lead to excessively feed wastage.
- ☆ After meeting the initial requirements of dimensions there are number of barrier namely tomb stones, diagonal or simple horizontal rails.
- ☆ At places where feeding of silage, hay and straw is done in big bale forms. It was found that 10% wastage of silage in conventional ring type feeders is there. The animals pull the silage and then trample it under feet.
- ☆ In case of improved feeders two big bales are held on a sloping base and slide forward when eaten (Fig 2).

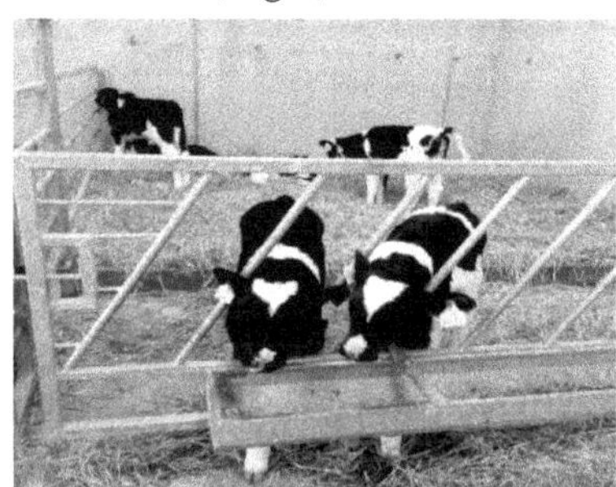

Fig. 2. Feed Barrier Design

Any feed dropped by the cattle falls into a secondary trough, adjacent to the limestone barrier. It can not be trampled under foot and thus feed wastage is eliminated.

C) Floor Design

The area of constant interaction between livestock and the building is the floor. So,

- Poorly designed floors can contribute to the lameness. Factors that may be involved include wetness, slippery or abrasive floors, poor foot hygiene, feeding of conserved forage and lack of exercise.
- Lameness in dairy cow building has been reviewed by a number of researchers[5]. They recommended texturing new floors or retexturing slippery and polished old concrete floor.
- Sensible overall design will alleviate this problem. Means avoiding sudden changes in the levels, eliminating dark and narrow passages and eliminating sharp and narrow passages and avoiding sharp and protruding objects.
- Avoid uneven or sloppy surface as these increase the risk of falling because cow often displays sense of defensive reflexes when confronted with such a situation and make sudden uncoordinated movements.
- Provide a bedded area in addition to the main cubicle complex. This is good for those small number of cows which may not be able to cope with hard floors and standings associated with the cubicle housing system.

D) Slopped Floor Housing

- This system is good for those farmers who are not willing to commit themselves to the high straw demands of a traditional bedded court.
- The basic principle involves confining cattle in pens in which the floor slopes away from the feeding trough. (Fig.3)

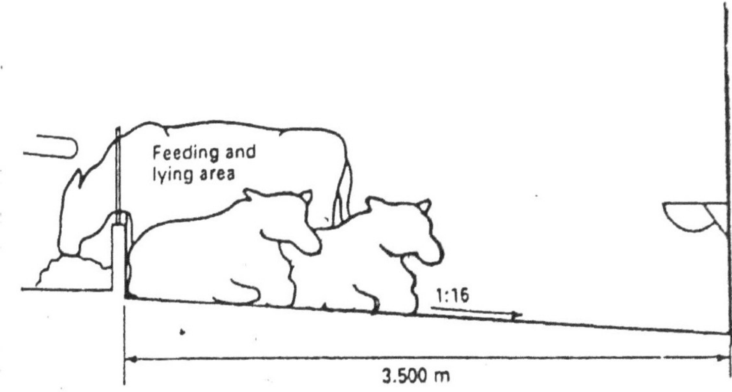

Fig. 3 Sloped Floor

- The slope encourages urine to run off, leaving the higher part clean and dry.
- Animal activity at the feed barrier will have cleaning effect, in providing brushing action as animal drag their feet away from the barrier.
- In small pens all animals are removed from their pens prior to the whole flow being scraped. This can be time consuming for larger units having a number of pens and dividing gates. But in the slopped floor houses, higher section of the floor remains clean and mechanical scrapping of the back of pen is practiced. (Fig.3)
- Experience of slopped floors indicates that injuries to stock are rare and no udder problems are been encountered with suckler cows.
- Feed type has an important baring on the success of the system as it effects both animal cleanliness and dung handling.
- Twice a day scrapping is recommended. Stocks can have faeces adhering to their coats, particularly in the early part of the housing period. However animal do perform well despite not always looking clean.

E) Slatted Floor

- Foot and leg injuries associated with cattle movement on slates continue to cause concern. Better management is needed in such houses (grouping animals in smaller groups and good feed and water access).
- It is harsh housing system because of the hardness of the floor and the injury problem that can occur as slats become worn and slippery.
- In order to improve this system rubber coated slats were used were used. Animals do feel more comfortable but more hoof growth due to absence of abrasion result which cause difficulties.
- Daily weight gain on slate with the rubber coatings is more in the cows.
- The animals kept on the slates they remain more clean. A scoring system was devised as shown in fig. 4 with a typical cleanliness score.

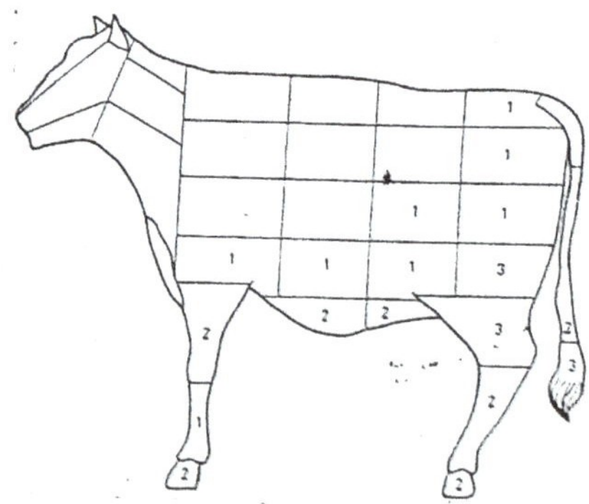

Fig. 4 Clean Scoring System

A clean area of the coat is given a score of zero while extremely dirty area can score upto twice. Poorly bedded courts can lead to very dirty animals, while animals on slates can be very clean, or moderately dirty depending upon many factors like cattle size, density of stocking, coat length, feed type, management and frequency of bedding and scrapping.

The Ventilation of Cattle Housing

A healthy environment for stock can be provided by improved ventilation in the dairy cattle houses.

- ✰ An open ridge design provide very good ventilation in the sheds.(fig. 5)

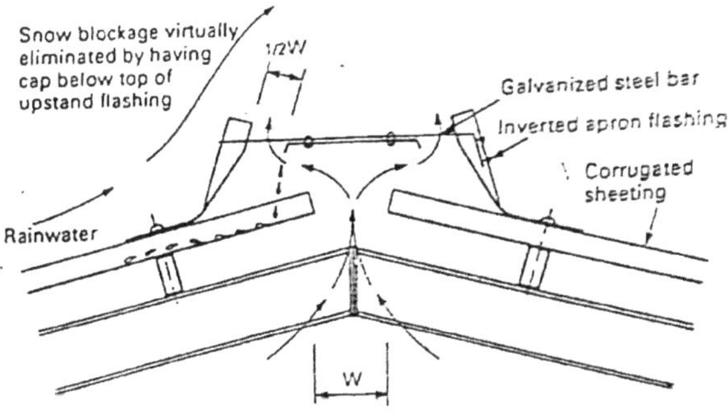

Fig.5 Open Ridge Design

- ✰ The design enables an outlet opening to be retained without a problem of rain ingress usually on a cential feed pass.
- ✰ The technique is the spaced or slotted roof. It is particularly applicable to wide span, multispan building, close proximity to others through which good air distribution can often be a problem.
- ✰ This technique involves the slotting or spacing of roof sheets to create openings approx. 20 mm wide down the length of the roof. This will act as both inlet and outlet. The opening is formed in the crown of the sheets so creating a channel either side in run off rain water.
- ✰ A bright, healthy, internal environment is created which is of benefit to both stock and management.

Advances in Bedding Options for Cattle Houses

The bedding plays an important role in all dairy operations. The best bedding choice will depend on the type of housing used, as well as local cost and availability of different bedding products. The different types of bedding materials could be chosen taking into consideration the animals comfort and the economic status of the farmer. Because cows are large animals, bedding must offer uniform support. It must be comfortable to lie on and provide coolness in summer and warmth in winter. Dry bedding is important both for comfort and for reduction in pathogen growth. Non-abrasive bedding promotes both comfort and injury reduction. In addition it should be cost efficient and labor efficient.

Different types of bedding materials		
1)	Organic bedding materials	Sawdust
		Wood shavings
		Paper based bedding materials
		Straw
2)	Inorganic bedding materials	Sand
		Limestone
		Gypsum

The organic bedding materials are readily available and absorbs moisture. They are compatible with manure handling systems. The different types of organic bedding materials include

1) **Saw-dust and Wood Shavings:** It is probably the most commonly used bedding products for dairy cows. They have the advantage over sand of being broken down by microorganisms in the disposal system, but they have the disadvantage of allowing growth of microorganisms (pathogens). Addition of lime to bedding may reduce growth of pathogens. The smaller particle size of sawdust makes it more absorbent than wood shavings and quicker to break down. However, small particle size is also associated with rapid growth of bacteria and other harmful pathogens. Cost and availability tend to be deciding factors in choice of material. Sawdust can be a highly variable material, but when screened and dried can provide an effective bedding material when managed properly. Unscreened materials are unsuitable as they can contain shards of wood and even nails and are likely to be very variable. Damp sawdust is an excellent medium for supporting many pathogens so it is essential to keep sawdust dry in storage; well-managed sawdust-based systems can give excellent results but when badly-managed there is considerable potential for problems to occur.

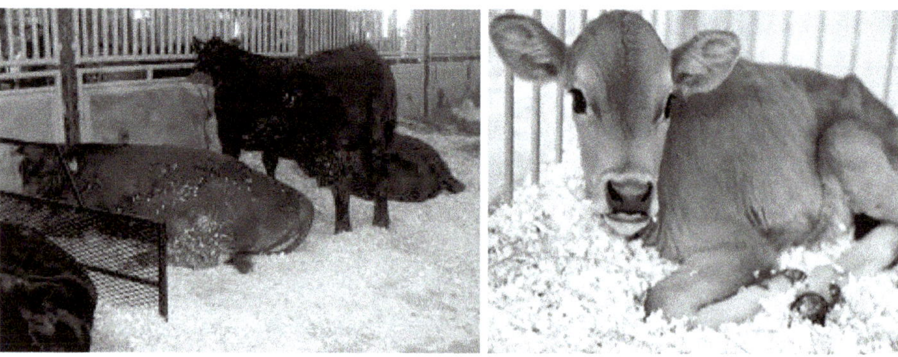

Fig.6: Sawdust and Wood Shavings as Bedding Material

2) Paper-Based Bedding Materials: A variety of paper-based products are used for livestock bedding, including shredded waste paper, paper pulp and specially-designed proprietary granulated bedding products. Specially-designed granulated materials can possess excellent characteristics that make them suitable as dairy cow bedding. The latent alkalinity of some paper-based products also has a disinfectant effect and can help to control pathogens. Paper pulp can set hard, and produce an undesirable uneven surface. When wet it can heat-up to provide good conditions for pathogens to flourish. Shredded paper is not widely used on farms as it is not particularly absorbent, and cattle bedded on this material can appear dirty.

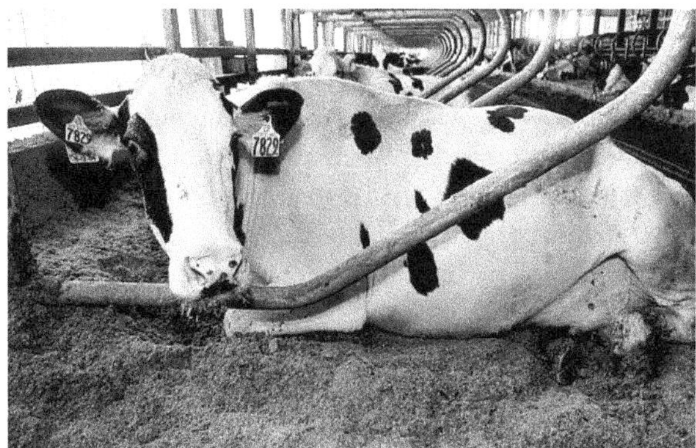

Fig.7: Paper Based Bedding Material

3) Straw: Chopped straw is a widely-used bedding material for cow housing, and when clean, dry, well-stored straw is used and managed correctly it can provide a comfortable environment for cattle bedding. However, where straw beds are allowed to become heavily soiled, particularly in deep-bedded yards, the bedding has the potential for becoming an effective medium for pathogens responsible for causing infectious foot problems. It composts well and reduces in volume when composted, better than sawdust or wood shavings. It is important when using straw as bedding that the particle size be small, preferably fitting through a ¾ inch screen, both to increase animal comfort and to shorten breakdown time. Bedding absorbency as well as comfort to animals varies according to the species as well as to the chop size.

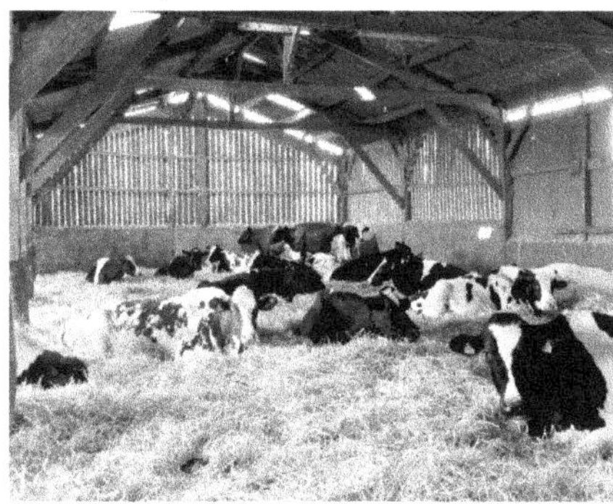

Fig.8: Straw as a Bedding Material

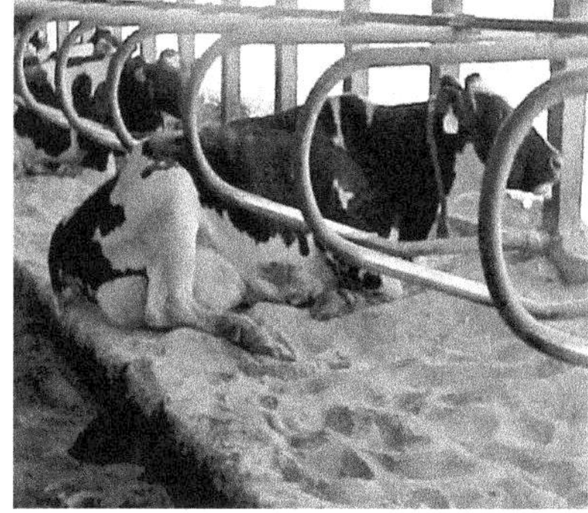

Fig.9: Sand as a Bedding Material

The inorganic bedding materials include:

1) Sand can be a good choice of bedding. Depth of 6-8 inches in a tie stall or free stall barn is recommended. Because sand is an inert material, it will not tend to promote growth of pathogens, though when mixed with manure, the manure will support pathogen growth. Particle size is of great importance. Too small particle size (or too much organic matter mixed in) will hold water too well. Large particles (> 3mm) will not be comfortable to lie on. Sand which is naturally occurring will have more rounded edges and be more comfortable as bedding than manufactured sand which comes from crushing rock. The potentially negative side of using sand as bedding is its disposal. In a liquid manure handling facility, sand must be settled out and disposed of. In this way we can reuse the clean sand.

2) Lime is used sparingly with other bedding materials. It has the potential to dry-out and damage teat and udder skin and so must be adequately covered with chopped straw or sawdust, but is very useful in drying-out soiled wet patches on cubicle beds and controlling bacterial levels.

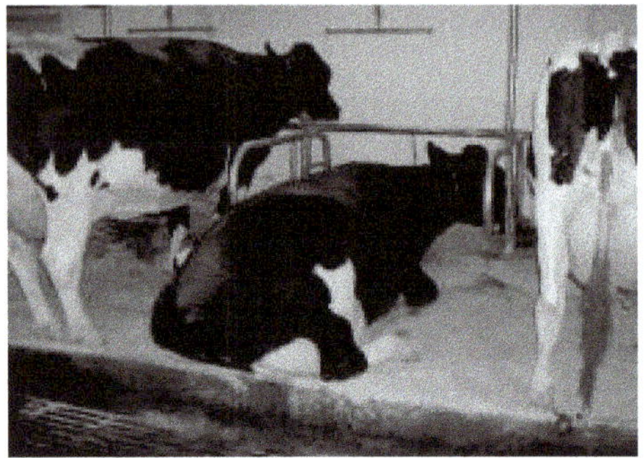

Fig.10: Use of Lime as a Bedding Material

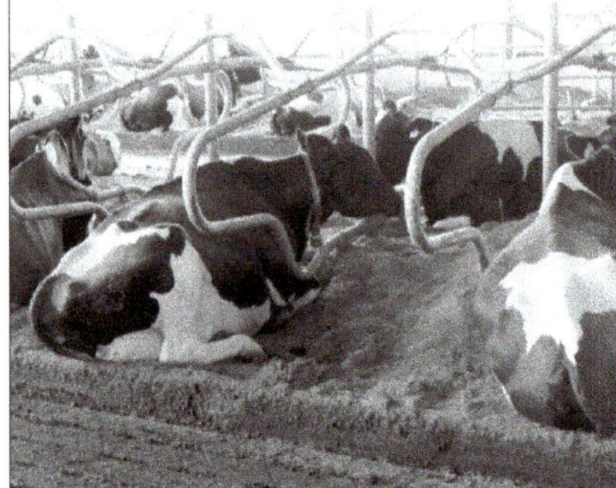

Fig. 11: Manure Compost Bedding

Manure Compost Bedding is another option. It is a renewable source that is readily available in large quantities and can be used liberally in free stalls. Undigested pieces of feed fibres can be separated from dairy manure and used for bedding. Use the bedding soon after processing and apply it several times per week to avoid reheating in the stalls. When the bedding becomes wet or soiled, scrape off the manure and bedding and replace it with clean compost bedding.

Recent Innovations

One of the recent innovation in bedding are **Geotextile Mattresses.** They are manufactured from a variety of materials that are commercially available. These may be used in either tie stall or free stall barns. These have waterproof exteriors, and are filled with a variety of materials including rubber crumbs, polyethylene foam, and water. They are marketed as requiring no bedding, but research has shown that added bedding makes the mattresses much more attractive to cows. Mattresses are generally installed in rows, attached to one another, and come in a variety of sizes to fit typical stall sizes.

Cow stall Mats is another Innovation. They are normally constructed of a 1.9 to 2.5 centimetre (¾ to 1 inch) thick industrial grade solid rubber or a multi-layered vinyl. Given their solid nature they offer the least improvement for cow comfort over a concrete base covered with bedding. However, these mats do provide a non-abrasive, non-skid surface that adds traction for cows, is impervious to water, bacteria and mold, while offering low maintenance and reduced bedding requirements. Stall mats properly installed on a sloped surface facilitate drainage of fluids keeping the cows drier. In addition, the mat offers a layer of insulation between the cold concrete stall base and the cow during winter temperature conditions. Stall matting is available in an individual mat or a continuous roll configuration. Individual mats can be utilized in tiestall barns with in-floor stall dividers with continuous mats lending themselves come in a range of sizes to fit standard sized cow stalls with some manufactures offering custom sized mats to fit non-standard sized stalls. The continuous roll design can cover a number of stalls with a single piece of matting reducing the number of seams. However, if an area of matting becomes damaged the individual mat configuration offers an easier repair via mat replacement whereas; the continuous mat requires a larger area to be replaced. The rubber mats are environmentally friendly. The bed also moves with the cow's skin, protecting her from abrasions. Both of these factors help minimize bacterial build up that might introduce mastitis-causing bacteria. While an added labour cost, many producers may also dust beds with a handful of sawdust or powdered lime once or twice per day.

Cow Mattress consists of an exterior envelope made of either synthetic materials or rubber, filled with an inner core of crumbled rubber, gel or water. In addition to the benefits of solid mats described above, mattresses tend to be much thicker than mats thus offering additional cow comfort. Mattresses filled with crumbled rubber often become firmer with time due to the compaction of the particle core. To overcome the compaction issue gel-mats have been developed where the core is made up of multiple compartments filled with a gel substance instead of a crumbled rubber. These mattresses are purported to remain softer for much longer periods as well as reducing pressure points on the cow's contact points with the mattress. Alternately, **dual chambered mattresses** filled with water, commonly referred to as **cow waterbeds**, have become more popular in recent years due to low incidence of hock joint abrasion, minimal bedding needs and the prolonged life of the mattress. One water filled chamber at the front of the mattress cushions the front of the cow while a rear chamber supports the rear weight of the animal. It is important that the stall surface over which the stall base is installed is adequately sloped to the rear to facilitate drainage of fluids off the base material.

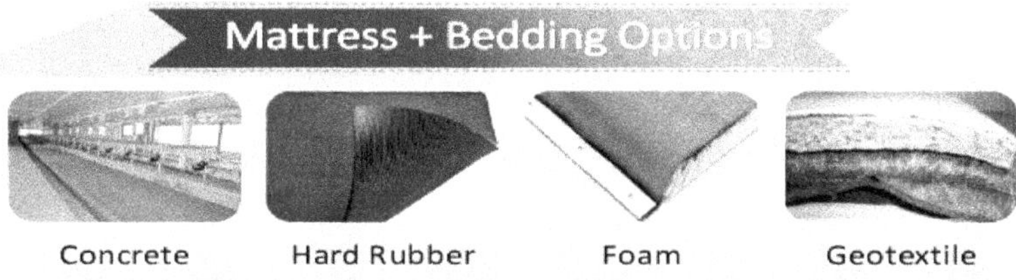

Fig.12: Different Types of Mattresses

Housing, Disease and Welfare

Because of close confinement, animals are more susceptible to spread of infections diseases. The housing environment may be a significant factor in the cause of disease. The main causes being lameness and mastitis.

Housing and Mastitis

- The change in loose housing, combined with keeping cows with larger groups led to significant increase in mastitis in many herds.
- The use of damp straw, less frequency of cleaning is also the cause of increased mastitis.
- It has been reported that the reducing stocking density from fifty four to forty five cows per yard, storing bedding straw and increasing its usage, combined with changed milking routine, reduce the incidence of clinical mastitis.
- Hygine in the houses is equally important, soiled bedding should be removed from the rear of the cubicle, twice daily, passage should be scrapped twice daily and the lying area rebedded once a day.
- The variation in bedding material do not have an affect on the bacterial population. Sand and shreaded paper support lower bacterial population.
- The application of few handful of line twice weekly prior to rebdding has been suggested. As a method of drying the bed or flooring and also reducing the number of bacteria.
- The passage should be cleaned prior to cows returing after milking. This reduces indirect faecal contamination of beds via the feet as the teat squinter does not fully close and see until thirty minutes after milking, keeping the cow standing out the bedded area is beneficial.

Housing and Lameness

Lameness is a major economic and welfare problem.

- The cows which spend excessive periods standing are worst effected.
- Compared two identically managed herds, both housed in identical cubicle showed that by increase use of straw bedding lying time increased, more first location heifers entered the cubicle house and the time between entry and lying was significantly decreased. The higher use of straw decreased the aberrant behavior and thus marked decrease in incidence of lameness.
- Overcrowding may cause trauma, in that cows do not spend sufficient time walking. This produces poor blood flow in the hoof and as such is similar to the 'trench foot' suffered by soliders in the First World War.
- Unsanitary conditions for example in adequately scraped yards, especially around feed areas can pre dispose to interdigital neurobacillosis heel erosion and digital dermatitis.

Housing and Welfare

So the welfare can be evaluated in terms of five basic freedoms.

1. Freedom from hunger and malnutrition
2. Freedom from thermal or physical distress.
3. Freedom to express most normal behavior.
4. Freedom from diseases and injury.
5. Freedom from fear.

Space allowance and design of feed area are important determinants of stress. It has been suggested that the cows in loose yards prefer to tie at least 1m from other cow and in tied system restricted movements had to stress because the animal is unable to establish its social position in the social hierarchy. So if there is shortage of space, it would have the adverse effects. If barriers exist between animals when feeding, this produces more even intake of feed between low and high ranking animals. Where there is no feed barrier and less feeding space, the animal spends time while walking and waiting.

Welfare problems do exist while handling the animals. For example while routine T.B testing or for loading into lorry for transportation. For such purposes proper design of the area should be there. Fig. 13 shows two possible handling systems.

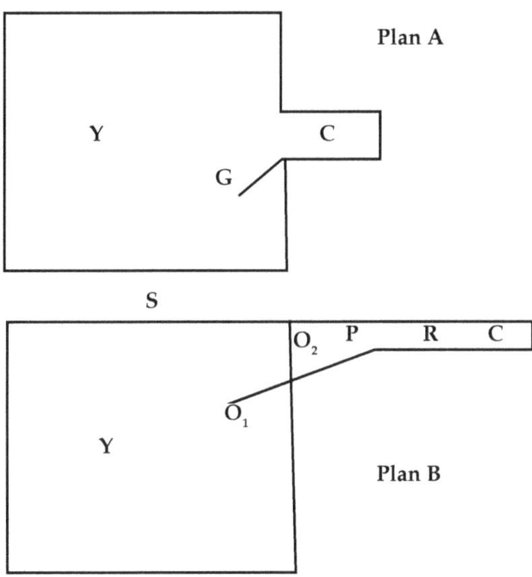

Fig. 13: Animal Handling System

Conclusions

1. The loose housing of dairy cows in cubicles will continue as the dominant housing system. A greater understanding of behavioural needs of cows has led to improved cubicle and feed barrier designs in recent years.
2. Coating on slopped floors tends to increase the comfort of the animals.
3. Good natural ventilation of cattle building is continually being promoted and computer aided design now assists greatly in determining outlet and inlet opening for a wide range of buildings, the slotted or spaced roof is a well proven concept which provides a breathening roof ensuring an excellent airflow distribution.

Transforming Rural Areas through Veterinary Science *Pages* **15–28**
Editor: Dipanjali Konwar, Shilpa Sood & Shahid Ahamad
Published by: **ASTRAL INTERNATIONAL PVT. LTD., NEW DELHI**

2 Strategies to Raise Income by Small Ruminants Rearing in the Hilly Areas

Dr. Suraj Amrutkar & Dr. Surinder K. Gupta

Introduction

Hill farming primarily rearing sheep and goat is an extensive farming in upland areas. Small ruminants (sheep and goats) are essential components of the mixed farming systems in the hills which found in all parts of country. They are mainly kept for meat; although wool, fibre and manure are also important products from these animals. A high proportion of sheep and goats are found in the hills because of their inherent ability to utilize mountain terrain, unsuitable for crop farming. Sheep and goat husbandry has no social, religious or cultural taboos, or caste restrictions. Poor farmers of the hills prefer small ruminants mostly because they can't invest large sums of money in cattle and buffalo. Small ruminants in the hills are reared either under a sedentary or a migratory system. Sedentary flocks may also be stall-fed, semi-stall-fed or completely grazed, while the migratory flocks are reared under an extensive management system. Many struggles have been made over the past three decades to increase production from sheep and goats.

Means of Maintaining Soil Fertility

Sheep and goats perform an important role in maintaining soil fertility particularly in the hills where the use of chemical fertilizer may not be permitted either by unavailability or cost or may be due to still unknown to the farmers. Goat and sheep manure is to be superior to that of other ruminants. Sheep and goat manures contain 0.61% and 0.83% nitrogen respectively on a fresh weight basis, compared to 0.25% and 0.33% in the faeces of cattle and buffalo. Nitrogen contained in the faeces produced by one sheep and goat in one year is around 1.4 kg and 1.5 kg, respectively. Nitrogen and potassium contains in sheep urine is 1.5–1.7% and 1.8–2.0%, respectively.

Producers of High Quality Skins

Sheep and goat has high quality skin which may be used for multiple purposes.

Efficient User of Available Resources

Small ruminants make very effective use of a variety of different grazing lands, including rocky mountain terrain and alpine pastures, which cannot be utilized by other domestic animals. They convert relatively inaccessible low quality forage and feed to high quality meat, wool and fibre. They can adapt to different climatic conditions because of their hardy nature. Depending on the availability of pasture land and the cropping pattern of an area, they can also be stall-fed, semi-stall-fed, or grazed. Goats can live and produce satisfactorily on vegetation which is not consumed by any other species of domestic livestock.

Economically Viable Enterprise

Rearing of sheep and goat is very economical. The economically value of sheep and goats is the factor in their popularity within smallholder farmers. The financial investment requirement for small ruminants, purchase of animals, equipment and buildings is very low. Even a poor farmer can invest for rearing of small ruminants because most of the equipment and buildings constructed from locally available raw materials. The animals start production at about 1-1½ years of age. Goats being prolific and produce many offspring per year. They give a good return per unit of capital invested due to the high turnover and so provide an economically profitable enterprise. Small ruminants provide a ready source of cash to the farmers. In the hills, crop production is often insufficient to meet family requirements. Small ruminants are in high demand because they can be sold at emergency condition. Family meat consumption can be reduced for more urgent necessities which may arise, so that sheep and goats are therefore regarded as a symbol of wealth.

Source of Employment

Farmers in the villages are involved as shepherds and in wool spinning work. Available time in the morning or evening is consumed by village women in wool spinning and weaving, which is also a source of additional income. People are involved in informal employment associated with the carpet industry, undertaking washing, carding, spinning, dyeing and weaving of wool on a household or cottage industry basis.

Management Practices

Migration

Flocks in hilly region of Jammu and Kashmir, Himachal Pradesh, Uttarakhand are small, and most are stationary. In Himachal Pradesh, 73% sheep are stationary and 27% of sheep are migratory. Stationary flocks generally do not cover more than five sheep and are kept as an additional occupation to crop farming. The migratory flocks have average of 22 numbers of sheep, although some can exceed 100. In the hilly regions of Uttar Pradesh, 86.8% of sheep are migratory and 13.2% are stationary. Migration may take place from the permanent home in the valley to the alpine pastures during summer only, or from the temporary home to the alpine pastures during summer and to the foothills and plains in the winter. Migration to the alpine pastures begins in April or May; and takes a month or more depending upon the vegetation available as well as the onset of the rains. The flocks start returning to their homesteads during September/ October and reach their destination by November. The permanently migrating flocks leave their homestead for the foothills in November and graze on crop residues in harvested fields, on natural vegetation on fallow lands and in forest areas, and on tree lopping's, until March/early April, when they start to return. Shepherds in the hill areas are not travelers, and only one or two members of the family accompany the flock. The economic condition of the shepherds in this region is better than that of their counterparts in the plains. During migration, the shepherds generally keep their flocks separate, and one person handles only 100 to 200 animals.

Grazing

The stationary flocks are grazed in harvested fields along waterways in forests and in permanent pastures on common grazing land. The sheep are allowed to graze for about 7 hours. About 14% of the flocks are given supplementary feeding, such as fodder and green leaves. Migratory flocks are primarily grazed on alpine pasture during summer and on the harvested fields, forest areas and other uncultivated fallow and barren lands during winter. Tree leaves and pods of fodder trees constitute an important feed resource during winter and early spring, when the flocks are in the foothills and the plains.

Breeding and Lambing Season

The animals are mostly bred when migration from the alpine pastures begins in September/October, so that lambing takes place in February/ March. To a limited extent, breeding also takes place in February/March. In Himachal Pradesh, most breeding takes place in October/November and January/March.

Shearing

Shearing takes place in January/March, June/July and October/November; somewhat less than half of the sheep are shorn three times a year, the remainder only twice.

Disease

The major cause of sheep mortality in stationary flocks is pneumonia (including lung-worm infestation), followed by liver-fluke, diarrhoea and dysentery (mostly due to internal parasites), sheep-pox and anthrax. In migratory flocks, the major causes are pneumonia, cold winds, diarrhoea and dysentery, anthrax and sheep-pox.

Sheep Breeds in the Northern Temperate Region

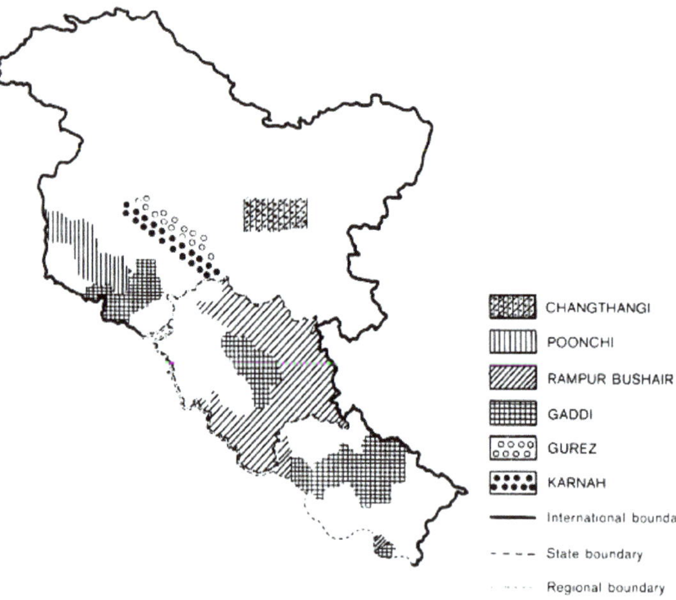

Goat Breeds in the Northern Temperate Region

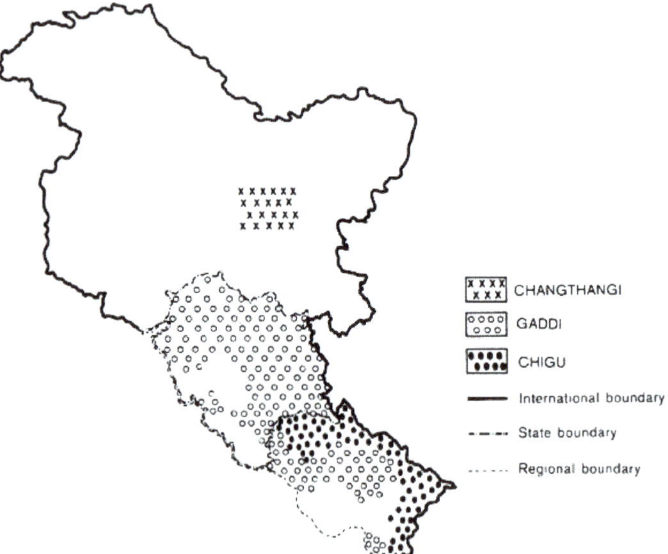

Population, Production and Important Breeds

India has second rank in goat population and third rank in sheep population. The total sheep in country is 65.07 million numbers in 2012, declined by about 9.07% over census 2007. The goat population has declined by 3.82% over the previous census and the total goat in the country is 135.17 million numbers in 2012. Sheep and goat population in J & K is 3.389 and 2.017 million number representing 5.21% and 1.49 % of that of the country as whole. It produces about 3.08 million kg of wool, 8.27% of the country's wool production. The important breeds of sheep are Rampur Bushair, Gaddi, Gurez, Karnah, Bhakarwal, Poonchi, Kashmir Merino and Changthangi; most of these have been involved over the last few years in cross-breeding with exotic fine-wool breeds for increasing apparel-wool production.

Sheep Breeds

Gaddi (also Known as Bhadarwah)

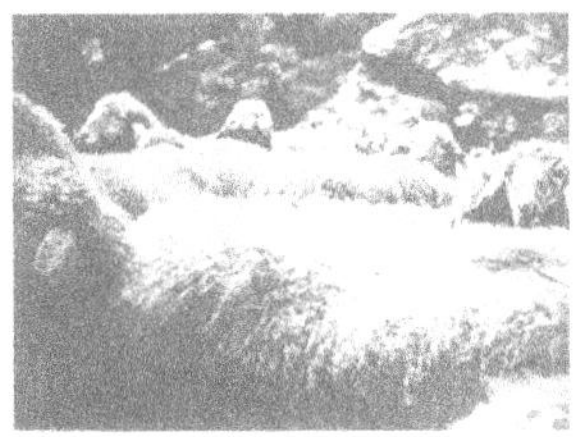

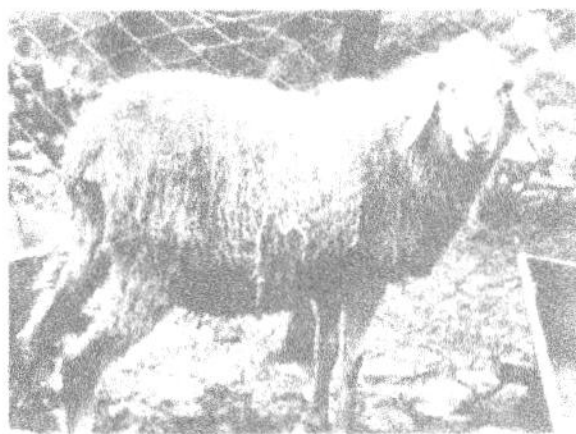

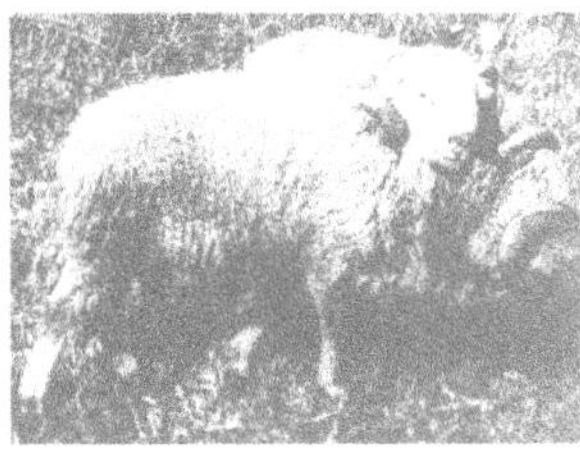

Adult Male **Adult Female** **Flock**

Distribution

Kistwar and Bhadarwah Tehsils in Jammu province of Jammu & Kashmir State; Hamirpur, Ramnagar, Udampur and Kulu and Kangra valleys of Himachal Pradesh; and Dehradun, Nainital, Tehrigarhwal and Chamoli districts of Uttar Pradesh.

Breed Characteristics

- ☆ **Size:** The body weight, body length, height at withers and chest girth are 26.59 kg, 57.45 cm, 56.14 cm and 70.42 cm respectively.
- ☆ **Conformation:** Medium-sized animals, usually white, although tan, brown and black and mixtures of these are also seen. Males are horned; 10 to 15% of females are horned. Tail is small and thin. The fleece is relatively fine and dense.
- ☆ **Reproduction:** Under farm conditions: Lambing percentage on the basis of ewes available: 58.9%; Litter size: Single.
- ☆ Mortality: 0 to 3 months: 20.5%; 3 to 6 months: 27.6%; 6 to 12 months: 42.4%; adults: 10.7%.
- ☆ **Breeding:** Pure breeding, except that, to a limited extent, cross-breeding with exotic fine-wool breeds (especially Rambouillet and Merino) is being carried out, primarily through natural service with exotic or cross-bred rams. The cross-breds show improvement in fleece production and quality over the pure breed.
- ☆ **Performance**
    - **Meat: Body weight (kg):** The body weight at birth, at weaning, at 6 months and at 12 months are 2.52, 7.44, 10.81 and 14.29kg, respectively.

- **Wool production and quality:** The average 6 monthly greasy fleece wool production is 0.78 kg. The staple length of wool is 5.70 cm. The average fibre diameter of wool is 28.52 µ. The modulation percentage of wool is 25.80%.

Rampur Bushair

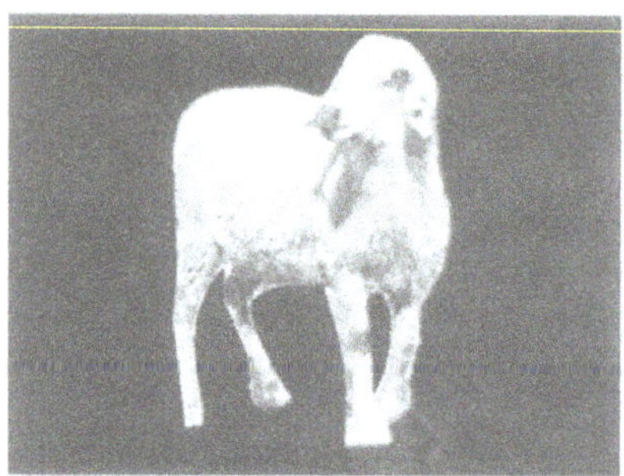

Adult Male

Distribution: Simla, Kinnaur, Nahan, Bilaspur, Solan and Lahaul and Spiti districts of Himachal Pradesh and Dehradun, Rishikesh, Chakrota and Nainital districts of Uttar Pradesh.

Breed Characteristics

- **Size:** The body weight, body length, height at withers and chest girth in male are 28.84 kg, 62.33 cm, 59.05 cm and 67.97 cm, respectively. The body weight, body length, height at withers and chest girth in female are 25.38 kg, 59.55 cm, 57.83 cm and 65.92 cm, respectively.
- **Conformation:** Medium-sized animals. The fleece colour is predominantly white, with brown, black and tan also seen on the fleece in varying proportions. The ears are long and drooping. The face line is convex, giving a typical Roman nose. The males are horned; most females are polled. The fleece is of medium quality and dense. Legs, belly and face are devoid of wool.
- **Reproduction:** Under farm conditions: lambing percentage varies from 52.9 to 88.3%.
- **Mortality:** In farmers' flocks: young: 8 to 15%; adults: 5 to 10%. Under farm conditions: 0 to 6 months: 13.9%; 6 to 12 months: 17% ; adults: 19.86%.
- **Breeding:** Pure breeding, except in limited areas where the State Department of Animal Husbandry has initiated cross-breeding with exotic fine-wool breeds (Rambouillet and Merino). The cross-breds show improvement in both fleece production and quality.
- **Performance:**
  - Meat: Body weight (kg): The body weights at birth, at weaning and at 12 month of age are 2.38, 12.69 and 17.84 kg.

- Wool production and quality: The annual greasy fleece weight of wool is 1.17 kg. The staple length, average fibre diameter and modulation of wool are 7.70 cm, 34.35 μ and 23.81%, respectively.

Bhakarwal

The name of the breed is derived from the nomadic tribe which rears these sheep.

Distribution: No distinct home tract; sheep are entirely migratory.

Breed Characteristics

- ☆ **Size:** Adult ewes weigh between 29 and 36 kg; rams can weigh as much as 55 kg. In adult females, height at withers: 62 cm; body length: 65 cm; chest girth: 82 cm.
- ☆ **Conformation:** Medium-sized animals, with a typical Roman nose. The animals are generally white, although coloured fleeces are occasionally observed. All animals are spotted fawn or grey. Rams are horned; ewes are polled. Ears are long and drooping. Tail is small and thin. Fleece is coarse and open.
- ☆ **Breeding:** Most of this breed has now been crossed with Merino for improving greasy-wool production and quality for apparel wool and only a very small proportion of flocks still contain pure Bhakarwal animals.
- ☆ **Performance:** The sheep are shorn three times a year. The total annual wool produced, per animal, ranges from 1 to 1.5 kg. The wool quality is from 36s to 40s, with an average fibre diameter varying from 36 to 38 μ.

Poonchi

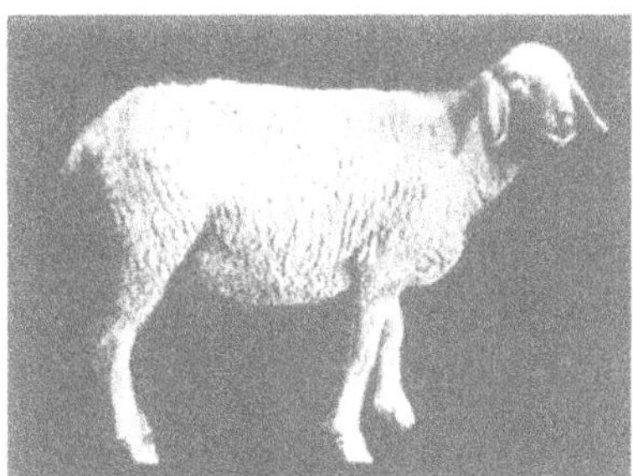

Adult Female

Distribution: Poonch and part of Rajori districts of Jammu province.

Breed Characteristics

- ☆ **Size:** The weight of the adult ram ranges from 35 to 40 kg, that of a ewe from 25 to 30 kg. Weight of females at 2½ years: 27.64 kg. Average height at withers of adult female: 57.0 cm; body length: 56.7 cm; chest girth: 72.6 cm.

- **Conformation:** Similar in appearance to Gaddi, but lighter. Animals are predominantly white in colour, including the face, but spotted sheep are also seen, varying from brown to light black. Ears are medium long. Tail is short and thin. Legs are also short, giving a low-set conformation.
- **Breeding:** Most of the flocks are being crossed with Merinos to improve greasywool production and quality for apparel wool and thus now contain cross-breds with a varying level of Merino inheritance.
- **Performance:** Wool is of medium to fine quality, mostly white in colour. Sheep are shorn three times a year and produce between 0.9 to 1.3 kg of greasy wool each per year. Fibre length ranges between 15 to 18 cm and average fibre diameter ranges between 22 and 30 μ.

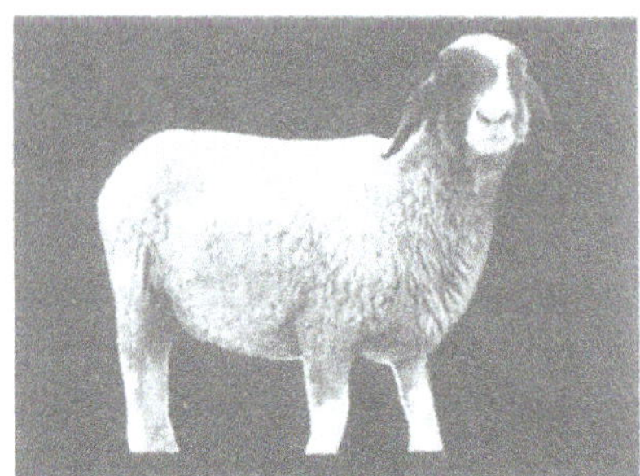

Adult Female

Karnah

Distribution: Distributed in Karnah, a mountainous tehsil in North Kashmir.

Breed Characteristics

- **Size:** The body weight in adult and adult female is 40-48 and 29-37 kg, respectively. The body length, the height at withers and chest girth in adult male are 72 cm, 70 cm and 102 cm, respectively. The body length, the height at withers and chest girth in adult female are 59-62 cm, 59-63 cm and 70-75 cm, respectively.
- **Conformation:** Large animals. The rams have large curved horns and a prominant nose line.
- **Breeding:** Cross-breeding with Merino has been introduced in Karnah, although the proportion of cross-breds is lower than for Gaddi, Bhakrawal and Poonchi.
- **Performance:** Wool is generally white in colour. The sheep are shorn twice a year, in spring and autumn, and produce between 1 to 1.5 kg of wool each per year. Staple length ranges from 12 to 15 cm and average fibre diameter between 29 and 32 μ.

Gurez

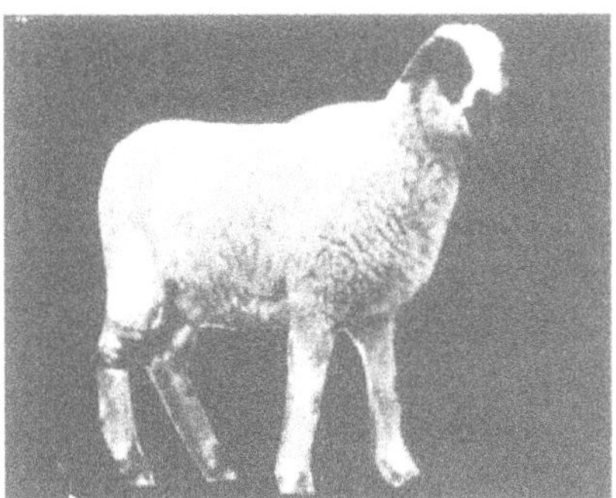

Adult Female

- ☆ **Distribution:** Distributed in the Gurez area of Northern Kashmir.
- ☆ **Conformation:** Largest of the sheep breeds in Jammu & Kashmir. Generally white in colour, although some animals are brown or black or have brown or black spots. A small proportion of the animals have small, pointed horns. Tail is thin and short. Fleece is generally coarse and hairy. Ears are long, thin and pointed.
- ☆ **Breeding:** This breed is being crossed with Merino for improving apparel-wool production and quality.
- ☆ **Performance**: The annual greasy-fleece weight varies from 0.5 to 1 kg per animal.

Kashmir Merino

This breed originated from crosses of different Merino types (at first Delaine Merinos, and subsequently Rambouillet and Soviet Merinos) with predominantly migratory native sheep breeds, such as Gaddi, Bhakarwal and Poonchi. The level of inheritance in the cross-bred animals included in Kashmir Merino varies from very low to almost 100% Merino; a level of from 50 to 75% predominates. The animals are highly variable because of the involvement of a number of native breeds, and no specific description of the breed can therefore be given. Some flocks of Kashmir Merino have been maintained by the State Department on their farms.

- ☆ **Performance**
  - **Meat: Body weight (kg):** The body weight at birth and at weaning are 3.37 and 21.80 kg, respectively.
  - **Wool production and quality:** The average 6-monthly greasy fleece weight of wool is 1.2 kg. The annual greasy fleece weight is 2.8 kg. The staple length of wool is 15.60 cm whereas average fibre diameter of wool is 20.4 μ.

Changthangi

- **Distribution:** Distributed in the Changthang region of Ladakh.

Breed Characteristics

- **Size:** The body weight of adult male and adult female is 38.64 and 34.0 kg, respectively. The body length, the height of withers and chest girth of male are 76.0, 69.0 and 97.5 cm, respectively whereas in female are 75.2, 67.0 and 89.0 cm, respectively.
- **Conformation:** Strongly-built, large-framed animals with good fleece cover which has an extraordinarily long staple.
- **Breeding:** Some cross-breeding with Merinos has been initiated for improving greasy-wool production and quality for fine apparel-wool.
- **Mortality:** In lambs: from 20 to 35%; in adults: from 10 to 20%.
- **Performance:** Animals are usually shorn twice a year, generally in May/ June and September/October, but in some cases shearing takes place only once a year, in July/ August. Greasy-wool production ranges from 1 to 1.5 kg per animal per year. The wool is of a good carpet/medium apparel quality.

Goat Breeds

Gaddi (also known as White Himalayan)

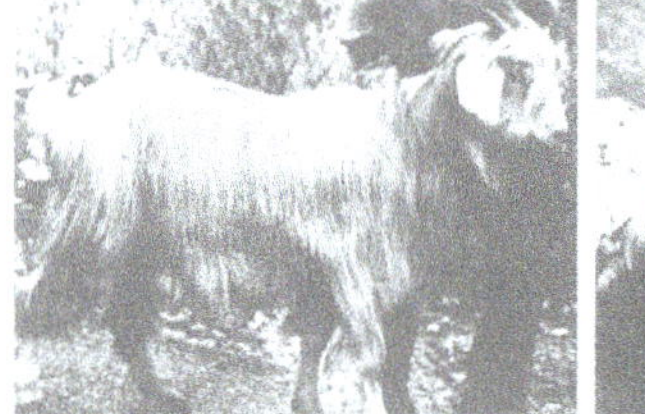

Adult Male

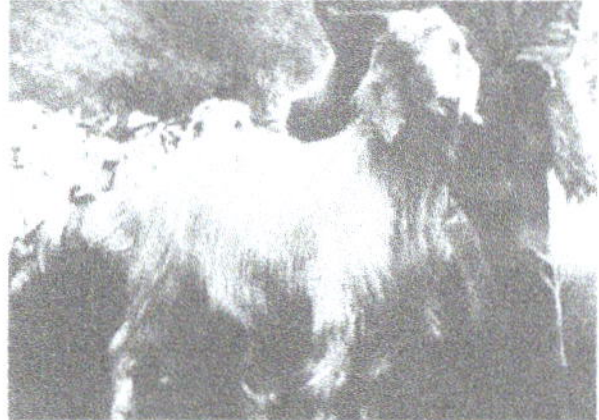

Adult Female

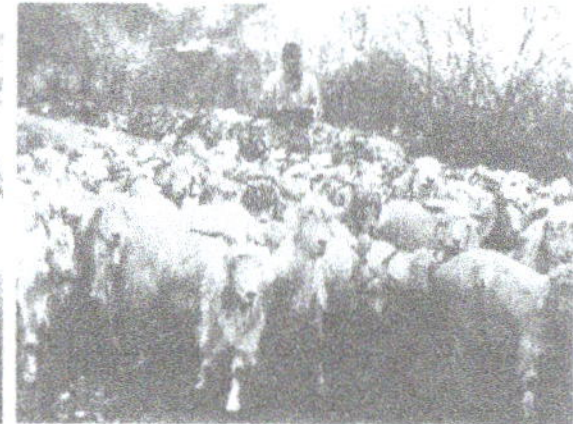

Flock

- **Distribution:** Chamba, Kangra, Kulu, Bilaspur, Simla, Kinnaur and Lahaul and Spiti in Himachal Pradesh and Dehradun, Nainital, Tehrigarhwal and Chamoli hill districts in Uttar Pradesh.

Breed Characteristics

- **Size:** The body weight of adult male and adult female is 27.25 and 24.72 kg, respectively. The body length, the height at withers and chest girth in adult male is 69.5, 61.3 and 72.2 cm, respectively whereas in adult female are 65.2, 58.1, 69.3cm, respectively.
- **Conformation:** Medium-sized animals. Coat colour is mostly white, but black and brown and combinations of these are also seen. Both sexes have large horns, directed upward and backward and occasionally twisted.

Ears are medium long and drooping. The nose line is convex. The udder is small and rounded, with small teats placed laterally. The hair is white, lustrous and long.

- ☆ **Reproduction:** Essentially single; twinning occurs in only 15 to 20% of births.
- ☆ **Mortality:** In farmers' flocks: kids: approximately 10%; adults: 5%. Under farm conditions: 0 to 3 months: 2.17%; 3 to 12 months: 1.24%; adults: 22.3%.
- ☆ **Breeding:** Pure breeding. There is little selection.
- ☆ **Performance**
  - **Milk:** Under farm conditions: milk yield: 308 g
  - **Wool Production and Quality:** The average wool yield per clip is 300 gm. The average fibre diameter of wool is 74.48 μ whereas modulation percentage of wool is 73.4%.

Changthangi

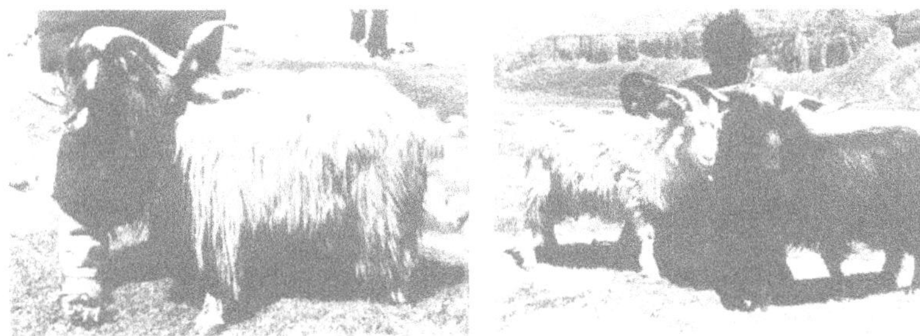

Adult Male **Adult Female**

- ☆ **Distribution:** Changthang region of Ladakh, at altitudes above 4 000 m.
- ☆ **Climate:** A cold arid region. Average annual precipitation: 9.26 cm, distributed throughout the year, with maxima during January/April. Summer and winter temperatures are extreme (+40°C to -40°C). Most cultivation takes place along the rivers.

Breed Characteristics

- ☆ **Size: Body Weight:** The body weight of adult male and adult female is 20.37 and 19.75 kg, respectively. The body length, the height at withers and chest girth in male is 49.8, 49.0 and 63.0 cm, respectively, whereas in adult female is 52.4, 51.5 and 65.2 cm, respectively.
- ☆ **Conformation:** Medium-sized animals. Half of the animals are white, the remainder black, grey or brown. Both sexes have horns, generally large (range: 15 to 55 cm), turning outward, upward and inward to form a semi-circle, but a wide variation exists in both shape and size.
- ☆ **Reproduction:** In farmers' flocks: kidding percentage: from 80 to 90%. Under farm conditions: kidding percentage: 65%.

- **Mortality:** In farmers' flocks: young: 25 to 35%; adults: 4 to 15%. Under farm conditions: young: 5.73%; adults: 1.9%.
- **Performance**
  - **Meat: Body weight (kg):** The body weight at birth, at 3 months, at 9 months and at 12 months are 2.18, 7.76, 9.18 and 11.80 kg, respectively.
- **Pashmina Production and Quality:**
  - The average fibre length of pashmina is 4.95 cm. Scouring yield of pashmina is 65.28%. The average fibre diameter of pashmina is 13.86 μ.
  - The pashmina is harvested once a year, generally in June/July, either by shearing or by combing. Average production is 214 g (range: 68 to 500 g).

Chigu

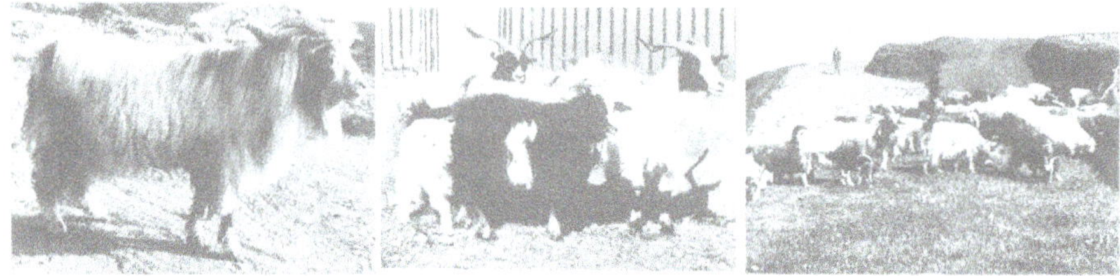

Adult Male **Adult Female** **Flock**

- **Distribution:** Lahaul and Spiti valleys of Himachal Pradesh, and Uttar Kashi, Chamoli, Pithoragarh districuts of Uttar Pradesh, bordering Tibet.
- **Climate:** Mountainous ranges with the altitude varying from 3500 to 5000 m. The area is mostly cold and arid.

Breed Characteristics

- **Size**
  - The body weight, body length, height at withers and chest girth in adult male is 39.32kg, 75.8 cm, 68.6 cm and 80.70cm, respectively.
  - The body weight, body length, height at withers and chest girth in adult female is 25.71kg, 69.3cm, 60.0cm and 73.7cm, respectively.
- **Conformation:** Medium-sized animals. The coat is usually white, mixed with greyish red. Both sexes have horns, directed upward, backward and outward, with one or more twists. These goats are not very different in conformation from Changthangi.
- **Reproduction:** Age at first kidding: 615.8 days; kidding interval: 272.8 days; kidding percentage: 65.4%; litter size: singles: 99.2%; twins: 0.8%.
- **Mortality:** In young : 44.2%.
- **Performance**

- **Meat: Body weight (kg):** Body weight at birth, at weaning, at 6 months, at 9 months and at 12 monthsa are 2.10, 8.41, 12.17, 14.75 and 18.46 gm respectively.
- **Pashmina Production and Quality:** The average production of Pashmina is 120.31gm. The average fibre length of pashmina is 5.9cm. The average fibre diameter of pashmina is 11.77 µ.

Transforming Rural Areas through Veterinary Science *Pages* **29-60**
Editor: Dipanjali Konwar, Shilpa Sood & Shahid Ahamad
Published by: **ASTRAL INTERNATIONAL PVT. LTD., NEW DELHI**

3 Transforming Rural Livelihoods through Scientific Dairying and Dairy Entrepreneurship

Dr. Pranav Kumar & Dr. Amandeep Singh

Indian dairying is emerging as a sunrise industry. It is crucial for rural economy and livelihood. India represents one of the world's largest and fastest growing markets for milk and milk products due to the increased disposable incomes among the 250 million strong middle class. With an annual growth rate of over 5 per cent the country's milk production is expected to exceed 250 million liters per day (92 million tons per year) as a result India emerging as the world's number one milk producer.

The country has achieved major breakthrough in milk production in the recent years. In India, dairying has been practiced as a rural cottage industry, since the remote past. Thus, entrepreneurial development is one of the ways to make rural people more competent in dairying. Dairy farming is not only an indispensable component of agriculture, but also the most suitable production system that has enormous potential to improve the socio-economic status of the large percentage of the rural population. While discussing the present status of the dairy farming in India, it has to be mentioned here that the bulk of milk production is in the hands of numerous land less, marginal and small farmers scattered all over the country. India has the largest cattle and buffalo population and is currently the largest producer of milk in the world.

The following characterizes India's dairy farming and its relevance to inclusive growth:

- Small and marginal farmers own 33 percent of land and about 60 percent of female cattle and buffaloes.
- Some 75 percent of rural households own, on average, two to four animals.
- Dairying is a part of the farming system, not a separate enterprise. Feed is mostly residual from crops, whereas cow dung is important for manure.
- Dairying provides a source of regular income, whereas income from agriculture is seasonal. This regular source of income has a huge impact on minimizing risks to income. There is some indication that areas where dairy is well developed have less incidence of farmer suicide.
- About a third of rural incomes are dependent upon dairying.
- Livestock is a security asset to be sold in times of crisis.

A well-developed dairy industry will enable millions of farmers to capitalize on the emerging opportunities and make a significant impact on rural incomes. On the flip side, weak efforts towards dairy development also can have a significant but negative impact on the dairy industry. The growth rate has been sluggish over the past few years. With an increase in demand on one hand and sluggish supply on the other, there is a likely shortfall in demand in the coming years.

General Facts

India ranks first among the world's milk producing nations since 1998 and has the largest bovine population in the world. Milk production in India during the period 1950-51 to 2014-15, has increased from 17 million tonnes to 146.3 million tonnes as compared to 137.7 million tonnes during 2013-14 recording a growth of 6.26 %, whereas FAO reported 3.1% increase in world milk production from 765 million tonnes in 2013 to 789 million tonnes in 2014. The per capita availability of milk in the country which was 130 gram per day during 1950-51 has increased to 322 gram per day in 2014-15 as against the world average of 293.7 grams per day during 2013. This represents sustained growth in the availability of milk and milk products for our growing population. Dairying has become an important secondary source of income for millions of rural families and has assumed the most important role in providing employment and income generating opportunities particularly for marginal and women farmers. Most of the milk is produced by animals reared by small, marginal farmers and landless laborers. About 15.46 million farmers have been brought under the ambit of 1,65,835 village level dairy corporative societies up to March 2015. Government of India is making efforts for strengthening the dairy sector through various Central sector Schemes like "National Programme for Bovine Breeding and Dairy Development", National Dairy Plan (Phase-I) and "Dairy Entrepreneurship Development Scheme".

Dairy activities have traditionally been integral to India's rural economy. The country is the world's largest producer of dairy products and also their largest consumer. Almost its entire produce is consumed in the domestic market and the country is neither an importer nor an exporter, except in a marginal sense. Despite being the world's largest producer, the dairy sector is by and large in the primitive stage of development and modernization. Though India may boast of a 200 million cattle population, the average output of an Indian cow is only one seventh of its American counterpart. Indian breeds of cows are considered inferior in terms of productivity. Moreover, the sector is plagued with various other impediments like shortage of fodder, its poor quality, dismal transportation facilities and a poorly developed cold chain infrastructure. As a result, the supply side lacks in elasticity that is expected of it. On the demand side, the situation is buoyant. With the sustained growth of the Indian economy and a consequent rise in the purchasing power during the last two decades, more and more people today are able to afford milk and various other dairy products. This trend is expected to continue with the sector experiencing a robust growth in demand in the short and medium run. If the impediments in the way of growth and development are left unaddressed, India is likely to face a serious supply – demand mismatch and it may gradually turn into a substantial importer of milk and milk products.

Why to Promote Entrepreneurship in Dairying?

It will not be less than correct to mention that entrepreneurship has become the buzzword of the day. Entrepreneurship has now become most important phenomenon for rapid progress in dairy. Today when there is growing concern for greater attention to our rural economy, the dairy sector offers big opportunity to transform our economy by bringing prosperity to the rural sector. The supporting income from animal husbandry and dairying is farmer's cash insurance against any distress caused by the crop failures. In our country 26 crore people still live below the poverty line. The dairy sector provides immense opportunities for eradicating poverty. There is an urgent need to make dairy development an area of core competence in the national programme of poverty reduction and rural prosperity. The fact that dairying could play a more constructive role in promoting rural welfare and reducing poverty by generating employment at farm level is increasingly being recognized Despite this upside fact about dairying, this sector in India has not picked up on commercial line. Tenth Plan proposal of Govt. of India, truly mention that animal husbandry and dairying will receive a high priority in the effort for generating income and employment, increasing animal protein availability in the food basket and for generating exportable surplus. A sustainable and financially viable dairy farming, which will generate income and self-employment through entrepreneurship, is need of the day. Market oriented milk production will be key livestock activities to generate income on a steady daily basis for resource poor households. In this context entrepreneur is one of the most important inputs for development of dairying, which may prove phenomenal for economic development of a country or of regions within the country.

Four P's of Successful Dairy Entrepreneurship

In addition to the SWOT analysis, the successful Dairy Entrepreneur must have a proper understanding of the **four 'P's:** Procurement, Production, Processing and Promotion.

1. **Procurement:** It covers collection of milk from rural producers or

contractors including setting up of chilling centers, provision of laboratory equipment and supplies, milking machines, cattle welfare, including feed and fodder and last but not the least the transportation.

2. **Production:** It includes activities of producing various types of liquid milks like the conventional whole, toned and standardized as well as innovative like milk with extra nutrition for school children, pregnant mothers, the aged and the infirm, low fat milk for the calorie conscious. The key is to sale milk also as a **fun product** and not merely as something, which is good for health.
3. **Processing:** Processing of products such as butter and cheese spread, pre-sliced butter and cheese, dairy whiteners, milk beverages (Plain and Carbonated), butter oil as a cooking medium, whip-and-serve milk shake powders, wet and dry *kulfi* and ice cream mix, high protein whey drinks for sports man, milk sweets, *shrikhand,* dried condensed milk, dried *khoa* and many more can be added the list.
4. **Promotion:** It covers activities like brand promotion, setting up of dairy parlors, buying milk in bulk and repacking to sell, distribution, devising attractive packaging and other such activities, which will result in building an image either nationally or even regionally and enhance the marketing of the products.

Scope of Entrepreneurship Development

1. Ration Balancing Advisory Services

Ration given to animals usually comprises one or two locally available concentrate feed ingredient(s), seasonal grasses and crop residues. This leads to imbalanced feeding which adversely affects the health and productivity of animals in various ways and also reduces the net daily income to milk producer from dairying. At times, overfeeding of animals can also raise the cost of milk production. Therefore, milk producers need to understand the implications of imbalanced feeding and recognize the importance of giving balanced ration to their animals. Keeping this in view, NDDB has developed software for ration balancing, which will guide the milk producer about scientific animal feeding.

Implementation of RBP optimizes milk production of milk animals at the least cost by proper utilization to available feed ingredients, so as to provide them adequate amounts of proteins, minerals, vitamins as well as energy. This requires creation of a delivery system that provides advices to the producers and also arranges sale of feed and feed supplements that helps in sustaining the activity.

2. Field Artificial Insemination Services

High levels of productivity in dairy cattle can be achieved by bringing larger proportion of breedable female bovines under artificial insemination (A.I.) services. This opens a wide opportunity for entrepreneurs who can become Mobile A.I. Technicians (MAITs). MAITs can provide quality A.I. services at the farmer's doorstep.

Other Opportunities

- Operating one's own dairy farm, involving milk production activities.
- Working as dairy farm managers.
- As dairy herdman.
- As milkers.
- As testers.
- As Stockman.
- As Manager in a Cooperative set up.
- Manufacture of cattle feeds and other value added products.
- Veterinary services for animal health and breeding.
- Import-Export (Machinery/Ingredients/Products).
- Use of automation and information technology.
- As fieldsmen for dairy organisations.
- As fieldsmen for pure breed associations.
- As technical staff for research organisations.
- Teachers.
- Dairy extension worker—imparting vocational training.
- Writers for technical journals/magazines.
- Opportunities for leadership.
- Miscellaneous-
  - (a) Consultancy services.
  - (b) Financial security is afforded.
  - (c) Wholesome environment provided.
  - (d) Savings are encouraged.
  - (e) Encouragement for improvement.

Prevailing Support System for Dairy Entrepreneurship

1. Technical support
2. Financial support

1. Technical Support

A. Institutes for Professional Skills in Dairy Based Enterprises

Several institutions offer training programmes in dairy based enterprises:

I. Society for Innovation & Entrepreneurship in Dairying (SINED): Society for Innovation & Entrepreneurship in Dairying (SINED) is registered under Societies Registration Act 1860, hosted by ***National Dairy Research Institute, Karnal*** for promotion of entrepreneurship in dairying. The major activity of the society is to administer a **Technology Business Incubator** which provides support for technology based entrepreneurship in Dairying.

The TBI is Designed to Support and Nurture Industries in the Following Areas

- ☆ Commercial Dairy Processing
- ☆ Commercial Dairy Farming
- ☆ Commercial Food Processing
- ☆ Commercial Feed Technology

Entrepreneurship Development Programme (EDP) Conducted by SINED-TBI at NDRI, Karnal

i. Entrepreneurship Development Programme on Commercial dairy Farming

ii. Entrepreneurship Development Programme on Clean Milk Production

iii. Entrepreneurship Development Programme on Milk and Milk Products Processing

II. State Agricultural Universities: SAU's through its directorate of extension education and KVK (Krishi Vigyan Kendras) organize several training programmes to farmers, dairy owners, and rural youth for skill development in agriculture including dairy farming.

III. State Animal Husbandry Department also have mandate for capacity building programmes for dairy owners.

IV. Indira Gandhi National Open University (IGNOU): Indira Gandhi National Open University IGNOU offers several diploma programmes on training in dairy entrepreneurship for farmers and rural youth. Some of these programmes are

i. Diploma in Dairy Technology

ii. Training skills in Dairy entrepreneurship

iii. Awareness Programme on Dairy Farming for Rural Farmers (APDF)

V. National Social Entrepreneurship Forum (NSEF) is a non-profit organization supporting youth-driven social innovations & entrepreneurship in India (http://nsef-india.org). National Social Entrepreneurship Forum was founded by Yashveer Singh and Srikumar in 2009 at Bangalore. Since its inception, NSEF has undertaken social entrepreneurial activities in several academic institutes and cities across India and has worked in collaboration with various organizations such as Villgro, Samhita Social Ventures, NASSCOM Social Innovation Honours, Ashoka Innovators for the Public, and Sankalp Forum to enable youth-driven social innovations and young social entrepreneurs. NSEF has trained thousands of students through its programs across India.

Programs

- NSEF Idea Conferences- A platform to educate students about social innovations and to provide them with a launch pad for their social entrepreneurial ideas.
- NSEF Authors of Change Program- A solutions delivery program for key challenges that social organizations are facing, by connecting them to student talent from across the country through internships.
- NSEF Fellowship- A support program for students who start social ventures after completing college, to connect them with the resources and network they would need to grow their ventures.

VI. Skill India is an initiative of the Government of India. It was launched by Prime Minister Narendra Modi on 16 July 2015 with an aim to train over 40 crore people in India in different skills by 2022. The initiatives include National Skill Development Mission, National Policy for Skill Development and Entrepreneurship 2015, Pradhan Mantri Kaushal Vikas Yojana (PMKVY) scheme and the Skill Loan scheme.

B. Institutes for Management and Strategic Skills

Several institutes help to build management and strategic skills required by a budding entrepreneur. Some of them are

National Level Training Institutes

- National Institute of Micro, Small and Medium Industry Extension Training (NIMSMIET), Hyderabad.
- National Institute for Entrepreneurship and Small Business Development (NIESBUD), at Noida, which conducts national and international level training programmes in different fields and disciplines.
- Indian Institute of Entrepreneurship (IIE), Guwahati. The main objective of the institute is to act as a catalyst for entrepreneurship development with its focus on the North East.

Other Associated Agencies

- National Small Industries Corporation (NSIC) for technology and marketing support
- Small Industries Development Bank of India (SIDBI) an apex bank set up to provide direct/indirect financial assistance under different schemes to meet credit needs of the small-scale sector and to coordinate the functions of other institutions in similar activities.
- Khadi and Village Industries Commission (KVIC) assist the development and promotion and disbursal of rural and traditional industries in rural and town areas.

State Level Institutional Support

- ✰ State Government executes different promotional and developmental projects/schemes and provides a number of supporting incentives for development and promotion of MSME sector in their respective States.
- ✰ These are executed through State Directorate of Industries, who has District Industries Centers (DICs) under them to implement Central/State Level schemes.
- ✰ The State Industrial Development & Financial Institutions and State Financial Corporations also look after the needs of the MSME sector.

2. Financial Support

Bank Support for Dairy Entrepreneurship in India

Setting up dairy enterprise be it a small dairy unit, goat unit, milk and meat processing plant, selling parlor requires capital. Lack of access to credit to expand the herd is a critical problem for farmers. There is little access to formal credit through the cooperatives or banks. Informal credit is available from private traders and agents of private companies, but the interest rate is very high. Keeping this situation in mind and to provide financial support from banks few major dairy entrepreneurship schemes have been developed and implemented by banks with the support of state animal husbandry departments across different parts of the country. National Bank on agriculture and Rural Development (NABARD) is the lead bank for financial support of such schemes.

1. Dairy Entrepreneurship Development Scheme

Dairy Entrepreneurship Development Scheme (DEDS) was started in September, 2010 with the objective for promotion of private investment in dairy sector in order to increase the milk production in the country and helping in poverty reduction through self-employment opportunities. This scheme is being implemented through NABARD which provides financial assistance to commercially bankable projects with loan from Commercial, Cooperative, Urban and Rural banks with a back ended capital subsidy of 25% of the project cost to the beneficiaries of general category and 33.33% of the project cost to SC & ST beneficiaries. The scheme has approved for continuation with certain modifications and the budget provision of Rs 1,400 crore during 12th five year plan. Since inception, against the total release of Rs 871.29 crore, NABARD has disbursed Rs 823.14 crore as back ended capital subsidy to the beneficiaries for setting up of 2,24,402 dairy units upto 31st December, 2014.

Under these scheme farmers, individual entrepreneurs, NGOs, companies, groups of unorganized and organized sector including self-help groups, dairy cooperative societies, milk unions and milk federations are eligible for financial assistance from banks to set up following type of dairy based enterprise:

1. Establishment of small dairy units with crossbred cows/ indigenous descript milch cows like Sahiwal, Red Sindhi, Gir, Rathi etc. or graded buffaloes upto 10 animals.

2. Bank supports cheap credit upto Rs 6.00 lakh (earlier Rs 5 lakh) for 10 animal units.
3. Rearing of heifer calves – cross bred, indigenous descript milch breeds of cattle and of graded buffaloes – upto 20 calves. Bank supports cheap credit upto Rs 5.30 lakh (earlier Rs 4.80 lakh) for 20 calf units
4. Vermicompost with milch animal unit (to be considered with milch animals and not separately), bank supports cheap credit up to Rs 22,000/- (earlier Rs 20,000/-)
5. Purchase of milking machines /milk testers/bulk milk cooling units (upto 5000 lit capacity, earlier 2000 lit capacity), bank supports cheap credit upto Rs 22 lakh
6. Purchase of dairy processing equipment for manufacture of indigenous milk products, bank supports cheap credit upto Rs 13.20 lakhs.
7. Establishment of dairy product transportation facilities and cold chain, bank supports cheap credit upto Rs 26.50 lakh (earlier Rs 24 lakh)
8. Cold storage facilities for milk and milk products, bank supports cheap credit upto Rs 33 lakh (earlier Rs 30 lakh)
9. Establishment of private veterinary clinic, bank supports cheap credit upto Rs 2.60 lakh (earlier Rs 2.40 lakh) for mobile clinic and Rs 2 lakh (earlier Rs 1.80 lakh) for stationary clinic
10. Dairy marketing outlet / Dairy parlor, bank supports cheap credit upto Rs 1 lakh (earlier Rs 56,000/-)

Dairy Entrepreneurship Development Scheme (DEDS)

S. No	*Component*	*Unit Cost*	*Pattern of Assistance*
I	*Establishment of small dairy units with crossbred cows/ indigenous descript milch cows like Sahiwal, Red Sindhi, Gir, Rathi etc / graded buffaloes upto 10 animals, (for SHGs, Cooperatives societies, Producer Companies unit size will be 2-10 animals per member)*	*Rs. 6.00 lakh for 10 animal unit-minimum unit size is 2 animals with a n upper limit of 10 animals*	*25% of the project cost (33.33% for SC/ ST farmers), as back ended capital subsidy. Subsidy shall be restricted on prorata basis to a maximum of 10 animals subject to a ceiling of Rs. 15,000 per animal, (Rs 20,000 for SC/ ST farmers) or actual whichever is lower.* *Beneficiaries may purchase animals of higher costs, however, the subsidy will be restricted to the above ceilings*
II	*Rearing of heifer calves – cross bred, indigenous descript milch breeds of cattle and graded buffaloes – upto 20 calves*	*Rs. 5.30 lakh for 20 calf unit with an upper limit of 20 calves*	*25 % of the project cost (33.33 % for SC/ ST farmers) as back ended capital subsidy. Subsidy shall be restricted on prorata basis to a maximum of 20 calf unit subject to a ceiling of Rs 6,600/- per calf (Rs 8, 800 for SC/ST farmers) or actual, whichever is lower.*
III	*Vermicompost with milch animal unit (to be considered with milch animals/small dairy farm and not separately)*	*Rs. 22,000*	*25% of the project cost (33.33 % for SC /ST farmers) as back ended capital subsidy subject to a ceiling of Rs. 5,500/- (Rs7300/- for SC/ST farmers) or actual whichever is lower.*

S. No	Component	Unit Cost	Pattern of Assistance
IV	*Purchase of milking machines / milkotesters / bulk milk cooling units (upto 5000 lit capacity)*	*Rs. 20 lakh*	*25% of the project cost (33.33 SC/ST farmers) as back ended capital subsidy subject to a ceiling of Rs 5.0 lakh (Rs.6.67 lakh for SC / ST farmers) or actual whichever is lower.*
V	*Purchase of dairy processing equipment for manufacture milk products.*	*Rs.13.20 lakh*	*25% of the project cost (33.33 % for SC/ST farmers) as back ended capital subsidy subject to a ceiling of Rs. 3.30 lakh (Rs. 4.40 lakh for SC/ST farmers) or actual whichever is lower.*
VI	*Establishment of dairy product transportation facilities and cold chain*	*Rs. 26.50 lakh*	*25% of the project cost (33.33 % for SC/ST farmers) as back ended capital subsidy subject to a ceiling Rs. 6.625 lakh (Rs. 8.830 lakh for SC/ST farmers) or actual whichever is lower.*
VII	*Cold storage facilities for milk and milk products*	*Rs 33 lakh*	*25% of the project cost (33.33% for SC/ST farmers) as back ended capital subsidy subject to a ceiling of Rs. 8.25 lakh (Rs. 11.0 lakh for SC/ST farmers) or actual whichever is lower.*
VII	*Establishment of private veterinary clinic*	*Rs. 2.60 lakh for mobile clinic and Rs 2.0 lakh for stationary clinic*	*25% of the project cost (33.33% for SC /ST farmers) as back ended capital subsidy subject to a ceiling of Rs. 65,000/- and Rs. 50.000/- (Rs. 86,600/- and Rs. 66.600/- for SC/ST farmers) respectively for mobile and stationary clinics or actual whichever is lower.*
IX	*Dairy marketing outlet / Dairy parlour*	*Rs.1.0 lakh/-*	*25% of the project cost (33.33 % for SC /ST farmers) or actual whichever is lower.*

Funding Pattern

1. 1. Entrepreneur contribution (margin) - 10 % of the outlay (minimum)
2. 2. Back ended capital subsidy of 25 %(33.33 % for SC/ST beneficiaries of the project cost.

Banking Requirement for the Scheme

Procedure for Sanction of project and availing subsidy through banks

Step 1: Beneficiary should apply to the bank for sanction of the project

Step 2: The bank shall approve the project of the eligible as per their norms and sanction the total outlay excluding the margin, as the bank loan.

Step 3: The loan amount is disbursed in suitable installments depending on the progress of the unit.

Step 4: The bank shall apply to the concerned Regional Office of NABARD for sanction and release of subsidy in the specified format, after the disbursement of first installment of loan.

Time Limit for Completion of the Project

It is maximum of 9 months from the date of disbursement of the first installment of loan which may be extended by a further period of 3 months, if reasons for delay are considered justified by the concerned financial institution

Process for Obtaining NABARD Dairy Farming Subsidy

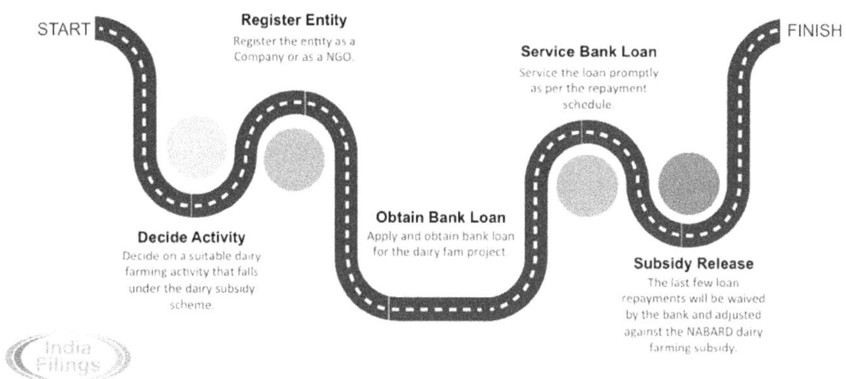

EDI (Entrepreneurship Development Institute) at State Level

EDIs run training courses for the successful running of dairy farms for the farmers who have a keen interest in this industry and are established by the state governments to cater needs of different sections of the society for entrepreneurship development.

Dairy Insurance

Dairy rearing is central to livelihoods and survival of millions of people of India. It is estimated that approximately 100 million people derive their live hood from dairy rearing as primary or secondary source of income. Dairy related activities help to maintain regular in flow of income for these households. Small farmers in India generate nearly half of their income from dairy and the value of cattle represents a significant part of their wealth, so the death of cattle poses a significant risk and affects farmers' net worth and income.

Type of Risks to Dairy Based Livelihoods

Large animals are expensive and thus carry higher risk exposure. Dairy losses due to the disease, accident, theft, natural calamity can cause significant losses to these household. Sometimes owners are forced to sell their animals due to loss due to incurable disease/ disorder/ fodder and water scarcity and they are unable to rebuild their stock. Many times animal losses force them into poverty trap from where they are unable to recover.

Risks faced by dairy owner's dairy dependent livelihoods can be classified into two broad categories

1. Production risk

2. Price risk

1. Production Risk- These Include

1. **Lack of Nutrition:** It may be due to non-availability of inputs (dry and green fodder for animals)
2. **Morbidity:** (Cattle disease like mastitis, FMD, HS result in reduction or stoppage of milk production, loss of animal value due to permanent loss in productivity, fertility and hide value of animal.
3. **Cattle Morality:** It may be accidental or natural loss of asset is biggest challenge for cattle owner as there is dramatic fall in income.

2. Price Risk

1. Fluctuation in the costs of cattle and its products during disease outbreaks
2. Changes in demand supply equation of dairy production leading to reduced demand/ lower price which results in income losses to farmers.

Dairy Insurance in Dairy Risk Management

Dairy risk management would involve two components-risk reduction and risk transfer. Risk reduction mechanisms through government owned veterinary services have limited impact due to shortage of manpower, timely nature of veterinary services, remoteness of famer's location, poor delivery of services etc. Therefore, role of risk transfer in the form of dairy insurance becomes importance. Dairy insurance would not only minimize the economic losses due to animal loss but also it may incentivize the dairy owner to rear quality animals in the wake of adequate risk protection mechanism through dairy insurance.

Dairy Insurance in India

Pioneering effort to create a market for dairy insurance was started by Government of India in 1971 with the help of Small Farmers Development agency (SFDA). Subsequently several scheme e.g. Integrated Rural Development Programmes (IRDP) were launched at the national level to provide safety nets for all dairy rearing farmers in the country. In these schemes cattle insurance was tied with rural credit delivery programs. Thus, insurance remained scheme driven and mandatory in nature with little awareness among the customers. Also, public players remained the only sources of dairy insurance in India till 2003. However, private players like ICICI Lombard, IFFCO Tokio etc. entered in dairy insurance since 2003.

Procedure of Dairy Insurance in India

1. Normally dairy insurance covers following category of animals whether indigenous, exotic or cross-bred.

    a) Milch Cows and Buffaloes

    b) Calves / Heifers

    c) Stud Bulls

d) Bullocks (Castrated Bulls) and Castrated Male Buffaloes.

2. Animals within a specified age group are accepted under the Standard Insurance Scheme.
3. Sum Insured under the policy will be the Market Value of the animal.
4. Indemnity under the policy will be the sum insured or market value prior to illness whichever less is. The indemnity is limited to 75% of Sum Insured in case of a Permanent Total Disability (PTD) claim.
5. The basic premium rate per annum is 4% of the Sum Insured. Long term policies are also issued with long term discounts.
6. The premium rates under the policy are concessional for covering animals under government subsidized schemes e.g. Dairy insurance.
7. Group Discounts are also available.

Insurance Coverage

The policy shall give indemnity for death due to

a. Accident (Inclusive of fire, lightning, flood, inundation, storm, hurricane, earthquake, cyclone, tornado, tempest and famine).
b. Diseases contracted or occurring during the period of this policy.
c. Surgical Operations.
d. Riot and Strike.

The Policy can also be extended to cover PTD on payment of extra premium;

i. Permanent Total Disability which, in the case of Milch Cattle result in permanent and total incapacity to conceive or yield milk.
ii. PTD which in the case of Stud Bulls results in permanent and total incapacity for breeding purpose.
iii. In case of Bullocks, Calves / Heifers and Castrated male buffaloes results in permanent and total incapacity for the purpose of use mentioned in the proposal form.

Major Exclusions

(A) Common Exclusions

i. Malicious or willful injury or neglect, overloading, unskillful treatment or use of animal for purpose other than stated in the policy without the consent of the Company in writing.
ii. Accidents occurring and /or Disease contracted prior to commencement of risk.
iii. Intentional slaughter of the animal except in cases where destruction is necessary to terminate incurable suffering on humane consideration on the basis of certificate issued by qualified Veterinarian or in cases where

destruction is resorted to by the order of lawfully constituted authority.

iv. Theft and clandestine sale of the insured animal.

v. War, invasion, act of foreign enemy, hostilities (whether war be declared or not), civil war, rebellion, revolution, insurrection, mutiny, tumult, military or usurped power or any consequences thereof or attempt threat.

vi. Any accident, loss, destruction, damage or legal liability directly or indirectly caused by or contributed to by or arising from nuclear weapons.

vii. Consequential loss of whatsoever nature.

viii. Transport by air and sea.

ix. Any non-scheme claim arising due to diseases contracted within 15 days from the date of risk are not covered.

(B) Specific Exclusions

i. Pleuropneumonia in respect of Cattle in Lakhimpur and Sibasagar Districts and newly carved out districts out of these two districts of Assam.

ii. All the claims received without ear tag.

Documents to Effect Insurance Coverage

a. Proposal Form.

b. Veterinary Health Certificate from a qualified Veterinarian giving the age, identification marks, health, and market value of the animal in the prescribed format.

Identification of Animal

a. All insured animals should be suitably identified by natural Identification marks and color should be clearly noted in the proposal form and Veterinarian's Report.

b. Ear tags made of suitable material are applied to the ear of the animals and the code number is entered into the Veterinary Health Certificate.

c. Photographs of animals may be insisted in case of high value animal.

Claim Procedure

In the event of death of an animal, immediate intimation should be sent to the Insurers and the following requirements should be furnished:

i. Duly completed claim form.

ii. Death Certificate obtained from qualified Veterinarian on Company's form.

iii. Postmortem examination report if required by the Company.

iv. Ear Tag applied to the animal should be surrendered. The condition of' No Tag- No claim' will be applied if the tag is not surrendered.

Claim Procedure for PTD Claim

i. A certificate from the qualified Veterinarian to be obtained.

ii. The animal will be inspected by the company's Veterinary Officer also.

iii. Complete chart of treatment, medicines used, receipts, etc., should be submitted.

iv. Admissibility of claim will be considered after two months of Veterinary Doctor / Company Doctor's report.

v. The indemnity is limited to 75% of Sum Insured.

Dairy Insurance Scheme by Government of India

The dairy insurance scheme is a centrally sponsored scheme, which was implemented on a pilot basis during 2005-06 of the 10th five year plan and in 2007-08 of 11th five year plan in 100 selected districts of India.

Objectives of Scheme

The Dairy Scheme has been formulated with the twin objective of providing protection mechanism to the farmers and cattle bearers against any eventual loss of their animals due to death and to demonstrate the benefit of the Insurance of dairy to the people and popularize it with the ultimate goal of attaining qualitative improvement in dairy and their products.

Features of the Scheme

1. Under the scheme, the crossbred and high yielding cattle and buffaloes are being insured at maximum of their current market price. The premium of the Insurance is subsidized to the tune of 50%. The entire cost of the subsidy is being become by the central Government.
2. The benefit of subsidy is being provided to a maximum of 2 animals per beneficiary for policy of maximum of three years.
3. Animal to be covered under the scheme and selection of beneficiaries:
4. All those female cattle / buffalo yielding at least 1500 Littre of milk per lactation are to be considered high yielding and hence can be insured under the scheme for maximum of their current market value.
5. Animals covered under any other Insurance scheme / plan scheme will not be covered under scheme.
6. Benefit of subsidy is to be restricted to two animals per beneficiary and is to be given for one time Insurance of an animal up to a maximum period of three years.
7. The farmer will have to be encouraged to go for a three year policy which is likely to be more economical and useful for getting the real benefit of on

occurrence of natural calamities like flood and drought etc, However , if a dairy owner prefers o have an Insurance policy for less than three years period for valid reasons, benefit for valid reasons, benefit of the subsidy under the scheme would be available to them also , with the restriction that no subsidy would be available of further extension of the policy.

8. The animal insured will have to be properly and uniquely identified at the time of Insurance claim. The ear tagging should, therefore, be fool proof as ear as possible. The traditional method of ear tagging or the recent technology of fixing microchips could be used at the time of taking the policy.
9. The cost of fixing the identification mark will be borne by the Insurance companies and responsibility of its maintenance will be mutually agreed by the beneficiaries and the Insurance Company.

The Veterinary practitioners may guide the beneficiaries about the need and importance of the tags fixed for settlement of their claim so that they proper care for maintenance of the tags.

Scientific Dairy Practices

Selection of Dairy Cattle

Proper selection is the first and the most important step to be adopted in dairying. Records are the basis of selection and hence proper identification of animals and record keeping is essential. Cross-breed animals with exotic inheritance of about 50 percent are preferable.

Bringing animals from different agro-climatic conditions causes problems due to non-adjustment in many cases. In case, purchase becomes absolutely essential it should be from similar environmental conditions as far as possible.

General Selection Procedures for Dairy Breeds

Selecting a calf in calf show, a cow in cattle show by judging is an art. A dairy farmer should build up his own herd by breeding his own herd. Following guidelines will be useful for selection of a dairy cow.

- ✰ Whenever an animal is purchased from cattle fair, it should be selected based upon its breed characters and milk producing ability.
- ✰ History sheet or pedigree sheet which is generally maintained in organized farms reveals the complete history of animal.
- ✰ The maximum yields by dairy cows are noticed during the first five lactations. So generally selection should be carried out during First or Second lactation and that too are month after calving.
- ✰ There successive complete milking has to be done and an average of it will give a fair idea regarding production by a particular animal.
- ✰ A cow should allow anybody to milk, and should be docile.
- ✰ It is better to purchase the animals during the months of October and November.

- ✰ Maximum yield is noticed till 90 days after calving.

Breed Characteristics of High Yielding Dairy Cows

- ✰ Attractive individuality with feminity, vigor, harmonious blending of all parts, impressive style and carriage.
- ✰ Animal should have wedge shaped appearance of the body.
- ✰ It should have bright eyes with lean neck.
- ✰ The udder should be well attached to the abdomen.
- ✰ The skin of the udder should have a good network of blood vessels.
- ✰ All four quarters of the udder should be well demarcated with well-placed teats.

High Yielding Breeds of Dairy Cattle And Buffalo

Cattle		*Buffalo*
Indigenous	Exotic	
Sahiwal	Holstein Friesian	Murrah
Red Sindhi	Jersey	Nili-Ravi
Crosses of HF and Jersey with indigenous breeds		

Economic Characters in Dairy Cattle and Buffalo

The various economic characters in Dairy Cattle and Buffalo management are:

Lactation Yield

- ✰ Normally in dairy cattle 30 - 40 % increase in milk production from first lactation to maturity is observed.
- ✰ After 3 or 4 lactation the production starts declining.
- ✰ After parturition the milk yield per day will be increased and reaches peak within 2-4 weeks after calving. This yield is known as peak yield.

Lactation Period

- ✰ The length of milk producing period after calving is known as lactation period.
- ✰ The optimum lactation period is 305 days.

Persistency of Milk Yield

- ✰ During lactation period the animal reaches maximum milk yield per day within 2-4 weeks which is called peak yield.
- ✰ The maintenance of peak yield for long period is known as persistency, slow decrease in dairy milk yield after reaching peak yield in necessary.
- ✰ High persistency is necessary to maintain high level of milk production.

Age at First Calving

- ✰ The desirable age at first calving in Indian breeds is 3 years, 2 years in cross breed cattle and 3½ years in Buffaloes.

Service Period

- ✰ It is the period between date of calving and date of successful conception. For cattle the optimum service period is 60-90 days.

Dry Period

- ✰ It is the period from the date of drying (stop of milk production) to next calving.
- ✰ A minimum of 2 - 2½ months dry period should be allowed.

Inter-Calving Period

- ✰ This is the period between two successive calvings.
- ✰ It is more, profitable to have one calf yearly in cattle and at least one calf for every 15 months in buffaloes.

Reproductive Efficiency

- ✰ The reproductive efficiency means the more number of calves during life time, so that total life time production is increased.

Efficiency of Feed Utilization and Conversion into Milk

- ✰ The animal should utilize the feed efficiently to convert into the milk.

Disease Resistance

- ✰ Indian breeds are more resistant to majority of disease compared to exotic cattle. Cross breeding helps to get this character.

Housing for Dairy Animals

General Housing Requirements

Dairy animals will be more efficient in the production of milk and in reproduction if they are protected from extreme heat, and particularly from direct sunshine. This can be achieved through provision of shade in tropical and subtropical climates. If dairy animals are confined, the area should be free of mud and manure in order to reduce hoof infection to a minimum. Concrete floors or pavements are ideal where the area per animal is limited. However, where ample space is available, an earth yard, properly sloped for good drainage is adequate.

Location of Dairy Buildings

The points which should be considered before the creation of dairy buildings animal houses are as follows:

Topography and Drainage

The houses should be well raised / elevated for the surrounding ground to offer a good slope for rainfall and more drainage of dairy wastes to avoid stagnation and for the spread of diseases. A leveled area requires less site preparation and thus lesser cost of building. Low lands and depressions should be avoided.

Exposure to the Sun and Protection from Wind

A dairy building should be located to a maximum exposure to the sun in the north and minimum exposure in the south and protect from prevailing strong wind currents whether hot or cold. Buildings should be placed such that direct sunlight can reach the platforms, gutters and mangers in the cattle shed. It is better to have, the long axis of the dairy barns set in the north-south direction to have maximum benefit of the sun.

Water Supply

Abundant supply of fresh, clean and soft water should be available.

Surroundings

Narrow gates, high manger curbs, loose hinges, protruding nails, smooth finished floor in the areas where the cows move should be eliminated.

Labor

Honest, economic and regular supply of labor should be available.

Marketing

Dairy buildings should be in those areas where selling of dairy products can be done profitably and regularly. Owner should be in a position to satisfy the needs of the farm within no time and at reasonable price.

Facilities

Cattle yards should be situated in relation to feed storages, hay stacks, silo and manure pits as to effect the most efficient utilization of labor. Sufficient space per cow and well-arranged feeding mangers and resting contribute not only to greater milk yield of cows and make the work of the operator easier also minimizes feed expenses.

Orientation

In deciding which orientation to build, the following factors need be considered:

a. With the east-west orientation the feed and water troughs can be under the shade which will allow the animals to eat and drink in shade at any time of the day. The shaded area, however, should be increased to 3 to 4 m^2 per animal. By locating the feed and water in the shade, feed consumption will be encouraged, but also more manure will be dropped in the shaded area which in turn will lead to dirty animals.

b. With the north-south orientation, the sun will strike every part of the floor area under and on either side of the roof at some time during the day. This will help to keep the floored area dry. A shaded area of 2.5 to 3m² per animal is adequate if feed and water troughs are placed away from the shaded area.

c. If it is felt that paving is too costly, the north-south orientation is the best choice in order to keep the area as dry as possible.

d. In regions where temperatures average 30°C or more for up to five hours per day during some period of the year, the east-west orientation is most beneficial.

e. The gable roof is more wind resistant than a single pitch roof and allows for a centre vent. A woven mat of local materials can be installed between the rafters and the corrugated iron roof to reduce radiation from the steel and lower temperatures just under the roof by 10°C or more.

Animal Shed

- ✰ The entire shed should be surrounded by a boundary wall of 5 feet height from three side and manger etc., on one side.
- ✰ The feeding area should be provided with 2 to 2 ½ feet of manger space per cow.
- ✰ All along the manger, there shall be 10″ wide water trough to provide clean, even, available drinking water. The water trough constructed can minimize the loss of fodders during feeding.
- ✰ Near the manger, under the roofed house 5″ wide floor should be paved with bricks having a little slope. Beyond that, there should be open unpaved area (40′X35′) surrounded by 5 feet wall with one gate.
- ✰ It is preferable that animals face north when they are eating fodder under the shade. During cold wind in winter the animals will automatically lie down to have the protection from the walls.
- ✰ Cow sheds can be arranged in a single row if the numbers of cows are small.
- ✰ In double row housing, the stable should be so arranged that the cows face out (tails to tail system) or face in (head to head system) as preferred.

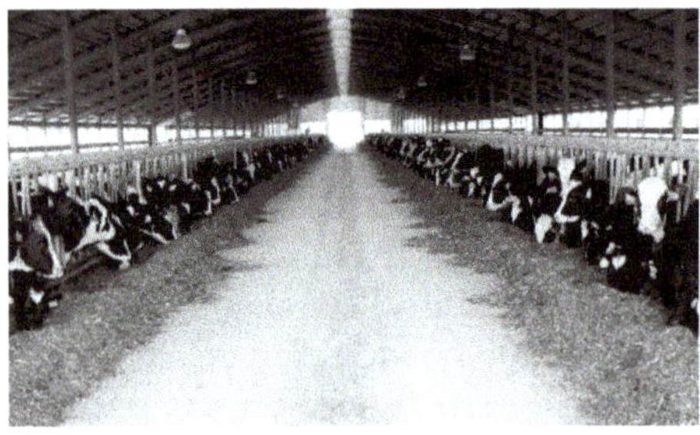

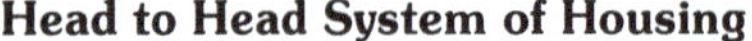

Head to Head System of Housing

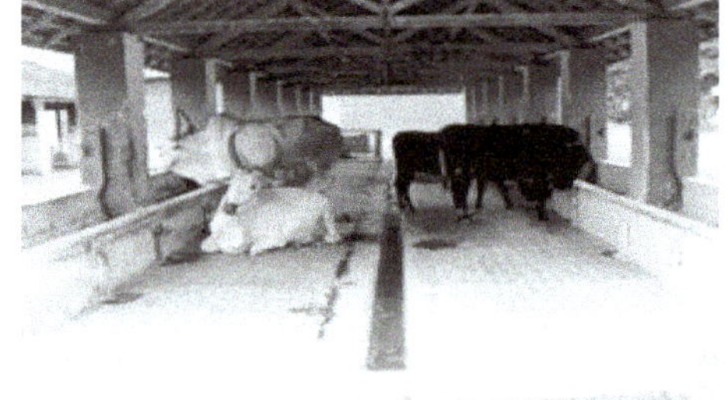

Tail to Tail System of Housing

Floor

The inside floor of the barn should be of some impervious material which can be easily kept clean and dry and is not slippery. Grooved cement concrete floor is still better. The surface of the cowshed should be laid with a gradient of 1″ to 14″ from manger to excreta channel. An overall floor space of 60 to 70 square feet per adult cow should be satisfactory.

Type of animal	*Floor space per animal (sq. feet)*		*Manger length per animal (in inches)*
	Covered area	*Open area*	
Cow	20-30	80-100	20-24
Buffalo	25-35	80-100	24-30
Young stock	15-20	50-60	15-20
Pregnant cows	100-120	180-200	24-30
Bull pen	120-140	200-250	24-30

Feeding of Dairy Animals

Feed

The important feed ingredients are carbohydrates, proteins, fats, minerals, vitamins and water. These ingredients are supplied through roughages and concentrates. Before embarking on a dairy farming enterprise it is important to find out the type of feeds available affordably in your area. Types of feeds can be divided into:

1. Forages (Roughages): these include Napier grass, hay, grass, maize (Stover and residues) plants, and banana pseudo stems. Fodder legumes like leucaene (Leucaena leucocephala), calliandra (Calliandra calothyrsus), sesbania (Sesbania sesban) and gliricidia (Gliricidia sepium).
2. Concentrates: these include wheat bran, maize germ, dairy meal, and pollard or maize bran. These types of feeds cannot be produced on small or medium scale farms, as they require large capital investments. Concentrates are usually used in small quantities, unlike forages.
3. Other byproducts: e.g. cotton seed cake, fishmeal, molasses, brewer's waste and poultry waste. These are usually by products of other industrial or farm enterprises, but are rich in nutrients that increase productivity of dairy animals.
4. Feed additives: e.g. minerals and vitamins, livestock salts, buffers, enzymes, probiotics yeast and urea. These also have to be purchased and are an essential component of costs in a dairy enterprise.

Guideline for Preparation of 100kg Concentrate Feed

1. Crushed maize: 42kg
2. Oats/wheat/rice bran: 35kg
3. Oil cakes: 20kg

4. Mineral mixture: 2kg
5. Salt: 1kg

Balanced Ration

- ☆ During formulation of dairy cow rations, the daily requirements for all the above nutrients must be taken into consideration.
- ☆ The available feed resources should then be mixed to meet the cow's nutrient requirements, which are dependent on bodyweight, milk yield, reproductive (pregnancy) requirements and growth.
- ☆ A balanced ration will consist of combined feed ingredients which will be consumed in amounts needed to supply the daily nutrient requirements of the cow, both in correct proportion and amount.
- ☆ A ration will be balanced when all the required nutrients are present in feed eaten by the cow during a 24 hour period.
- ☆ When a ration is not balanced, the cow eats some nutrients in excess or in insufficient amounts.
- ☆ Some excesses and deficiencies, if not checked, can lead to death (e.g. calcium deficiency resulting in milk fever).
- ☆ A properly balanced ration will therefore be a mixture of all the ingredients.

Practical Feeding

During the formulation of rations for lactating dairy cows, the quality of the ration should be commensurate with the requirements of the cow. The requirement is directly related to the milk yield, which is in turn dependent on the stage of lactation. Cows in the same stage of lactation will have almost similar requirements and can therefore the rations can be formulated according to the phase (stage) of lactation.

Phase 1: (1-70 days)

- ☆ During this phase, milk production increases more rapidly than feed intake resulting in higher energy demand than intake leading to a negative energy balance.
- ☆ The health and nutrition of the cow during this phase is critical and affects the entire lactation performance.
- ☆ Excessive weight loss may be detrimental to cow's health and reproductive performance (cow may not come on heat at the optimum time) leading to long calving intervals.
- ☆ Concentrates should be added to the basal diet to increase the energy and protein content as forage alone will not be sufficient.
- ☆ Cows that are poorly fed during this early phase do not attain peak yield and milk production drops from 1st week.
- ☆ If excessive concentrates are added too rapidly (non-accustomed cows) to the ration, they can lead to digestive disturbances (rumen acidosis, loss

of appetite, reduced milk production, low milk fat content). It is therefore recommended that concentrates should be limited to 50-60% of diet dry matter, the rest being forage to ensure rumination (proper function of the rumen).

- If high amounts of concentrate are fed during this time buffers (chemicals that reduce the acid in the rumen and available commercially) can be helpful.
- At this stage, high protein content is important since the body cannot mobilize all the needed protein and bacteria protein (synthesized in the rumen by bacteria) can only partially meet requirements.
- A ration with protein content of 18%CP is recommended for high yielding cows. If the cow is underfed during this stage, milk production cannot recover even when balanced rations are fed at later stages.

Phase 2: (70-150days)

- During this phase the dry matter intake is adequate to support milk production and either maintain or slightly increase body weight.
- Feeding should be to maintain production peak as long as possible.
- Decline of 8-10%/month in milk production are common after peaking.
- The forage quality should still be high and a CP content of 15-18%.
- Concentrates high in digestible fiber (rather than starch) e.g. wheat or maize bran can be used as energy source.

Phase 3: (151-305days)

- During this phase feed intake and milk production decline.
- The body weight increase is due to replenishment of body reserves and, towards the end of lactation, due to increased growth of fetus.
- It has been shown that it is more efficient to replenish body weight during late lactation than during the dry period.
- The animals can be fed on lower quality roughage and limited amounts of concentrate compared to the other two phases.

Phase 4: (Dry Period: 305-365days)

- During this phase the cow continues to gain weight primarily due to weight of fetus.
- Proper feeding of cow during this stage will help realize the cow's potential during next lactation and minimize health problems at calving time (milk fever and ketosis).
- At the time of drying, cows should be fed a ration to cater for maintenance and pregnancy but two weeks before calving, the cow should be fed on concentrates in preparation for next lactation.

- This extra concentrate (steaming) enables the cow to store some reserves to be used in early lactation and to adapt rumen microbial population to digest concentrates in early lactation to minimize digestive disturbances.
- During this phase the cow can be fed good quality forage or poor quality supplemented with concentrate to provide 12% CP.
- The cows should not be fed high amounts of concentrate to avoid over conditioning. If the diet is rich in energy, intake should be limited.
- Bulky roughages can be fed to help increase rumen size to accommodate more feed at parturition.
- The amount of calcium and phosphorous fed should be restricted during the dry period to 0.4% and 0.25% to minimize incidences of milk fever.

Guidelines for Concentrate Feeding

- It should be noted that feedstuffs available in the market e.g. bran (wheat or maize), pollard or maize germ are not similar to the mixed concentrate as they are low in protein and minerals and should be used in combination with other ingredients when supplementing forages.
- The maximum amount of milk that can be produced without concentrate supplementation will depend on the quality of the pasture or forage. This has been reported to vary from 7-20 kg milk per day.
- Several guidelines have been suggested on the amount of concentrate that should be fed to a cow. The only accurate one is the one calculated based on the cow's nutrient requirements and the quality of the basal diet by a nutritionist.
- The example below is one of the many guidelines:

Up to 7 kg of milk comes from the basal forage diet.

For every extra 1.5kg milk above 7kg, give 1kg dairy meal should be given.

Examples of Nutrient Content of Common Feedstuffs used for Feeding Dairy Animals

Feed name (live weight kg)	*Energy (ME in Mcal)*	*TDN (kg)*	*Total crude protein (g)*	*Calcium (g)*	*Phosphorous (g)*
Alfalfa hay	2.36	0.63	200	15.4	2.2
Napier grass	2.0	0.55	87	6	4.1
Rape fresh	3.16	0.81	164	-	-
Oats	2.73	0.6	140	-	-
Sorghum fresh	2.36	0.63	88	4.3	3.6
Sorghum silage	2.14	0.58	62	3.4	1.7
Maize silage	2.67	0.7	81	2.3	2.2
Wheat straw	1.51	0.44	0	1.8	1.2
Rape seed	2.93	0.76	390	7.2	11.4
Cotton seed cake	2.71	0.71	448	1.9	1.2
Wheat bran	2.67	0.7	171	11.8	3.2

Feed name (live weight kg)	*Energy (ME in Mcal)*	*TDN (kg)*	*Total crude protein (g)*	*Calcium (g)*	*Phosphorous (g)*
Molasses	2.67	0.7	103	11	1.5
Urea	0	0	281	0	0

Examples of Feeding Regimes for a Lactating Dairy Animal Weighing 550 kg

Milk yield (7% fat)	*4% FCM*	*Kg dry matter of roughage*	*Kg dry matter of concentrate*
4kg	5.8kg	3.5 alfalfa hay + 3.2 maize silage + 4 wheat straw or	2 wheat bran
5kg	7.40kg	2 alfalfa hay + 4 maize silage + 4 fresh sorghum	
7 kg	10.15 kg	5.3 alfalfa hay + 5.5 maize silage or 4.5 alfalfa hay + 5 maize silage + 2 wheat straw or 3.5 alfalfa hay + 5.5 maize silage and	2 wheat bran
9 kg	13.05 kg	5.6 alfalfa hay + 5.5 maize silage + 3 wheat straw or 4.5 alfalfa hay + 5.5 maize silage and	2.5 wheat bran
10 kg	14.50 kg	6 alfalfa hay + 7 maize silage or 9 alfalfa hay + 3 maize silage and	1 cotton-seed-cake
12 kg	17.40 kg	7 alfalfa hay + 5 maize silage + 2 wheat straw and	1.5 wheat bran
15 kg	21.75 kg	7.5 alfalfa hay + 6 maize silage and	2.2 wheat bran + 0.5 molasses + 0.3 urea

Calf Starter Mixture

Feed source	*Amount*
Crushed barley	50%
Groundnut cake	30%
Wheat bran	8%
Skim milk powder	10%
Mineral mixture	2%
To increase palatability, add per 100kg of starter:	
Molasses	5-10kg
Salt	500g

Reproductive Management

Breeding of Heifers

- Regardless of age, puberty is reached when a heifer weighs approximately 40% of her mature body weight.
- Breeding however, is recommended when a heifer has reached 60% of her expected mature body weight. This is normally achieved when the heifer is 14 to 16 months old.
- Smaller breeds may be bred one or two months earlier than large breeds because they mature faster.

- Heifers in good condition and gaining weight at breeding time generally show more definite signs of estrus and have improved conception rates over heifers in poor condition and/or losing weight.
- Over-conditioned or fat heifers have been reported to require more services per conception than heifers of normal size and weight.
- Heat Detection

This is an extremely important exercise as a missed heat translates into a wasted 21 days while efficient heat detection makes it possible to serve the animal at the right time. The average heat interval is 21 days with a range of 18 to 24 days. Duration of heat is 24 to 36 hours in exotic and crossbred cows. Several methods are used to detect heat. The most commonly used by farmers are behavioral signs and physical changes.

Symptoms of Heat

The various symptoms of heat are

1. The animal will be excited condition.
2. The animal will be in restlessness and nervousness.
3. The animal will bellow frequently.
4. The animal will reduce the intake of feed.
5. Peculiar movement of lumbo-sacral region will be observed.
6. The animals which are in heat will lick other animals and smell other animals.
7. The animals will try to mount other animals.
8. The animals will standstill when other animal try to mount. This period is known as standing heat. This extends 14-16 hours.
9. Frequent micturition (urination) will be observed.
10. Clear mucous discharge will be seen from the vulva, sometimes it will be string like mucous will be seen stick to the near the pasts of vulva.
11. Swelling of the vulva will be seen.
12. Congestion and hyperarmia of membrane.
13. The tail will be in raised position.
14. Milk production will be slightly decreased.
15. On Palpation uterus will be turgid and the cervix will be opened.

Mating

Once heat has been detected, cows should be mated.

When to Serve

Present the cow for insemination at the right time to increase the chances of conception. Below is a guide as to the best time to present the cow for insemination:

AM – PM Rule:		
Standing heat observed:	Before 9 am	Late evening the same day
Present for insemination:	Late afternoon or evening	Early next morning.

Milking of Dairy Animals

Milking Hygiene

Good Practice

- ☆ Washing hands with soap and water before milking each cow.
- ☆ Washing the udder and each teat vigorously with soap and water and dry them with a clean cloth.
- ☆ Direct the first milk outside the milking bucket into separate container and throw away.
- ☆ Have a clean, dry, floor preferably of rough surfaced concrete without sharp points for the milking area.
- ☆ Keep calves where cows can see them during milking.
- ☆ Use clean containers for milking and before re-using the milk container, rinse it, scrub it with warm water and detergent or soap, rinse it again leave it to air-dry.
- ☆ After milking, cover the milk to avoid contamination and place in a clean and cool area.
- ☆ Keep the area clean and safe for animals.

Bad Practice

- ☆ Using Milk from sick cows can transmit diseases to humans.
- ☆ Using unclean plastic containers.
- ☆ Leaving milk uncovered.
- ☆ Keeping the milk in the sun or outdoors.

Methods of Milking

- ☆ Hand milking, and
- ☆ Machine milking

Hand Milking

- ☆ Many milkers during milking tend to bend their thumb against the teat. The method is known as knuckling which causes injury to teat tissues.
- ☆ Thus milking should always be done with full hand unless the teats are too small or towards the completion of milking.
- ☆ The first few strips of milk from each quarter should not be mixed with the rest of the milk as the former contains highest number of bacteria.

Machine Milking

Modern milking machines are capable of milking cows quickly and efficiently, without injuring the udder. The milking machine performs two basic functions:

- ☆ It opens the streak canal through the use of a partial vacuum, allowing the milk to flow out of the teat cistern through a line to a receiving container.
- ☆ Massages the teat, preventing congestion of blood and lymph in the teat.

Advantages

- ☆ Easy to operate, costs low, saves time as it milks 1.5 liter to 2 liters per minute.
- ☆ It is also very hygienic and energy-conserving as electricity is not required.
- ☆ All the milk from the udder can be removed.
- ☆ The machine is also easily adaptable and gives a suckling feeling to the cow and avoids pain in the udder as well as leakage of milk.

Care and Management of Calf

The feeding and care of the calf begins before its birth. The dam should be dried 6-8 weeks before expected calving and should be fed well. Underfed animals will give weak and small calves.

A) Early Management

1. Immediately after birth remove any mucous or phlegm from those nose and mouth.
2. Normally the cow licks the calf immediately the birth. This helps to dry off the calf and helps in stimulating breathing and circulation. When the cows do not lick or in cold climate, rub and dry the calf with a dry cloth or gunny bag. Provide artificial respiration by compression and relaxing the chest with hands.
3. The Naval should be tied about 2-5cm away from the body and cut 1cm below the ligature and apply Tr. Iodine or boric acid or any antibiotic.
4. Remove the wet bedding from the pen and keep the stall very clean and dry in condition.
5. The weight of the calf should be recorded.
6. Wash the cow's udder and teats preferably with chlorine solution and dry.
7. Allow the calf to suckle the first milk of the mother i.e. Colostrum.
8. The calf will be standing and attempts to nurse within one hour. Otherwise help weak calves to stand.

B) Feeding of Calves

1. Feed colostrum *i.e.* the first milk of the cow for the first 3 days.
2. Whole milk should be given after 3 days it is better to teach to drink the

milk from the pail or bucket. Feed twice a day which should be warmed to body temperature. For weak calves feed thrice a day.

3. The limit of liquid milk feeding is 10 % of its body weight with a maximum of 5-6 liters per day and continues liquid milk feeding for 6-10 weeks. Over feeding causes 'Calf Scours'.
4. The milk replacers can be given to replace whole milk.
5. Give calf starter after one month of age.
6. Provide good quality green fodder and hay from 4th month afterwards.
7. Feeding of antibiotics to calves improves appetite, increases growth rate and prevents calf scours. E.g. aureomycin, Terramycin etc.

Other Management Practices

1. Identity the calf by tattooing in the ear at birth, and branding after one year.
2. Dehorn the calf within 7-10 days after birth with red hot Iron or caustic potash stick or electrical method.
3. Deworm the calf regularly to remove worms using deworming drugs. Deworm at 30 days interval.
4. Fresh water should be given from 2nd week onwards.
5. House the calves in individual calf pens for 3 months afterwards in groups. After six months males and females calves should be housed separately.
6. Weigh the calves at weekly interval upto 6 months arid at monthly interval afterwards to know the growth rate.
7. Mortality in calves is more in first month due to pneumonia, diarrhea (calf scours) and worms. House them under warm condition, clean condition to avoid above condition.
8. Extra teats beyond 4 should be removed at 1-2 months of age.
9. 8-9 weeks of age, males should be castrated.
10. Keep the body clean and dry to avoid fungal infection.
11. Mineral-blocks should be provided, so that the calves lick and no chances for mineral deficiency occur.
12. Wean the calf from the mother and feed through pail feeding system.

Health

It is a state of freedom from disease. It may also be stated as a condition of an animal in which all the body organs are normal and are functioning to their optimum capacity in relation to animal's age, sex, work, and production with optimum pulse, temperature and respiration rates appropriate to the species, sex and environment.

Signs of Healthy Animal

1. Wet muzzle.
2. Shining skin and eyes.

3. Rosette pink mucous membranes.
4. Normal rumination (Ruminal movements: 3 per 2.5 minutes).
5. Normal gait and eating behavior.
6. Active reflexes.
7. Urination and defecation normal.
8. Well-kept head.
9. No abnormal discharge from any natural orifice.
10. No abnormality in milk and milk composition.

Signs of Illness in Animals

- ☆ General posture of animals, its behavior, movements and expressions change.
- ☆ Animal show dull dejected appearance and stands in isolation with head downwards.
- ☆ Loss of appetite and cessation of ruminal movements.
- ☆ Skin becomes dry, hair coat becomes dull, and hair may become brittle and fall off.
- ☆ Muzzle becomes dry.
- ☆ Sunken, glued eyes, staring look, discharge from eyes.
- ☆ Any abnormal discharge from natural orifices, pus from the organ involved shows septic changes.
- ☆ Blood or dark colored urine with repulsive odor.
- ☆ Change in color and consistency of feces.
- ☆ Change in quality and quantity of milk production.
- ☆ Change in voice of animal i.e. grunting, groaning or grinding of teeth by animal shows that animal is in pain.
- ☆ Nervous signs, edema of any body part, abnormal gait, inflammatory conditions.
- ☆ Change in respiration, body temperature, and pulse rate. Normal data is given as:

S.no.	*Species*	*Body temperature (°F)*	*Pulse rate (per minute)*	*Respiration rate (per minute)*
1.	Cattle : Calf Adult	101.3-104.4 101.5	90-120 50-60	27-50 20-25
2.	Buffalo	98.3 (winter) 103 (summer)	40-50	15-20

Deworming Schedule for Cattle and Buffaloes for Good Health

S.No.	*Type of worm*	*Deworming Schedule*
1.	Roundworms	First dose at 3 days of age and thereafter at monthly interval upto 6 months. Thrice a year in animals above 6 months of age.
2.	Liver flukes	Twice a year in endemic areas (before and after monsoon).
3.	Tapeworms	Twice a year i.e. in January and June in calves in problematic herds.

Sanitation in Dairy Farm

Sanitation is necessary in the dairy farm houses for elimination of all micro-organism that are capable of causing disease in the animals. The presence of organisms in the animal shed contaminates the milk produced thus reducing its shelf life, milk produced in an unclean environment is likely to transmit diseases which affect human health.

Cleaning of Animal Sheds

The easy and quick method of cleaning animal house is with liberal use of tap water, proper lifting and disposes all of dung and used straw bedding, providing drainage, to the animal house for complete removal of liquid waste and urine.

Sanitizers

Sunlight is the most potent and powerful sanitizer which destroy most of the disease producing organism. Disinfection of animal sheds means making these free from disease producing bacteria and is mainly-carried out by sprinkling chemical agents such as Bleaching Powder, Iodine and Iodophore, sodium carbonate, Washing soda, Slaked Lime (Calcium hydroxide), Quick Lime (Calcium oxide) and Phenol.

1. **Bleaching Powder:** This is also called calcium hypochloride. It contains upto 39 % available chlorine which has high disinfecting activity.
2. **Iodine & Iodophores:** This is commercially available as lodophores and contains between 1 and 2 % available Iodine which is an effective germicide.
3. **Sodium Carbonate:** A hot 4 % solution of washing soda is a powerful disinfectant against many viruses and certain bacteria.
4. **Slaked Lime and Quick Lime:** White washing with these agents makes the walls of the sheds and the water troughs free from bacteria.
5. **Phenol:** Phenol or carbolic acid is a very potent disinfectant which destroys bacteria as well as fungus.
6. **Insecticides:** Insecticides are the substances or preparations used for killing insects. In order to control flies and disease transmitting ticks, insecticides are used in dairy farms. Ticks usually hide in cracks and crevices of the walls and mangers. Smaller quantities of insecticide solutions are required for spraying. Liquid insecticides can be applied with a powerful sprayer-hand sprayer, a sponge or brush, commonly used insecticides are BHC, DDT, Gamaxane wettable powders, malathion, surriithion, Sevin 50 % emusifying concentration solutions.

These are highly poisonous and need to be handled carefully and should not come in contact with food material, drinking, water, milk etc.

Disposing of Waste and Carcasses

Before handling a carcass, consider the diseases that can be passed to humans (anthrax, brucellosis, rabies, ringworm and mange are the most common ones). If the animal died unexpectedly, a post-mortem will reveal the cause of death and guide the means of disposal.

How to burn a carcass:

- ✰ Dig two trenches (2 m long, 40 cm wide and 40 cm deep) in the form of a cross. The trenches will provide oxygen to the fire.
- ✰ Place two iron bars so they lie across one of the trenches.
- ✰ Place strong wooden posts across the bars.
- ✰ Place the carcass and a heap of fuel (wood and straw soaked in waste oil) on the wooden posts.
- ✰ Light the fire and burn the carcass.

Disposal by Burying

1. Dig a hole 2 m long by 1.5 m wide and 2 m deep.
2. Put the carcass in the hole and cover with soil and logs or large stones to stop wild animals or dogs digging it up again.

Suggested Readings

Characteristics of cattle and buffalo breeds by Indian Council of Agricultural Research.

Dairy cattle production selected readings by BAIF Development Research Foundation.

Field Manual on Scientific Dairy Practices by Pranav Kumar, S.A. Khandi, Mudasir Sulatana & Amandeep Singh. Division of Veterinary & Animal Husbandry Extension Education, Faculty of Veterinary Sciences & Animal Husbandry, Sher-E-Kashmir University of Agricultural Sciences & Technology of Jammu, R.S. Pura-181102 (J&K). Field Manual: (6) AU/FVSJ/AHE/15-16/542 (2016).

http://agritech.tnau.ac.in/animal_husbandry/animhus_index.html

http://www.elearnvet.net/

http://www.nbagr.res.in/

Livestock and Poultry Improvement and Management by National Bureau of Animal Genetics Resources.

Transforming Rural Areas through Veterinary Science *Pages* **61-72**
Editor: Dipanjali Konwar, Shilpa Sood & Shahid Ahamad
Published by: **ASTRAL INTERNATIONAL PVT. LTD., NEW DELHI**

4 Commercial Broiler Farming in Jammu Province

Dr. Suraj Amrutkar & Dr. Surinder K.Gupta

Introduction

Chicken meat is an important source of high quality proteins, minerals and vitamins. Commercial broilers are now available with the ability of quick growth and high feed conversion efficiency. Now a day, broiler farming can be a main source of family income and gainful employment to farmers throughout the year. Poultry manure has high fertilizer value and can be used for increasing yield of all crops as well as it used in compost formation for production of mushroom.

Advantages of Broiler Farming

- ☆ Faster income from the investment
- ☆ Initial investment is a little lower as compared to layer farming
- ☆ Marketing age is 4 to 5 weeks only
- ☆ Multiple flocks can be taken in the same shed
- ☆ Broilers have high feed conversion ratio
- ☆ Poultry meat has more demand compared to sheep/Goat/pig meat.

Scope for Broiler Farming and its Importance

In the last two decades, India has made considerable progress in broiler production. Today in our market; High quality chicks, equipments, vaccines and medicines are available easily. Technical and professional training is available to the farmers in all KVK of Jammu area. Disease and mortality incidences are much reduced due improved management practices. Many institutions as well as KVK are providing training to entrepreneurs. Increasing assistance from the Central/ State governments, poultry corporations and NABARD is being given to create infrastructure facilities so that new entrepreneurs take up this business. Considerable importance has been given to commercial broiler farming in the national policy and it has a good scope for further development in the years to come.

Present Status of Poultry in India

Today in India, Poultry is one of the fastest growing segments of the agricultural sector. Commercial broiler industry has influenced by demands of human being upon the meat. Poultry industries are the source of income and food. The National Institute of Nutrition has recommended 180 eggs and 11 kg meat per capita consumption for our country. Poultry sector has shown a healthy increase by 12.39% over the previous census (2007) and the total poultry in the country was 729.2 million numbers in 2012. China has the 1st rank in poultry population in world. India has 5th rank in poultry population and 4th rank in poultry meat production. Per capita availability of egg in India is 58 eggs. Per capita availability of meat in India is 2.93 kg.

Table 1. All India Livestock Census in 2007 and 2012 (Birds in Thousands)

Species	*2007 census*	*2012 census*	*% change*
Fowl	617734	692646	12.13
Ducks	27643	23539	-14.85
Turkey and others	3452	13025	277.32
Total poultry	648829	729209	12.39

Fig 1. Percentage Share of Poultry Birds in Poultry Population

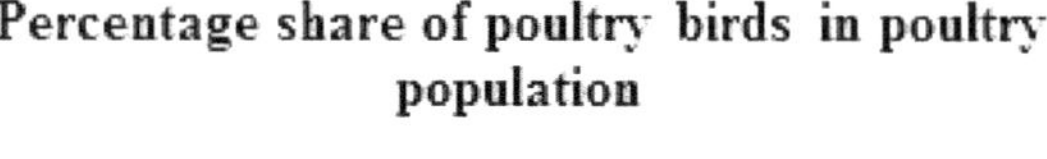

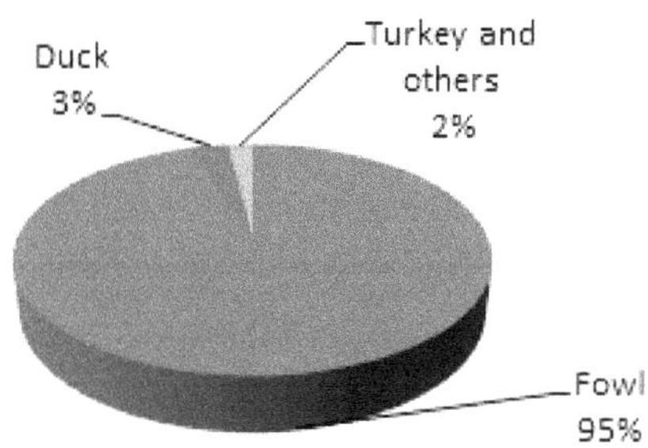

Andhra Pradesh is highest in the meat production of poultry in all states with 0.499 million tonnes per year. The second and third highest average productions of meat are reported by Maharashtra and Tamilnadu, respectively.

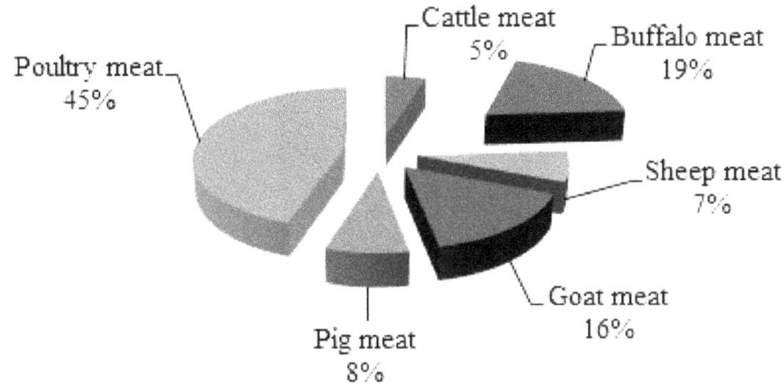

Present status of Poultry in Jammu & Kashmir

The Indian Livestock census is an exercise conducted every fifth year in the entire country. The 19th Livestock census was conducted with 15th October 2012. The poultry population is mainly contributed by fowls in Jammu & Kashmir with total poultry population of 8.27 million numbers in 2012. The changes in the poultry population over previous 3 census (2003, 2007 and 2012) are 5568, 6683 and 8273 (values in thousands), respectively. The total poultry population is showing increasing trend over 2003-2012. The birds have increased from 5.56 million numbers in 2003 to 8.27 million numbers in 2012. There is an increase of 23.8% in the poultry population during the inter census period (2007-2012).

The population of fowls has been increasing continuously since 2003. The fowls have increased from 5.32 million numbers in 2003 to 0.12 million numbers in 2012. The duck population has decreased by 35.98% over the previous census. The turkey and other birds have increased from 0.006 million in 2003 to 0.018 million in 2012 and registered a drastic increase during inter censuses period (2007-2012).

Table. 2. Recent Trends in Change of Population of Fowl, Duck, Turkey and others in J & K States (Note: Values in Thousand)

Species	*2003*	*2007*	*2012*	*% change from 2007-2012*
Fowl	5325	6487.4	8134.35	25.39
Ducks	237	190.30	121.84	-35.98
Turkey and other poultry	6	5.86	17.53	199.35
Total poultry	5568	6683	8273.71	23.8

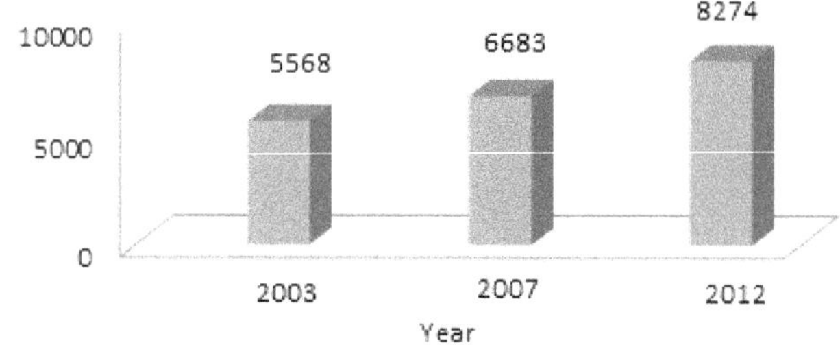

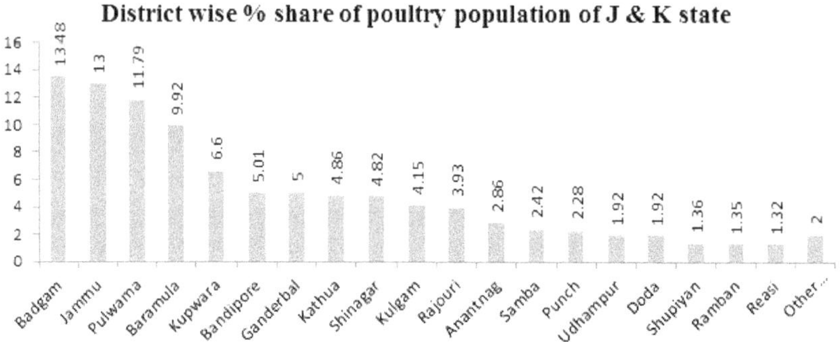

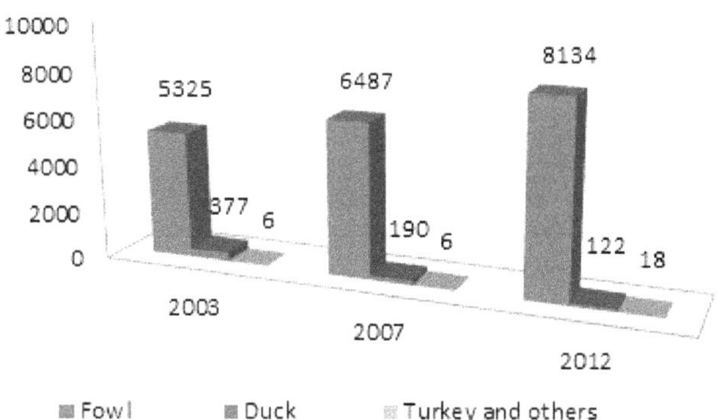

Breeds of Broilers Reared for Meat Production

Broiler breeds	Cari rainbro, Caribro vishal, Caribro Dhanraja, Caribro mrityunjai, Caribro Tropicana, Colour broiler, Hy-Bro, Ven-Cobb, Bab Cobb, Krishibro
Dual Purpose Breed	Red Vanaraja, Cha-bro, Kalinga brown, Kuroider dual, Cari Debendra, Cari shyma, Hitcari, Rhode Island

Common Management Practices Recommended for Poultry Farmers in Jammu Province

Some of the major management norms and recommended practices are given below:

Poultry Housing

- ☆ Poultry sheds should be at well raised land. Hard rock or "murram Land is more suitable. Water logging and flooding near the sheds should avoid.
- ☆ Facility for water, electricity, approach road, supply of chicks, feed should be ensure adequate
- ☆ Before starting a farm, must obtain training/experience in broiler farming. You should be prepared to stay on the farm and have constant supervision.
- ☆ Provide adequate floor space, feeding space and watering space to all birds.
- ☆ Sheds should construct in such a way that the end walls face East-West direction and the side walls face North-South direction, so that direct sun rays will not enter the sheds.
- ☆ Provide hard flooring and strong roof. Plinth of the shed should raise at least one feet above the outside ground level.
- ☆ Overhang of the roof should providc 3 to 4 feet to avoid entry of rainwater inside the shed.
- ☆ Distance between two sheds should be at least 50 feet.
- ☆ Adequate light and ventilation and comfortable housing conditions should provide during all seasons (cool in summer and warm in winter). Sheds should construct in such a way that predators (cats/dogs/snakes) will not enter the shed. Entry of rats should avoid by constructing rat proof civil structures.
- ☆ The shed should keep clean and free from flies/mosquitoes etc.
- ☆ After disposal of every batch of birds the dirty litter material and manure should be removed, walls and floors should be cleaned, white washed with lime and disinfected with 0.5% malathion or DDT insecticide spray.
- ☆ If deep litter system is followed, always use dry and clean litter material (sawdust, paddy husk, rice husk etc.). Spread 4" layer of litter on the floor, keep clean/disinfect brooding, feeding and watering equipment and then introduce chicks in the house.
- ☆ The litter material should be always kept loose and dry. Stir the litter twice a week. Any wet litter/droppings should be removed and replaced with fresh/clean dry litter.

Poultry Equipment

Scientifically designed cages and equipment should use for brooding, feeding and watering purposes. BIS specifications for equipment are available. A good design can be shown and manufactured locally, so that cost can be reduced.

Chicks

Chicks should purchase of improved strain of one day old healthy broiler type chicks from a reputed hatchery. Usually 2-5% extra chicks are supplied. Clean, wash and disinfect all equipments with 0.5% malathion spray after every batch of birds is disposed off.

Brooding Management

Brooding is an art and science of rearing large number of baby chicks in the absence of a broody hen. A newly hatched chick has not developed the thermoregulatory mechanism fully and takes about two weeks to develop this mechanism and homeostasis. Therefore, they can not maintain the body temperature properly for the first few weeks of life and may be subjected to chilling, if not properly taken care of. Hence, artificial brooding is mainly aimed at, providing the right temperature to the chicks. In addition to the temperature, adequate floor, feeder space, water space, relative humidity, ventilation and light should be provided for optimum comfort and growth of the chicks.

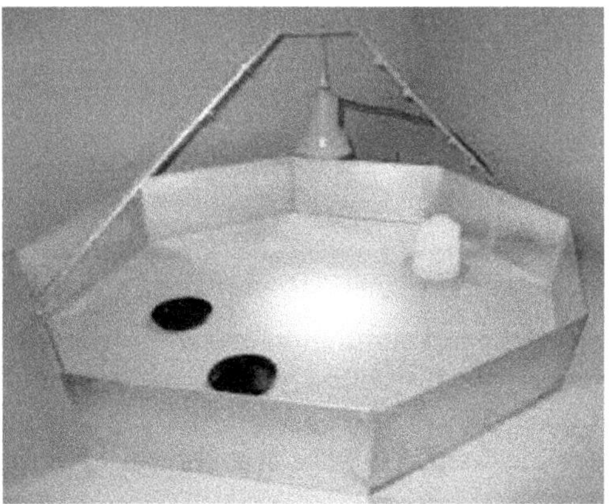

- Maintaining the correct temperature, light, ventilation, space, feeding, watering *etc.*
- Of these, the temperature is the most important criterion
- Room temperature of about 35°C has to be maintained during the first week of age
- Gradually reduced by about 3°C every week until the room temperature or 18-20°C is reached

Behaviors of Chicks

- If they crowd under or near the source of heat, then the warmth given is not sufficient.
- If the chicks have moved to the periphery and are reluctant to come to the center under heat source, then temperature in the environment is higher than required.
- If the chicks feel comfortable at a given temperature, they walk actively

throughout the area unmindful of heat provided and some take rest setting their head down on the side, the posture being given the name as "Chick comfort".

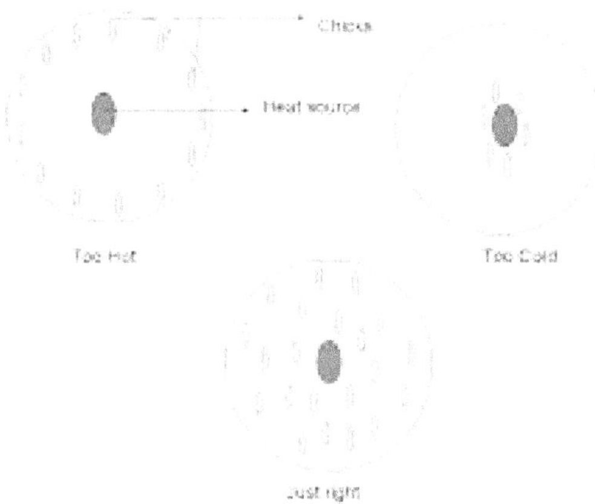

Types of Brooders

- ☆ Incandescent bulbs and other types of bulbs
- ☆ Heater coil with thermostat
- ☆ Gas brooder
- ☆ Kerosene stove
- ☆ Charcoal stove
- ☆ Biogas brooder
- ☆ Battery brooder
- ☆ Centralized heating system

Feeding

- ☆ With proper knowledge/experience, the feed can be prepared at the farm with high quality balanced feeds
- ☆ Store the feed in clean, dry, well ventilated room. A wet feed may bring fungus infection.
- ☆ Properly designed feeders should use
- ☆ Rats should kill to avoid feed wastage.
- ☆ Keep proper records on feed consumption per bird for each batch. Compare with the standard feed consumption pattern.
- ☆ Too low feed consumption may be due to disease condition, low quality/ unpalatability of feed, high temperature in poultry shed.
- ☆ Watering of Birds

- Always give fresh and clean drinking water. Water should be always available at birds.
- Use properly designed watering equipment. Provide adequate watering space per bird.
- Always keep water-pots clean. Avoid birds entering inside pots.
- Provide cool water during summer. Store the water in tanks that are not exposed to hot sun in summer.

Disease Prevention/Control

- Healthy chicks, clean sanitary conditions of poultry sheds and equipment, balanced feed, fresh clean water are essential to prevent diseases.
- Entry of visitors to farm should avoid especially inside the sheds. If visitors come, ask them to dip their feet in a disinfectant solution, wash and clean hands and to wear apron/boots provided by the farm.
- Use proper vaccination schedule
- Use high quality vaccines purchased from reputed manufacturers. Keep vaccines in cool, dry conditions away from sunlight.
- Any left-over vaccine should be properly disposed off. Vaccines should not be used after their expiry date is over.
- Any dead bird should be immediately removed from the shed and sent to laboratory for post-mortem or buried/burnt suitably away from the poultry sheds.
- The waste of farm should be suitably disposed off.
- Any bird showing advanced signs of a disease should be removed from the shed and culled. It can be sent to laboratory for diagnosis.
- Birds showing advanced signs of a disease should be shown to a qualified veterinarian and suitable medication/treatment is given as per his/drug manufacturers recommendations.
- Poultry manure, if infected, can spread disease, from one batch to another. Keep the litter dry, remove it after flock is sold and dispose the manure properly and quickly.
- Keep proper records on mortality and its causes and the treatment given to birds. Dates of vaccination for each flock should be properly recorded.
- Rats are important carriers of poultry disease. Avoid rats. Use suitable rat poisons/rat traps.
- Many poultry medicines can be given in drinking water. When medication is to be given, remove the waterers in poultry sheds on the previous evening. Next morning give medicine in measured quantity of water, so that entire medicine will be quickly consumed and there will be no wastage of medicines.
- Mild infection of disease may not cause mortality but it will reduce growth.

Keep sample record of body weight and mortality rate. Study the possible causes; if weight is low take steps to improve the management of the subsequent batches. A Constant vigil and analysis of records/results is necessary to keep up the efficiency in farming.

Processing/Marketing

- ☆ Should ensure the constant and steady demand for broiler meat is available and the market is nearer to the farm.
- ☆ Study the market demand for particular live weight of the birds.
- ☆ Birds should not be kept on the farm beyond 5-6 weeks of age, as their feed efficiency will go down considerably.
- ☆ If birds are sold after dressing (processing) use clean dressing hall and processing equipment. Dressed birds should be chilled in the ice-cold water for 3-4 hours and excess water removed. Birds should then be packed in clean plastic bags and the mouth of bag sealed.
- ☆ Processed birds should be marketed as early as possible. If they have to be preserved, deep freezing equipment (-10 to -20°C) be used. Refrigerated vans may be required for long distance transportation.

Floor Space, Feeding Space and Watering Space Data for Broiler Chicks

Age weeks	*Floor space Sq.ft./Chick*	*Feeding space inches/chick*	*Watering space inches/ chick*
1	0.2	1.5	0.5
2	0.2	2.0	0.7
3	0.3	2.0	0.7
4	0.4	2.5	0.8
5	0.6	2.5	0.8
6	0.8	3.0	1.0

Body Weight, Feed Consumption and Feed Conversion of Broiler Chicks

Age		*Body weight & gain (kg)*		*Feed consumption(kg)*		*Feed conversion*	
Weeks	*Days*	*Average weight*	*Weekly gain*	*Weekly*	*Cumulative*	*Weekly*	*Cumulative*
1	7	0.17	-	0.1	0.1	0.81	0.81
2	14	0.28	0.15	0.23	0.34	1.53	1.21
3	21	0.48	0.2	0.34	0.67	1.64	1.4
4	28	0.73	0.25	0.47	1.14	1.93	1.50
5	35	1.00	0.29	0.63	1.77	2.16	1.77
6	42	1.32	0.33	0.74	2.51	2.26	1.89

Composition of Broiler diets

Ingredients	*Formulations*	
Types of ration	Type 1	Type 2
Maize	51	58.5
Wheat bran	10	2.5
Groundnut cake/ Soyabean meal	25.2	25
Fish Meal	10.8	11
Dicalcium Phosphate	1	1
Lime Stone	0.5	0.5
Salt	0.5	0.5
Premix (added per 100 kg feed)	1	1
Total	100	100
Crude protein %	22.1	22
ME. KCal/Kg. diet	2,800	3,000

Premix (added per 100 kg feed)

Particulars	*Chemical*	*Quantity*
Vitamin (gm)	Vitabland (A1B2D3)	25
	Folic acid	0.1
	Vit.E	4
	Niacin	10
	Pyridoxine	1
	Choline Chloride	30
Mineral (gm)	Ferrous sulphate	20
	Zinc Sulphate	25
	Copper sulphate	25
	Manganese Sulphate	25
	Potassium iodate	0.1
Amino acid (gm)	L-lysine hydrochloride	220
	DL - Methionine	160

Vaccination Schedule for Broilers

Name of disease	*Name of Vaccination*	*Days/weeks of vaccination*	*Route of inoculation*	*Remarks*
Marek's disease	Herpes virus turkey vaccination	1 day old	Sub cutaneous	Life long immunity
Ranikhet disease	RD vaccine (Lasota 'F' strain)	4-7 days old	Intra-nasal Intra-ocular	Immunity is up to 10 weeks old
Fowl pox	Chick embryo adopted fowl	6-8 weeks of age	Wing web method	If the disease is prevalent in the area. Once vaccinated gives life long immunity

During chick rearing, the disease most likely to occur is coccidiosis. Its organisms thrive on wet litter and so keep the litter dry. The feed mixed with coccidiosis should be used. In case of an outbreak, the Coccidiocidal drug in drinking water should be used at recommended level.

Financial Assistance Available from Banks/NABARD for Broiler Farming

NABARD is an apex institution for all matters relating to policy, planning and operations in the field of agricultural credit. It serves as an apex refinancing agency for the institutions providing investment and production credit. It promotes development through formulation and appraisal of projects through a well-organized technical service.

Loan from banks with refinance facility from NABARD is available for starting broiler farming. For obtaining bank loan, the farmer should apply to the nearest branch of a commercial or cooperative or regional rural bank in their area in the prescribed application form which is available in the branches of financing bank. The technical officers attached to or the manager of the bank can help or give guidance to the farmers in preparing the project report to obtain bank loan.

For poultry farming schemes with very large outlays detailed project reports are required to be prepared. The items of finance would include construction of broiler sheds and purchase of equipments. Cost of one day old chicks, feed, medicine and labour cost for the first 7 weeks period for the first cycle, are also considered. Facilities such as land development cost, fencing, water and electricity, essential servant's quarters, godowns, transport vehicles, broiler dressing, processing and cold storage facilities can also be considered for providing loan. Cost of land is not considered for loan. However, if land is purchased for starting a broiler farm, its cost can be treated as party's margin money upto 10% of the total cost of project.

Scheme Formulation for Bank Loan

A scheme can be prepared by the beneficiary after consulting local technical persons of State veterinary department, Poultry Corporation or private commercial broiler hatcheries. If possible, they should also visit the progressive broiler farmers in the area and discuss the profitability of farming. A good practical training and experience on a broiler farm will be highly desirable, before starting a broiler farm. As broilers have to be sold after attaining 4-5 weeks of age, a regular and constant demand for broiler meat and nearness of the farm to the market should be ensured.

The scheme should include information on land, water and electricity facility, marketing aspects, training facilities and expertise of entrepreneurs and the type of assistance available from State government, poultry corporations, local hatcheries. It will also include data on proposed capacity of the farm, total cost of the project, margin money to be provided by beneficiary and requirement of bank loans, estimated annual expenditure, income and profit and the repayment of loan and interest.

Transforming Rural Areas through Veterinary Science *Pages* **73-92**
Editor: Dipanjali Konwar, Shilpa Sood & Shahid Ahamad
Published by: **ASTRAL INTERNATIONAL PVT. LTD., NEW DELHI**

5 Transformation of Rural Areas through Modern Sheep and Goat Farming

M. Rashid, Dr. Asma Khan & Dr. Nazam Khan

Small ruminant sector, after agriculture, is the second largest means for economic sustainability and livelihood in India. Sheep and goat husbandry is a tool for poverty alleviation of the rural masses because of wide adaptability with low investments, high fertility and fecundity, low feed and management costs, higher feed conversion efficiency, quick pay off and low risk in comparison to large ruminants. The above traits of small ruminants need to be exploited for economic upliftment of rural areas.

In India due to lack of supportive policies, the sector remained ignored and the farmers deprived of the attainable economic benefits. The ICAR Institutions like Central Sheep and Wool Research Institute and Central Institute of Goat Research have been putting on good efforts to trigger a positive change in spite of low budgetary provisions, but lack of an organized technology transfer infrastructure restricts sustainable development in this sector. Thus there is a tremendous scope/ potential for increasing the small ruminant production through profitable farming. Various technical aspects regarding above are presented underneath in detail.

Sheep

Sheep farming in India is one of the traditional occupations of some people of India. People of some regions are raising sheep as domestic animal for fulfilling family livelihood and business purpose from the ancient time. Sheep is a small sized calm animal and grows rapidly. Indian climate is very suitable for setting up sheep farming business in India. Sheep farming require little investment and we can get the returns of investment within a very short period.

Sheep farming in India can be a great source of handsome income for the marginal and landless farmers. There are numerous sheep breeds available in our country and many people are taking the opportunities of sheep farming business. However, in this chapter will describe some important drivers for transformation of this sector for getting maximum output. The main advantages of sheep farming in India and the steps for starting this business domestically or commercially are based on four pillars of management system: Heading, Feeding, Breeding and Weeding:

Heading: In a farming system this is the first consideration, which includes housing, health, hygiene and sanitation. Normally sheep and goats do not require elaborate housing facilities, but minimum provisions will definitely increase productivity, especially protection against inclement weather conditions and predation. Often, the flocks are penned in the open during fair weather and some temporary shelters are made use of in monsoon and winter. Sheep can be economically reared under ranch system. Requirements of building units are more or less the same for sheep and goats, except that additional buildings are required for milch goats. The shed site should be easily approachable and spacious, dry, elevated, well-drained and protected from strong winds. An East-West orientation ensures cooler environment. A "lean-to" type of shed, located against the side of an existing building, is the cheapest form of building. Loose housing is more advantageous as compared to conventional/stall-fed sheds because it is suitable for semi-arid regions and large-sized flocks, it involves less expenditure, it provides more comfort to the animals, it is less labour-intensive, and it provides freedom of movement and gives the benefit of exercise. Stilted housing is common in areas with heavy rainfall.

Floor Space Requirements

Sl. No.	*Type of animal*	*Minimum floor space (m2)*
1.	Ram or buck in groups	1.8
2.	Ram or buck, individual	3.2
3.	Lamb or kids in groups	0.4
4.	Weaner in groups	0.8
5.	Weaner, individual	0.9
6.	Yearling, individual	0.9
7.	Yearlings in groups	0.9
8.	Ewe or doe in groups	1.0
9.	Ewe or doe, individual	1.2
10.	Ewe with lamb	1.5

Types of Sheds

Sl. No.	*Type of shed*	*Size (m)*	*Height (m)*	*Maximum animals*
1.	Ewe/doe shed	15 x 4	3	60
2.	Ram/buck shed	4 x 2.5	3	3
3.	Lambing/kidding shed	1.5 x 1.2	3	3
4.	Lamb/kid shed	7.5 x 4	3	75

Sl. No.	Type of shed	Size (m)	Height (m)	Maximum animals
5.	Weaner shed	7.5 x 4	3	75
6.	Yearling shed	10 x 5	3	50
7.	Sick animal shed	3 x 2	3	1
8.	Shearing shed and store room	6 x 2.5	3	
9.	Shepherd's room	6 x 4	3	

Advantages of Sheep Farming in India

Sheep farming business is very profitable. It is a great business idea for the marginal and landless farmers to earn some extra income. The main advantages of sheep farming in India are listed below.

- Sheep are strong animal and well adapted to environment.
- They require less care and management.
- Rate of sheep meat in India is increasing day by day as there are are no religious binding in consumption.
- Sheep require less place for living. In domestic rearing one can keep sheep with other livestock animals. But for commercial production we must have to build a house or shelter for them.
- Labour costs for sheep farming in India is also very low, so economically sheep farming could be done.
- Sheep can survive by eating various types of grasses, weeds, plants, spinach, roots, plant roots and different types of low quality foods.
- Sheep do not damage the plants like goats while eating.
- They also help the farmer by eating unwanted plants.
- Their production is not for a certain period. They continuously produce valuable wool, meat, skin and manure throughout the year.
- Sheep meat has a huge demand and there are no religious taboos of consuming sheep meat in India.
- Sheep dung is a good fertilizer, that can be used for increasing organic crop production.
- Domestic sheep farming in India can yield extra income opportunities for the poor families.
- Commercial sheep farming business can generate employment opportunity for the unemployed educated youths. Thus the unemployed educated people can earn their livings through sheep farming and contribute in the national income.
- Easy bank loan for sheep farming business is available under different schemes in India.
- Along with those advantages, there are many advantages of sheep farming in India.

Feeding

Sheep in India are mostly maintained on natural vegetation on common grazing lands, wastelands and uncultivated (fallow) lands, stubbles of cultivated crops and top feeds (tree loppings). Rarely are they kept on grain, cultivated fodder or crop residue. Sheep are mostly reared for wool and meat. Sheep skins and manure constitute important sources of earning, the latter particularly in southern India. Milk from sheep is of limited importance and that too in very limited areas of Jammu and Kashmir, Rajasthan and Gujarat. Indian sheep are not regarded as dairy sheep.

Classification of Indigenous Breeds Based on Utility

Apparel wool breeds	*Superior carpet Wool breeds*	*Coarse carpet Wool breeds*	*Hairy Meat breeds*
Hissardale	Chokla	Malpura	Nellore
Niligiri	Nali	Sonadi	Hassan
Kashmir merino	Marwari	Muzzafarnagri	Mecheri
Avivastra	Magra	Jalauni	Kilakarsal
Bharat Merino	Jaisalmeri	Deccani	Madras Red
Hissardale	Pugal	Bellary	Trichy Black
	Pattanwadi	Coimbatore	Kenguri
	Tibetan	Chottanagpuri	Mandya
	Bonpala	Balangir	Vembur
	Gaddi	Ganjam	
	Rampur Bushari	Bhakarwal	
	Poonchi	Shahabadi	
	Karnah		

Exotic Breeds

Fine wool breeds	*Mutton breeds*	*Dual purpose*	*Pelt breeds*
Merino	Suffolk	Corriedale	Karakul
Rambouillet	Southdown		
Polworth	Dorset		

The feeding and grazing conditions of sheep vary from place to place. The most favorable grazing time is soon after the onset of monsoon till the onset of winter. Grazing resources become extremely poor during summer months. During this period supplementary feeding should be done. Sheep generally thrive well on pasture. Attention should be paid on pasture improvement and management. Rotational grazing should be followed to avoid worm infection and unthriftiness, and to ensure availability of good pasture all the time. The fodder should be conserved in the form of hay and silage for the lean period. Fodder trees should be planted in the pasture to provide shade and fodder during the lean period to the grazing flocks. Supplementary feeding of concentrate should be done depending upon the physiological status and availability of grazing resource in the pasture.

Water

Water requirement of sheep depend upon its physiological status and ambient temperature in different seasons. The sheep should be offered water at least once a day at the rate of 2-3 litres per head per day. The requirement of water for crossbreds during summer months may range between 5-6 litres. The younger ones may require 1-2 litres of water every day. Sheep breeds in arid regions have good adaptation to water restriction upto 48 hrs. Watering should be done in metallic troughs or cements channels. The flock should be weighed at least once in a week to the extent of at least 10% prior to being turned out for grazing. This work may be distributed over the week.

Feeding Lambs up to Two Weeks: There is no feed equal to the ewe's milk for putting rapid gains on young lamb because dam's milk yield is closely related to early growth of lamb. Lambs depend entirely on dam's milk upto 2 weeks. Colostrum is rich in fat, protein, vitamins etc. and contains antibodies to protect the lamb from infections. If the ewes are fed good ration during the last six weeks of gestation, it enhances milk production as well as health lambing.

Feeding Lambs Beyond Two Weeks: The Recommended Rations are Given Below

Feed ingredients (%)	*Pre-weaning period (upto 3 months)*	*(3-6 months)*	*Finisher*
Ground maize	65	27	25
Groundnut cake	10	35	20
Wheat bran	12	35	52
Fish meal	10	-	-
Common salt	1	1	1
Min. mix.	2	2	2
Expected growth rate per day (gms)	110-125	100-120	100-120

Rate of feeding/day (approx)

	Body weight	*Concentrate (gms)*		*Roughage*
		Legume is Available	*Legume Not Available*	
1	12-15	50	300	ad lib
2	15-25	100	400	ad lib
3	25-35	150	600	ad lib

Feeding Suckling Ewes: During suckling period, ewes should be fed good legume hay or oat hay with little or no grain for a week. After she's milking freely and her bowels are functioning normally with no sign of constipation, the amount of grains may be increased. If pasture is available, hay is not needed. The following rations can be used:-

	Feed ingredients	*Ration-I*	*Ration-II*
1	Grain mixture	400gm	400gm
2	Legumes hay	700gm	1400gm
3	Green fodder/silage	1400gm	-

Feeding Adult Sheep

Roughage part may be taken care by grazing, but 150 gm of concentrate to suckling ewes with mineral mixture and salt must be fed.

Energy: Adult – Non pregnant sheep – 93 K cal. ME / kg. W 0.75

Lactating - 102 K cal. ME / kg. W 0.75

Protein – DCP requirement – 1 g for every 1kg live weight (adult non pregnant) Increases by 50% during pregnancy and 100% during lactation.

Flushing

Ewes which are to be bred should be underfed for about 45 days prior to breeding in order to prevent fat accumulation which reduces fertility. Two weeks prior to breeding, the ewes should be fed about 150-200 gm concentrate mixture daily along with good quality forages (cowpea, oat, doob grass, berseem). It conditions the animal and induces maturation of more number of follicles, and thus improves conception and twinning rate.

Feeding Breeding Rams

Good quality green fodders like maize, cowpea, oat, doob grass, lucerne, berseem etc. would meet all requirements of breeding rams. If forages fed are of poor quality like straw or sorghum hay, then 150-200 gms concentrate should be fed daily.

Area-Specific Mineral Mixture: Area specific mineral mixtures (ASMM) for sheep and goats of semi-arid region of Rajasthan have been developed for improving health, reproduction and production level. The ASMM is available in both pelleted and powder form. The later is having advantage of delivering the micronutrients in more complete and in quantifiable manner.

Complete Feed Block (CFB)

The complete feed block of roughage and concentrate mixture was prepared in 70:30 ratios with 5% of molasses for easy binding. The blocks have many advantages like ease in transport, palatable in nature, lower in space requirement for storage and reduced losses during transport.

Vaccination in Sheep

Disease	*Age and booster doses*	*Route*	*Remarks*
FMD	6-8 weeks;repeat every 6-9 months	s/c or i/m depending on the vaccine	-
H.S	3-4 months;repeat annually	1 ml s/c	May/ June
Sheep pox	3 months	s/c	-
Tetanus	Tetanus toxoid	0.5 - 1 ml s/c or i/m	-
Anthrax	4-6 months; repeat annually	0.5 ml s/c at tail fold	In endemic areas
Enterotoxaemia	3-4 months, repeat after 15 days and then annually.	2.5 ml s/c	First two doses before august

Grazing Management of Sheep

Purpose: As pasture is a valuable fodder for sheep and the cheapest source of nutrients necessary for maintenance and production, proper grazing management and care of pastures is essential for ensuring higher yields.

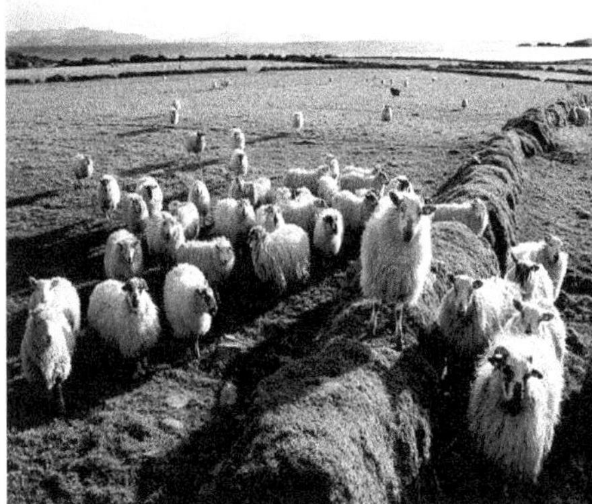
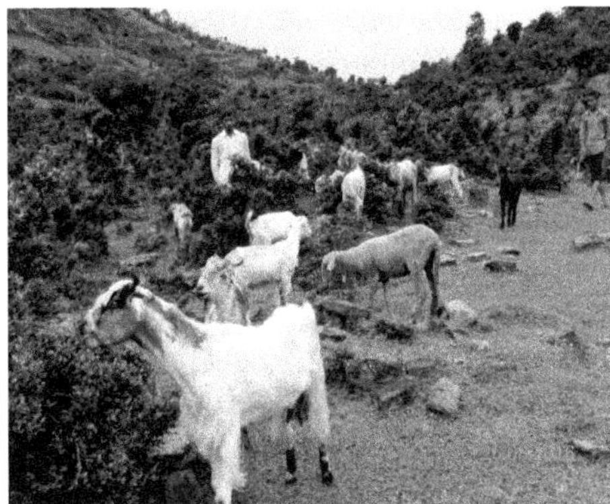

Grazing management of Sheep and Goat

Characteristics of Sheep Feeding under Range Conditions

Sheep have a small muzzle and split upper-lip which enables them to nibble tiny blades of vegetation which cannot be eaten by larger animals. Sheep prefer small, tender grasses and chew food more thoroughly than cattle. The capacity of the sheep stomach is 15-16 litres and excess feeding can cause indigestion and they do not relish ripe grass. Sheep on pastures may consume 10-15 % more dry matter compared to stall feeding and daily grazing for 10-12 hours should be permitted to meet the dry matter requirements. Sheep usually relish leguminous fodder such as Lucerne, cowpea, berseem etc. and rotation of pastures should be adopted to prevent under- or over-grazing. Growing lambs should be allowed to graze first, followed by pregnant and lactating ewes, and dry stock at the last (If cattle, sheep and goats are to graze on the same pasture, it will be desirable to allow goats first, followed by cattle and sheep, in that order). Even a good pasture does not meet the dietary requirements of advanced pregnant and lactating ewes, and hence additional concentrate feed of 250-300 gm/day should be given.

Pasture Improvement and Management

Pasture lands in India are poor and meager and need to be improved by protecting them from biotic factors, conserving good natural grasses, choosing the best fodder trees and shrubs, removing nonedible grasses, weeds and shrubs, and re-seeding with nutritious and perennial grasses and legumes. Natural legumes like Rhynochosia minima, Indigoferaendecaphylla and Tribulusterrestris are very useful and should be preserved. Grazing lands should be re-seeded with nutritious perennial grasses like Cenchrusciliaris, Cenchrussetigerus, Lasirussindicus and Dichanthiumannulatum in arid and semiarid plains; Sehimanervosum in sub-humid plains; and fescue, rye grass and kikyu grass in the temperate and sub-temperate regions. Perennial legumes like Dolichos lablab, Clitoriaternatea, Macropteliumatropurpureum, Atylosiascarabacoides and Stylosanthus species should be incorporated in the regenerated or reseeded pastures. Combined production of grass and legumes can increase forage production by 20-30 % as compared to that of grass alone. The legumes, besides being rich in protein content, are more palatable and digestible, enrich the soil by nitrogen fixation, and help in checking soil erosion. During the first year of pasture establishment, grazing should not be allowed; the fodder must be harvested, conserved as hay, and fed during the lean period. Rotational grazing, *i.e.* dividing the pasture into four equal compartments and allowing grazing sequentially, helps the grasses to regenerate, checks soil erosion caused by over-grazing and allows agricultural operations to be carried out. Pastures should be top dressed with sufficient quantities of farmyard and inorganic fertilizers at regular intervals. Protection of pasture, removal of undesirable bushes and weeds, soil and water conservation, application of fertilizers, proper stocking rate and grazing system (rotational or deferred rotational) are essential components of good pasture management.

Silviculture

1. Fodder trees serve as a potential source of feed for sheep during December to June when the grazing resources become scarce.
2. Fodder trees also provide shade during summer, check soil erosion and improve soil texture.
3. Fodder trees should be planted in well-managed pastures after the first monsoon rains at a spacing of 20 x 10 metres (approx. 50 trees/hectare).
4. Lopping can be done twice a year in Oct-Nov and May-Jun (fed green) in such a manner that the top branches are left in situ; yielding about 8-10 quintals of good quality green fodder.
5. The pods of many trees, especially babool (Acacia arabica) and khejri (Prosopis cineraria) are very nutritious and palatable, and serve as a good source of feed for flushing ewes.

Reproductive Management in Sheep

Reproductive management, comprising of detection of estrus, mating, identifying pregnant animals, care of pregnant animals, care at parturition and care of the male, plays a major role in the profitability of a sheep or goat farm. Effective managerial interventions can increase reproductive health, incidence of twinning/ triplets and lamb/kid livability.

Age at Mating: Sheep normally attain good growth at about 24 months (range 18-36) of age. Breeding too young ewes results in more weaklings and higher lamb losses. It is desirable to use rams for mating from the age of 2 years till the age of 7 years.

Mating Season and Estrus Cycle: Sheep are seasonally polyestrus. In India, there are three main breeding seasons viz. summer (Mar-Apr), autumn (Jun-Jul) and post-monsoon (Sep-Oct). In general, higher fertility is observed in autumn season in the plains and in summer season in the hilly areas. The ewes usually come in heat about 2 months after lambing. The duration of the estrus cycle is 17 days (range 14-19) and heat period lasts for 27 hours (2-60). Ovulation occurs about 12 hours before the end of heat period.

Preparations for Breeding

1. Flushing: Feeding extra grain or lush pasture 2-3 weeks prior to the breeding season for the purpose of increasing the number of ova shed from the ovary and increase the incidence of twinning. Feeding about 250 gms grains daily to each ewe results in an increase in the lamb crop by about 10-20 per cent.
2. Tagging: This refers to the shearing the locks of wool and dirt from the dock of the ewes, thus facilitating mating by the ram.
3. Eyeing: This refers to the clipping of excess wool around the eyes to prevent wool blindness in some breeds.
4. Ringing: This refers to shearing of wool from the body of the ram, especially in the neck, belly and sheath region prior to the breeding season.

Detection of Estrus: As sheep in heat show few external indications of estrus other than standing to be mounted, heat is generally detected with the help of a teaser. Wet paint (dye mixed in grease or linseed oil) can be smeared on the brisket of the teaser ram to spot the ewes in estrus. The colour of the dye should be changed every 16-18 days so that the repeaters can be discovered. Other indications of estrus are vulvar swelling, frequent urination, restlessness and reduced appetite.

Mating: As far as possible, rams should be kept away from the ewes and the two should be brought together only for breeding. Natural breeding is done either by flock mating, pen mating or hand mating.

- In flock mating, breeding rams are usually turned out in the flock during the mating season at the rate of 2-3 per cent of the ewes all through day and night.
- In semi-flock breeding or pen mating, rams are turned out for service with the flock in the pen during night, and confined and stall-fed or grazed separately during the day time in order to conserve their energy and give them rest.
- Hand mating is practiced when exotic purebred sires are used, or when it is considered desirable to extend the services of the ram over much larger flocks.

Identifying Pregnant Ewes: Identification of pregnant ewes is essential for the re-breeding of empty ewes and efficient management of pregnant ewes. Pregnancy can be diagnosed by observing for cessation of estrus cycle, abdominal ballotment (from third month onwards) and by means of a chemical test.

Procedure: Mix 5 ml of urine sample and 5 ml of 1% Barium chloride solution. Turbidity indicates pregnancy whereas clear solution indicates non-pregnant condition.

Common Diseases and their Control

Morbidity and mortality are the two important factors resulting in heavy losses in sheep production and improvement programmes. Prevention is always better than cure. This has special significance with sheep as they seem to respond less to treatment when sick than other livestock species. So the disease must be controlled by adopting certain tactic strategies which are not in the preview of this chapter but can be dealt separately.

Economics of Sheep Farming

A model economics for sheep farming with a unit size of 100 sheep is given below. This is indicative and the applicable input and output costs and the parameters observed at the field level may be incorporated.

Sr. No	*Parameter*	*Cost/ Amount in Rs.*
I	Land and Building	
1	Land fencing and partitioning	
A	Fencing for compound 850 R Ft @ Rs. 15 per R Ft. in 5 rows	12750
B	gates	5000
	Total	17750
2	Civil structure	
	Shed @ 10 sq.ft for ewe,20 sq.ft for ram and 4 Sq.ft for kid 100 ewes,4 rams and assuming 120 lambs maximum (10*100)+(20*4)+(4*110)= 1520 Sqft @ Rs. 100 per sq.ft	15200
3	Equipment	
	First aid equipment	1000
	Feeders and waterers	1040
	Total	11400
II	Animals	
A	Ewes 100 @ Rs 4500 per animal- 9-12 months age	450000
B	Rams 4 @ Rs. 5500 per animal - 12-15 months age	22000
	Total	472000
III	Working capital	
A	Feed of	
	Adult female	77315
	Adult male	3093
	Kids	12600
	Medicines	6800
	Insurance	18720
	Total of III	118528
	TFO	771678
	Bank lone	578758
	Margin money	192919

Goats

Goat is a multi functional animal and plays a significant role in the economy and nutrition of landless, small and marginal farmers in the country. Goat rearing is an enterprise which has been practiced by a large section of population in rural areas. Goats can efficiently survive on available shrubs and trees in adverse harsh environment in low fertility lands where no other crop can be grown. In pastoral and agricultural subsistence societies in India, goats are kept as a source of additional income and as an insurance against disaster. Goats are also used in ceremonial feastings and for the payment of social dues. In addition to this, goat has religious and ritualistic importance in many societies.

The total number of goat in the Jammu and Kashmir state as per 19ths census (2012) is 2.01 million number. There is a 2.44% decline in number of goat population during the inter censuses period (2007-12). The total number of female goat population has decreased from 1.53 million in 2003 to 1.51 million in 2012. The female goat population has decreased by 0.58% over the previous census. The male goat population has also decreased from 0.52 million in 2003 to 0.50 million in 2012. The population of male goat has decreased by 7.58% during the inter censuses period (2007-2012). Rajouri has the major contribution in goat population of 15.16%. The second and third highest contributors are Leh (Ladakh) and Kathua with share of goat population of 11.00 and 10.54%, respectively.

Advantages of Goat Rearing

1. The initial investment needed for Goat farming is low accompanied with small body size and docile nature, housing requirements and managemental problems with goats are also less.
2. Goats are prolific breeders and achieve sexual maturity at the age of 10-12 months gestation period in goats is short and at the age of 16-17 months it starts giving milk. Twinning is very common and triplets and quadruplets are rare.
3. In drought prone areas risk of goat farming is very much less as compared to other livestock species.
4. Goats are ideal for mixed species grazing. The animal can thrive well on wide variety of thorny bushes, weeds, crop residues, agricultural by-products unsuitable for human consumption. Goats are 2.5 times more economical than sheep on free range grazing under semi arid conditions.
5. The goat meat is more lean (low cholesterol) and relatively good for people who prefer low energy diet especially in summer and sometimes goat meat (chevon) is preferred over mutton because of its "chewability".
6. Goat milk is easy to digest than cow milk because of small fat globules and is naturally homogenized. Goat milk is said to play a role in improving appetite and digestive efficiency. Goat milk is non allergic as compared to cow milk and it has anti-fungal and anti bacterial properties and can be used for treating urogenital diseases of fungal origin.

7. No religious taboo against goat slaughter and meat consumption prevalent in the country

Brief Description of Important Breeds of Goats

Indian Breed				Exotic Breeds
Himalayan Region	**Northern Region**	**Central region**	**Southern region**	
Pashmina	Jamnunapari	Berari	Surti	Toggenberg
Chegu	Beetal	Kathiiawari	Osmanabadi	Sannen
	Barbari		Malarbar	Alpine
				Nubian
				Anglo Nubian
				Angora

Feeding of Goats

Goats generally produce more milk than a cow from the same quantity of nutrients. The nutrient conversion efficiency for the production of milk in goats is 45.71 per cent, whereas a dairy cow averages 38 per cent. It has been observed that goats are 4.04 per cent superior to sheep, 7.90 per cent superior to buffaloes, and 8.60 per cent superior to cows in crude fibre utilization. The goat uses more useless feeds for its maintenance than a cow.

The secret of successful feeding is in devising a cheap and efficient ration. While preparing a ration for goats, factors like bulk, palatability, availability, price and digestibility should be considered along with the nutritive quality of the feed. Abundant clean, fresh water, changed every morning and evening should be made available to goats at all times. Some of the most serious diseases of goats result from the drinking of dirty water from shallow pools. Water troughs should be thoroughly washed at least twice a month. Goats in milk require more water than dry goats and should be watered regularly at least three times a day.

Feeding Habits: Goats are sensitive animals with peculiar feeding habits. By the means of their mobile upper lips and very prehensile tongue, goats are able to graze on very short grass and to browse on foliage not normally eaten by other domestic livestock. Unlike sheep, goats relish eating aromatic plants in areas of scarce food supply and hence can penetrate deep into deserts. They are fastidious about cleanliness and like frequent change in the feed. Feeds given must be clean and fresh, since goats eat nothing that is dirty or foul-smelling. They dislike wet, stale or trampled fodder. For this reason, it is advisable to feed them in hay-racks or hang the feed in bundles from a peg in the wall or from a branch of a tree. Double-sided portable hay-racks are the most suitable and convenient for stall feeding. It is preferable to serve them small quantities at a time; when served in large quantities at a time, they waste a lot of it by trampling.

Goats are very fond of leguminous fodders. They do not relish fodder like sorghum/maize silage or straw. Goats do not relish hay prepared from forest grasses, even if cut in early stages, but very much relish hay prepared from leguminous crops. Some of the common green roughages liked by goats are : lucerne, berseem, napier grass, green arhar, cowpea, soyabean, cabbage and cauliflower leaves, shaftal, senji, methi, shrubs and weeds of different kinds; and leaves of trees such as babul, neem, ber, tamarind and pipal. The common dry fodders liked by goats are straws of arhar, urid, mung, gram, dry leaves of trees, and lucerne/berseem hays (which are the main forage crops for milch goats).

Nutrients Required: The nutrients needed may be divided into maintenance, production and pregnancy requirements:-

a) Maintenance Ration: As goats have a higher BMR than cattle, their maintenance requirements are higher. The maintenance requirement is 0.09 per cent DCP and 0.09 per cent TDN. For its size, a goat can consume substantially more feed than cattle or sheep, viz. 6.5-11 per cent of its body weight in dry matter when compared with 2.5-3 per cent for cattle or sheep. This means that the goat can satisfy its maintenance requirement and produce milk from forage alone.

b) Production Ration: Requirements for the production of 1 litre of milk with 3 % and 4.5 % fat is 43 gm of DCP and 200 gm of starch equivalent (SE), and 60 gm of DCP and 285 gm of SE, respectively. The nutritional requirement of a goat weighing 50 kg and yielding 2 litres of milk with 4% fat may be met by feeding 400gm of concentrate mixture and 5 kg of berseem or lucerne. The ration should have 12-15 % protein content.

The following concentrate mixtures may be used to feed the goat : (i) 1 part of wheat bran, 2 parts of maize grain, and 1 part of linseed cake, or (ii) 2 parts of maize grain, 1 part of barley, 2 parts of mustard-cake, and 2 parts of gram husk, or (iii) 1 part of wheat bran, 2 parts of barley grain, and 1 part of groundnut cake, or (iv) 2 parts of gram grain and 1 part of wheat bran. The above mixtures should also contain 2 % each of mineral mixture and salt.

c) Pregnancy Ration: The foetal growth in the last 2 months of pregnancy is rapid and the metabolic rate of the goat rises rapidly. During this period, the content of ration should be increased to the level of production ration. A week before she kids, the doe should be provided with more succulent type of food. For three or four days after kidding, the level of diet should be lowered and made more fibrous. This is necessary to minimize the shock to the goat's udder. After this period, the feeding should be done at a normal rate.

d) Feeding of Kids: Immediately after birth feed the young ones with colostrum and up to 3 days of birth keep dam with young ones for 2-3 days for frequent access of milk. After 3 days & up to weaning feed the kids with milk at 2 to 3 times a day. At about 2 weeks of age the young ones should be trained to eat green roughages and at one month of age the young ones should be provided with the concentrate mixture (Creep feed).

Composition of ideal creep feed:

- Maize - 40%
- Ground nut cake -30 %
- Wheat bran – 10 %

- ✰ Deoiled rice bran- 13 %
- ✰ Molasses – 5%
- ✰ Mineral mixture- 2%
- ✰ Salt – 1% fortified with vitamins A, B_2 and D_3 and antibiotic feed supplements.

Feeding Schedule for a Kid/Lamb from Birth to 90 Days

Age of kids/lambs	Dam's milk (ml)	Creep feed (grams)	Forage, green/day (gm)
1-3 days	Colostrum-300 ml, 3 feedings	-	-
4-14days	350 ml, 3 feedings	-	-
15-30 days	350 ml, 3 feedings	A little	A little
31-60 days	400 ml, 2 feedings	100-150	Free choice
61-90 days	200 ml, 2 feedings	200-250	Free choice

e) Mineral Mixture: The requirements of calcium and phosphorous for maintenance are 6.5 and 3.5 gm, respectively, per 50 kg body weight. Goats require slightly larger quantities of calcium than sheep. The mineral mixture may be included in the concentrate ration at the rate of 2 per cent.

f) Salt: Salt licks or lumps of rock salt of fairly good size should be hung up in some suitable place where the goats can easily get them. This is important as goats secrete a good amount of sodium and chloride ions in the milk.

g) Vitamins and Antibiotics: Goats particularly need vitamins A, D and E. Vitamin A can be supplied by feeding green forage and yellow maize; 1 kg of lush-green fodder will provide 1500 IU. Vitamin D can be obtained by exposure to sunlight. Vitamin E is present in adequate amounts in most normal rations. Synthetic vitamins A and D may be supplemented in the ration of growing kids. Feeding of aureomycin or terramycin increases the growth rate of young kids, reduced the incidence of scours and other infectious diseases and improves the general appearance of the kids.

Housing

Housing of goats is not a serious problem. It is enough if the goats are provided with a dry, comfortable, safe and secure place, free from worms, and affording protection from excessive heat and inclement weather. In Indian villages goats are mostly kept under widespread shady trees when the climate is dry, provided the goats are safe from thieves and predatory animals such as wolves and panthers. The kids are kept under large inverted baskets until they are old enough to run along with their mothers. Males and females are generally kept together.

It is worth while to design a cheap house for goats which may result in increased milk and meat production. Some kind of housing is necessary if herds of goats are maintained in cities and at organized farms; adequate space, proper ventilation, good drainage and plenty of light should be provided for while constructing houses. Successful goat dairying largely depends on the site where goats are kept. Goats do not thrive on marshy or swampy ground. Grazing areas should be free from pits and shallow pools, for goats contract parasitic infection mainly from such places.

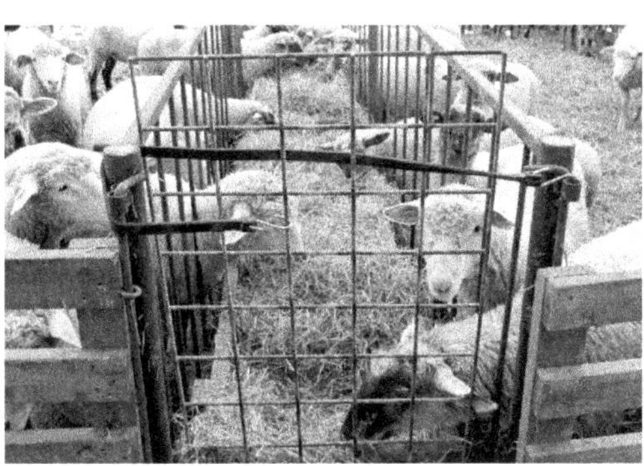

'Lean-to' Type Shed

The cheapest form of building is the 'lean-to' type shed located against the side of an existing building. Such a shed for a family of two goats should be 1·5 m wide and 3·0 m long. This length provides 0.3 m for the manger and 1·2 m for the goats; the remaining 1·5 m space is sufficient for two milking does with a stub wall between them. The height nearest the wall should be 2·3 m and on the lower side 1·7 m giving a slope of 0.6 11 to the roof, which may be tiled or thatched. An open-framed window of good size on the lower side and an open-framed door should be provided. Arrangements for storing hay or dried feed can be made overhead.

The plan for a house varies with the climatic conditions and the type of flock to be sheltered. In dry climates with a rainfall of 50 to 75 cm a long shed open on the sides, little exposed to weather and built on well drained ground makes an excellent shelter. A goat, when reared singly, can be housed in any building provided it is dry, free from draft and well ventilated. The space allowed should be 1·8 m x 1·8 m. A plain board, 28 cm wide and 2·5 cm thick with two circular holes sufficiently large for receiving two small galvanized iron pails, may be used in place of the manger or a trough for food. It should be raised 50 to 60 cm from the floor, supported on wooden or iron brackets fixed to the wall. These pails, one for water and the other for food, are preferred to the manger, as the accumulated residue of feed can be easily removed from them.

In the tropics because of high temperature, heavy rainfall and the susceptibility of goats-to parasitism, the most practical goat houses are those which are raised above the ground level, are well ventilated, and have long eaves to prevent heavy rain showers to splash in from the sides. The floor must be strong (wooden strips with small slits in between) and the roof material should provide effective insulation from the solar radiation. The roofing material would be made of bamboo or tree leaves or earthen tiles which are cheap and practical. Provision must be made for collection of dung and urine periodically.

Shelter for Buck

The buck should be housed separately. A single stall measuring 2·5 m x 2·0 m with the usual fittings for food and water would be suitable for the bucks. Two bucks should not be kept together, particularly during the breeding season, because they might fight.

Space for Goats in Stanchions and Confinement

The size of the stanchion where the goat is kept should be 0·75 m wide and 1·2 m long. Goats kept longer in a pen should have a floor space of $2m^2$.

Loose Stalls for Pregnant Does and Kids

Kids should be provided with separate loose stalls, away from adult females. The walls and doors of these stalls should be about 1·3 m high. A box barrel or a log is provided for exercise. One stall measuring 1·8 m^2 can accommodate up to 10 kids. Such loose stalls are also suitable for goats at the time of kidding. All stalls should be provided with an enclosure in which the animals can be let loose during the day. This loose housing system reduces the housing cost and labour.

Exercise Paddock for Stall-fed Goats

An enclosure measuring I2 m x 18 m is adequate for 100 to 125 goats. Such an enclosure or exercise paddock should be well fenced with strong woven wires which should not be far apart near the bottom. The exercise paddocks should be made bigger than the enclosures and should have some shade trees if the stock is to be maintained constantly in confinement. An extra-strong woven wire should be used, as goats have the habit of climbing fences and also of rubbing their bodies against them. Barbed wire should not be used so as to avoid injury to the udder and teats. It will be good if a box of 1 m x 1 m and 60 cm high and a stationary steel-drum or a log of 30 cm x 2·4 cm size is provided for their exercise.

Segregation Shed

When the herd is large, provision for a small segregation shed, about' 3·6 m x 5 m, is very desirable. It should be built in the farther comer of the farm and provided with a well-fenced yard; it should be divided into two or three sections. Each stall as well as the yard should have separate watering arrangement.

Recommended Floor and Trough Space for Goats in Intensive Production Related to Live Weight

	Weight	Floor Space			Trough Space
		Solid Floor	Slatted Floor	Open Yard	
	kg	m^2/animal	m^2/animal	m^2/animal	m/animal
Doe	35	0.8	0.7	2	0.35
Doe	50	1.1	0.9	2.5	0.40
Doe	70	1.4	1.1	3	0.45
Kid	-	0.4 - 0.5	0.3 - 0.4	-	0.25 - 0.30
Buck	-	3.0	2.5	-	0.5

Tethering

When one or two goats are to be kept and facilities for grazing are limited, tethering is convenient. This simple device has the advantage of keeping goats out-of-doors, and at same time on a limited area, although frequent changes of location become necessary. The animal is provided with a shelter with in its reach so that it may turn to it in the event of extreme heat or heavy rains. Goats have strong dislike for rain and for getting wet. The shelter should be temporary and preferably a portable one. The rope or chain used for tethering should be about 35 to 50cm long. The peg should be tethered only in the morning and evening, and kept in the shed during the mid-day. Tethering has also an important advantage of grazing the animal on a plot which is definitely known to be free from parasitic infections.

Elevated Platform

The floor must be strong (wooden strips with small slits in between) and the roof material should provide effective insulation from the solar radiation. The roofing material would be made of bamboo or tree leaves or earthen tiles which are cheap and practical. Provision must be made for collection of dung and urine periodically. In the tropics because of high temperature, heavy rainfall and the susceptibility of goats-to parasitism, the most practical goat houses are those which are raised above the ground level, are well ventilated, and have long eaves to prevent heavy rain showers to splash in from the sides.

Farming Systems

Extensive System

- ✰ Grazing the sheep and goat in the entire pasture and leaving them there for the whole season is the extensive system of rearing.
- ✰ In this method feed cost is very much reduced.
- ✰ It is not conducive to make the best use of the whole grasses. So we can preferably practice the rotational grazing method.

Rotational Grazing Method

- ✰ Rotational grazing should be practiced under which the pasture land should be divided by temporary fences into several sections.
- ✰ The animals are then moved from one section to another section. By the time the entire pasture is grazed, the first section will have sufficient grass cover to provide second grazing.
- ✰ Parasitic infestations can be controlled to a great extent.
- ✰ Further, it helps to provide quality fodder for most part of the year.
- ✰ Under this system, it is advisable to graze the lambs first on a section and then bring in ewes to finish up the feed left by the lambs.

Semi-Intensive System

- ✰ Semi-intensive system of sheep / goat production is an intermediate compromise between extensive and intensive system followed in some flocks having limited grazing.
- ✰ It involves extensive management but usually with controlled grazing of fenced pasture.

- It consists of provision of stall feeding, shelter at night under shed and 3 to 5 hour daily grazing and browsing on pasture and range.
- In this method, the feed cost is somewhat increased.

Advantages

- Meeting the nutrient requirement both from grazing and stall feeding
- Managing medium to large flock of 50 to 350 heads and above
- Utilizing cultivated forage during lean period
- Harvesting good crop of kids both for meat and milk
- Making a profitable gain due to less labour input

Intensive System (Zero Grazing System)

- It is a system in which sheep goats are continuously kept under housing in confinement with limited access in which they are stall fed.
- It implies a system where goats are not left to fend for themselves with only minimum care.
- Intensive operation of medium sized herd of 50 to 250 heads or more oriented towards commercial milk production goes well with this system particularly of dairy goats.
- It merits exploitation of the system of feeding agro-industrial by products as on fodder grass with carrying capacity of 37 to 45 goats per hectare.
- This system of management requires more labour and high cash input.
- However, this has the advantage of close supervision and control over the animals.
- In this method, the dung is collected in one place and used as a good fertilizer.
- Less space is sufficient for more number of animals.

Economics of Goat Farming– Techno-Economic Parameters

		No. of bucks *No. of does*	***10*** ***200***
A		*Production Traits*	
	i	Age at Maturity (months)	8-42
	ii	Kidding Interval (months)	8
	iii	Kidding percentage	80%
	iv	Twinning percentage	76%
	v	No. of Kidding per year	1.5
	vi	Sex ratio	1:1
	vii	Mortality (%) Adults	5
		Kids	10
	viii	Saleable age of Kids (months)	5-9

		No. of bucks *No. of does*	***10*** ***200***
	ix	Culling of does (% per year) from second on month	20
B		*Expenditure Norms*	
	i	Space Requirement (sft. Per head) Buck Doe Kids	 20sft. 10sft. 4sft
	ii	Cost of Construction (/Sft.)	Rs.85
	iii	Cost of equipment (`. Per adult animal)	Rs.100
	iv	a) Cost of green folder cultivation (`. Acre/season) b) No. of Acres	Rs.12500
	v	**Concentrate Feed** Adult does one month before and after kidding i.e., per kidding i.e., Buck (two months per breading season) Kids for (30 days)	 6.75kg month 7.5 kg/month 3.75kg month
	vi	Cost of Feed (/ Kg.)	10
	vii	Labor wages (Rs. Per month) 2 x Rs.5000	120000
	viii	Insurance (as percentage of the cost of breading stock)	25
	ix	Veterinary aid (Adult / year)	10
	x	Water, electricity and other misc. expenses (/ Adult)	
C		*Income Norms*	
	i	Sale price of buckling	3400
	ii	Sale price of Doe lings	3000
	iii	Sale of Adult does	4000
	iv	Sale of Adult Bucks	5000
	v	Sale value of male / female	3000

In the absence of fertile lands and assured irrigation which are controlled by a small population of rich farmers and lack of employment in the industrial and service sectors, most of the rural families belonging to socio-economically weaker sections of the society maintain different species of livestock to supplement their income. While the land owners prefer cattle and buffaloes, the landless prefer to own sheep, goat and poultry. With the policy of the State Animal Husbandry Department to extend free breeding, vaccination and veterinary services and permit free grazing on community lands, the farmers can be encouraged to expand their herd size without any major financial burden. Thus concluding that more concrete steps from lab to farmer approach needs to be adapted and a lot can be done in small ruminant industry.

Transforming Rural Areas through Veterinary Science *Pages* **93-102**
Editor: Dipanjali Konwar, Shilpa Sood & Shahid Ahamad
Published by: **ASTRAL INTERNATIONAL PVT. LTD., NEW DELHI**

6 Giant Freshwater Prawn: Farming Technology for Increasing Economic Returns of Fish Farmers

Dr. Akhil Gupta, Dr. Sahar Masud & Dr. Raj Kumar

Introduction

Freshwater prawn farming is fast gaining popularity. There are more than 100 species of freshwater prawn and out of these the giant freshwater prawn *Macrobrachium rosenbergii* is the largest prawn known in the world. The Giant freshwater prawn (GFP) *Macrobrachium rosenbergii*, also known as Scampi, farming is gaining popularity all over the world. It is the most preferred species for culture because it has fast growth rate, better meat quality, resistance to disease, omnivorous feeding habit, compatibility for polyculture with Indian and Chinese carps, adaptation to varying environmental conditions, easy breeding and good demand in domestic and international markets.

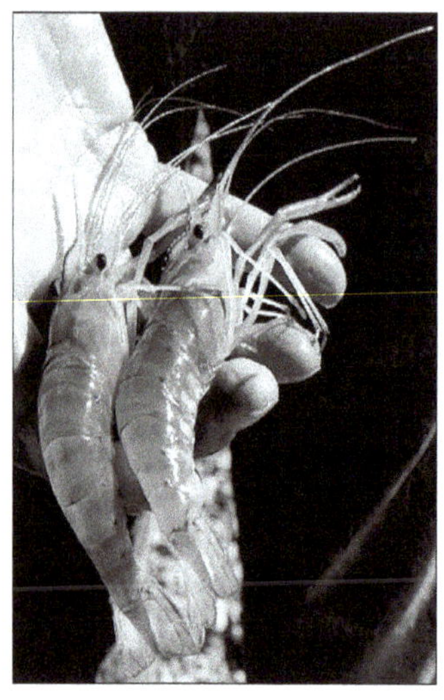
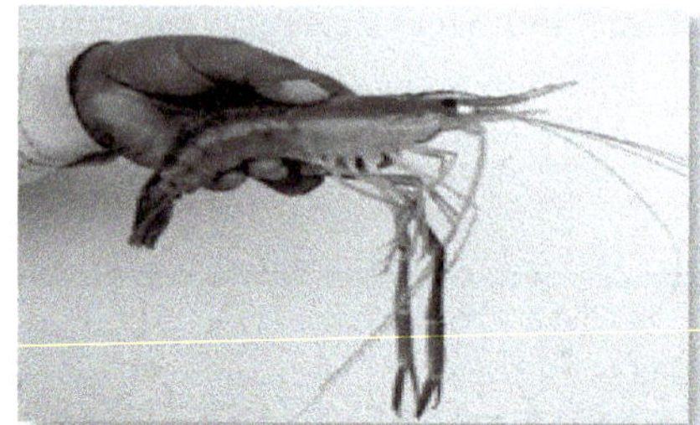
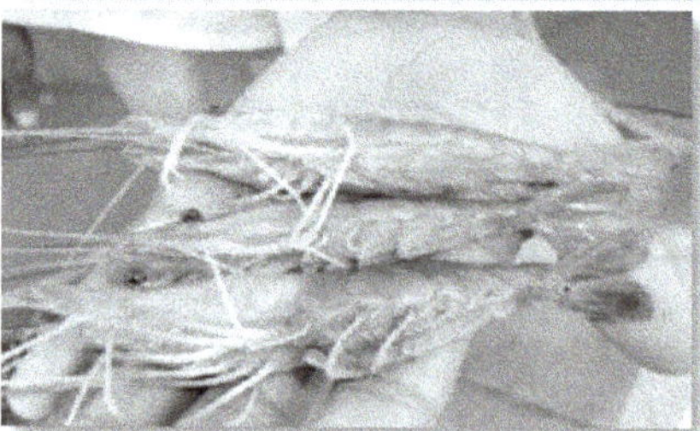

Freshwater Prawn Macrobrachium Rosenbergii

Culture Technology of Giant Freshwater Prawn

Culture of prawn can be carried out in earthen ponds, cement cisterns, in pens or in cages. However, most of the operations are being carried out in earthen ponds. It can be reared in mono-culture or poly-culture with carps. The standard practices of scampi farming include site selection, pond construction, water source and quality, management practices, etc.

a) Site Selection: The proper site selection is essential to obtain best results. The selected site should have the following major qualities: Supply of good quality, pollution free freshwater; Soil having a pH of more than 6.5 and good water retention capacity; and Warm climate for nearly 8 months (Temperature - > 25 ^{0}C).

b) Pond Construction: Ponds should have an inlet and an outlet; Pond bottom should have a gradient slope towards the out let; Pond bunds should have a suitable slope (1 :2); Pond size - 0.2 -< 1.0 ha (0.2-0.5 ha); Depth - 2 m, Shape – Rectangular; and Soil - Clay loam, sandy loam

c) Water Source and Quality: A permanent source of water is must before planning freshwater prawn farming. It includes tube well water, canal water, water from nearby river/reservoir/lake, etc. Water used for culture should be free from toxic chemicals and pollutants. The optimum range of few most important water quality parameters for freshwater prawn culture are salinity (freshwater/ <5 ppt), temperature (28 – 32 ^{0}C), pH (7.0-8.5), total hardness (50-100 mg/I), dissolved oxygen (> 5ppm).

d) Seed Quality: Selecting the best quality seed for stocking is one of the most important tasks in scampi culture. Stocking wild seed should not be resorted to, especially in scampi ponds since wild seed come in a mixture of species, mostly slow growing undesirable ones; are of non-uniform size; poor health because of crude methods of collection, packing and transport; and may bring diseases from unknown sources. The colour of the PL may not always give a reliable idea about their health. Some of the characteristics of healthy seed are described below.

- healthy PL swims with straight bodies
- display common appendages (particularly the two long antennal flagellae)
- respond rapidly to external stimuli
- actively swims against the current when the water is stirred
- clear shell without any fouling and damage or loss of appendages

The PL brought to the farm need to be acclimatized to the pond water. In any case, the PL should be acclimatized to the temperature as well as pH of the pond water. Many farmers consider only the former by simply floating the seed bags in the pond before releasing the seeds. The, water in the seed bag and the pond water should be gradually mixed to avoid pH shock to the PL.

e) Nursery Rearing: There are many advantages to the nursery rearing of scampi PL. The PL are stocked, in small nursery ponds at high densities and reared for 1.0 to 1.5 months. Providing a nursery area ensures that the PL are adequately fed during the first two months of culture. About 10-15% of the total pond area can be allocated for nursery ponds. Very high stocking densities up to 100/m^2 could be adopted in nursery ponds, provided sufficient food, aeration and additional substratum are ensured. However, the common practice is to stock nursery ponds at 2.0-2.5 lakh PL/ha.

The PL should be fed a pellet diet or other suitable diet for at least 3 to 4 times a day. Zooplankton are an important food source for prawns, especially during the first few weeks after stocking. The nursery reared PL grow to juveniles and weigh about 3-5 g depending on the stocking density employed and management practice. These juveniles are used for stocking in grow-out ponds. Preparation of the nursery ponds just before stocking is the most important aspect for successful rearing. The weed fishes should be totally cleared, and then the pond protected by fencing to avoid the entry of pests like frogs, turtles, crabs, predatory birds etc. which in most cases would serve as the carriers of many diseases.

f) Pond Management: The important management practices needed includes pond preparation, feeding, water quality measurement, prawn sampling and finally harvesting.

i) Pond Preparation: The steps involved in pond preparation includes, eradication of predators and competitors, application of lime and application of fertilizers (organic and inorganic). Bleaching powder and urea @ 300 and 100 kg/ha respectively can be applied to kill all predatory species in the pond. For this first urea and after six hours bleaching powder has to be applied. Stocking of prawn seed can be done two weeks after eradication of pests and predators.

Lime is applied @200-600 kg/ha depending on the soil pH. The lime used should be agricultural lime ($CaCO_3$) or dolomite ($CaMg\ CO_3$). The lime should be spread over the whole pond bottom and up to the top of the dyke.

Lime helps to correct the pH and disinfects the pond bottom. Lime is also a source of calcium, which is very important for exoskeleton formation of prawns. Cow dung @ 500 kg/ha and urea @ 10-30 kg/ha and super phosphate @ 20-60 kg/ ha may be applied to initiate a plankton bloom. After the initial fertilization water can be filled up to the desired level (4-5 feet).

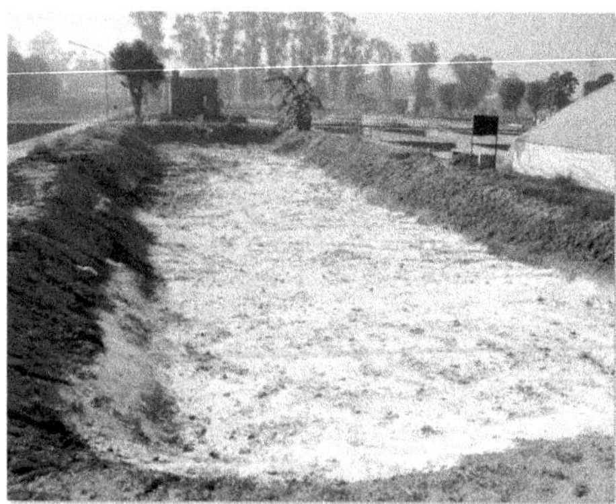

Liming of Freshwater Prawn Pond

ii) Provision of Hide Out: It is desirable to provide hideouts and more surfaces for clinging. Cut branches of trees, nylon screen, earthen/ plastic pipes etc. can be used as hideouts.

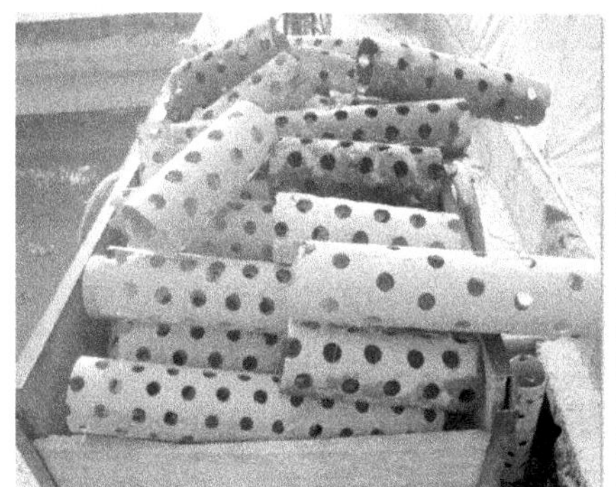

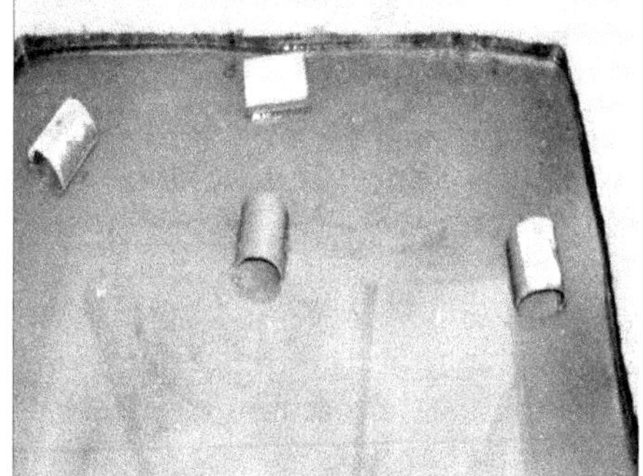

Plastic Pipes as Hideout

iii) Stocking: Prior to stocking the pond water quality should be tested and necessary correction should be made. Care should be taken to acclimatise the post larvae to the temperature of the pond by floating the transport bags in the ponds for 20 min. Early morning and late evening are considered ideal period for stocking the seed.

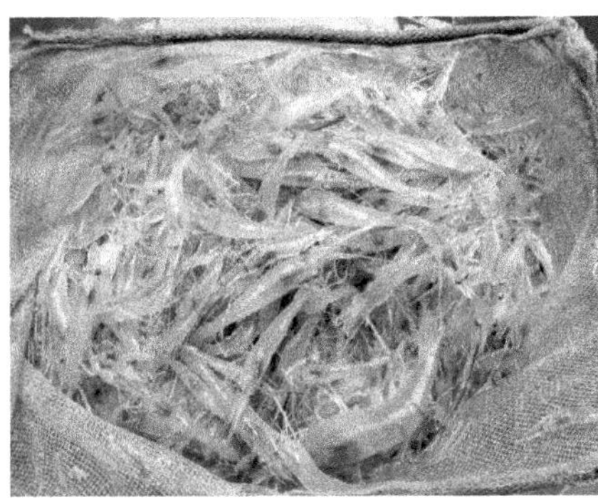
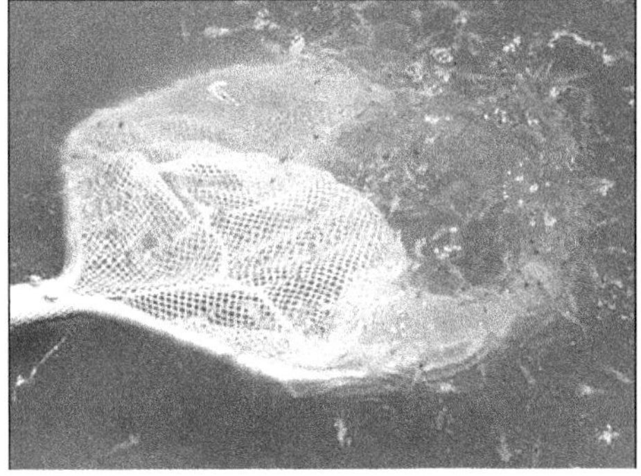

Stocking of Juvenile Prawns in Fertilized Ponds

For semi-intensive culture a stocking rate of 5-7/m^2 is desirable. In poly-culture stocking density of prawn is reduced to 50% *i.e.* @ 25000/ha and compatible carp species such catla, rohu, silver carp and grass carp are also stocked @7000/ha.

Table: Different Fish Species Combinations for Poly-Culture of Freshwater Prawn

Fish species	*Three species combination*	*Four species combination*	*Six species Combination*
Catla	2000	2000	1000
Silver carp	-	-	1500
Rohu	3000	3000	2000
Grass carp	-	-	1000
Mrigal	2000	1000	750
Common carp	-	1000	750
Total	7000	7000	7000

iv) Food and Feeding: Pellet diets containing 35% crude protein are preferred for feeding freshwater prawn. Feed should be spread evenly along the peripheral area of pond. Feeding through feeding tray (6 no. of tray/ha) results in better growth and save total feeding cost. Feeding should be done during late evening and early morning. Monthly sampling should be done to know the average body weight of prawn to adjust the feed quantity.

Table: Daily Feed Requirement of Freshwater Prawn

Prawn wt. (g)	*%age of body wt. feed daily*
<1	<20
2-5	15
5-10	10
10-30	5
>30	2

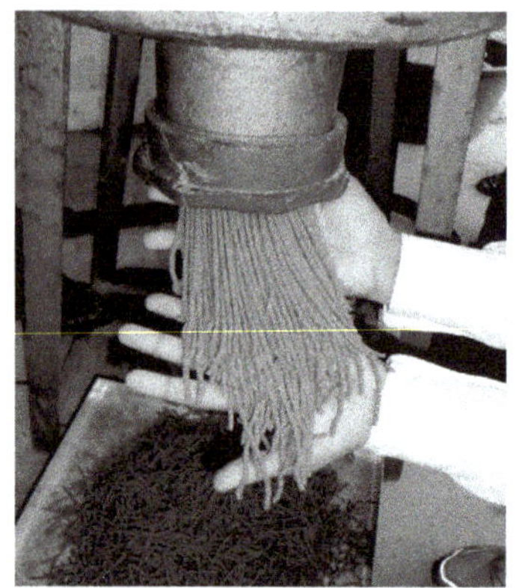

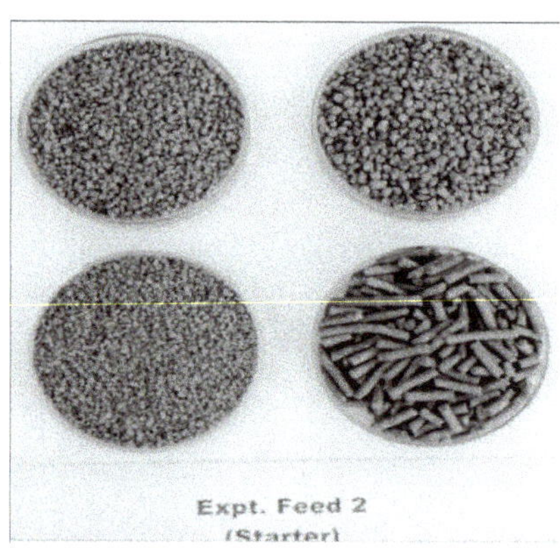

Pellet Feed of Different Grades for Feeding Freshwater Prawn

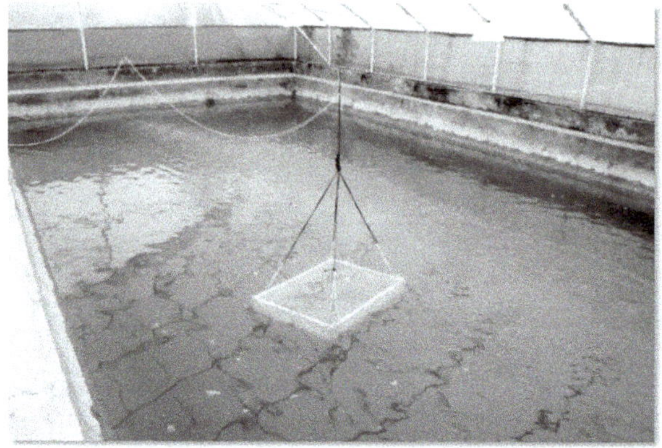

Feeding of Prawn through Feeding Tray

v) Water Quality Management: Daily monitoring of critical water quality parameters such as dissolved oxygen, pH, and temperature is essential to prevent any loss of stock due to poor water quality. Dissolved oxygen should be monitored during early morning. On cloudy days and rainy days depletion of oxygen may occur during daytime also. Phytoplankton bloom and decaying waste material are the main reasons for dissolved oxygen depletion usually seen in prawn ponds. When the oxygen level in pond water is critically low then prawns come to the surface along the periphery of the pond. Immediate remedial actions such as water exchange or operation of pond aerators should be taken to avoid mortality of stock.

Visibility and colour of the pond water gives a visual assessment of the condition of the pond ecosystem. In unproductive ponds the visibility can be up to the bottom. In highly blooming and or turbid ponds the visibility will be up to a few centimetres <10 cm. Visibility should be maintained in the range of 30-40 cm to avoid water quality deterioration.

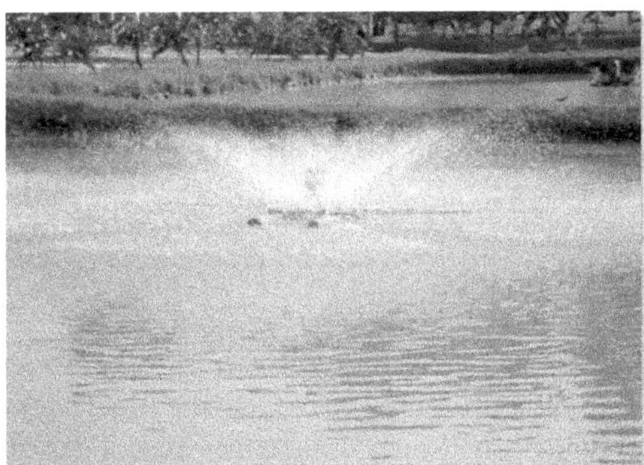

Aeration of Prawn Pond Water through Splash Aerator

vi) Stock Monitoring: Growth of the animal is assessed by regular monthly sampling with cast nets or small mesh seine nets. The growth rate and survival of a population of prawn depends on many factors including density, predation, feed and temperature.

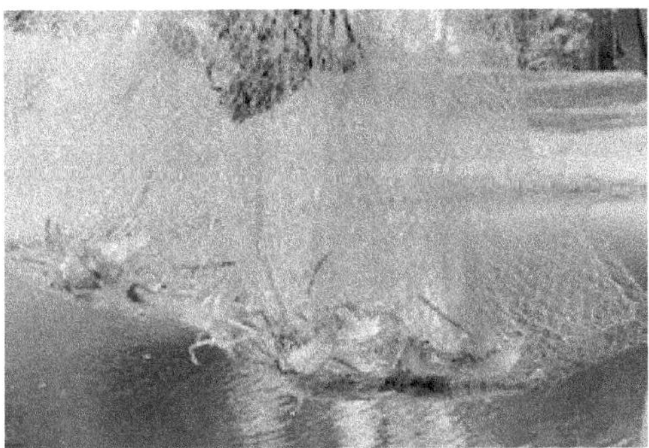

Periodically Check on Prawn Growth Progress through Cast Net

vii) Health management: Although *M. rosenbergii* is less vulnerable to disease than penaeid shrimps, this now seems to be an old story. The so-called disease resistance might have been due to the lower stocking densities used and less transfer of brood stock. A variety of diseases have been reported in larval, juvenile and adult scampi, which include fouling protozoans such as *Vorticella* and *Epistylis;* fungal pathogens such as *Fusarium;* bacteria such as *Vibrio, Aeromonas, Leucothrix, Enterococcus* etc., and also non-pathogenic diseases such as stress and neurotic symptoms, moult failures and so on. The most common problem encountered with scampi ponds in India seems to be the symptoms associated with poor water quality and pond bottom conditions such as shell erosion, cut in the appendages and abnormal exoskeleton due to irregular moulting. Another alarming news is the detection of white spot virus of penaeids from farmed scampi in Taiwan. The white tail disease (WTD) had been causing severe losses to scampi farmers for the last two years, especially during the hot summer seasons. The symptoms are very obvious, and mainly appear during the nursery-rearing phase. The PL becomes dull and inactive, and drifts in the hatchery tanks, while the healthy PL swim actively. The diseased prawns displayed poor growth, anorexia and inactivity besides the opaque musculature, leading mortality. Health management measures are: Maintaining a good rearing practice, avoid high density stocking and over feeding; Provide hideouts to increase the total surface area of the pond and to reduce cannibalism; Pelleted feed with 35% protein content is must for better production; Regularly check feeding tray to ensure consumption of the feed; Drying out the ponds between production cycles so that the beds can be re-oxidized; Exchange water regularly which induces moulting; Periodic harvesting is always preferred to reduce the heterogeneous growth pattern; Protozoan parasites, bacteria and fungi cause diseases. Loss of appendages, brown or black coloration of the exoskeleton, etc. can be seen in disease affected prawns. They may not accept feed; If disease symptoms are noted water should be replaced; and Water quality should be tested to determine the DO; pH and ammonia levels and necessary corrections should be made

Harvesting, Processing and Marketing

Growth of the animal is assessed by regular monthly sampling with cast nets or small mesh seine nets. The growth rate and survival of a population of prawn depends on many factors including density, predation, feed and temperature. Because of the heterogeneous growth pattern of freshwater prawn, individual weight is highly variable for prawns of the same age. Periodic harvesting is always preferred. After four months bigger size prawns (>30g) can be removed by using a seine net of suitable mesh size. Selective harvesting should continue once every 3-4 weeks for another 3-4 months and finally the pond may be harvested by complete draining. An average survival of 60% can be expected from a properly prepared pond, stocked with quality seed, fed with quality feed and monitored regularly to maintain optimum water quality. The average expected body weight of prawns after 6-7 months of culture is about 40-60 g. Yield may range from 1-1.5 tonnes/ha/6-7 months.

Scampi has got excellent international market. It is exported mainly to Europe as a luxury item served in elite restaurants. The tail weight percentage is less (about 50 %) than that for marine shrimp. This is also lesser for males than that for females, and also decreases with prawn size. Also there is a high rate (5%) of hanging meat. Dipping prawns in iced water ('kill chilling') prior to blanching at 65°C for 15-20 seconds, before icing and transport to market significantly improves quality. Beheading and intensive washing decreases initial microbial load and improves post storage quality. The market rate for 1 kg of freshwater prawn is about Rs. 500-700, depending on number per kilogram. Lesser the number greater will be the cost.

Over Wintering of Prawn

The culture period of freshwater prawn in Northern States is short i.e. only during summer from April to October. Most of the farmers are not be able to sale their stock at once after harvesting and mortality will occur due to decrease in temperature. In poly-house, temperature above 18 ^{0}C is maintained for better survival of the stock.

Economics

Economics of Monoculture of Giant Freshwater Prawn

S.No	Item	Amount (in Rs.)
I.	*Expenditure*	
A.	*Variable Cost*	
1.	Pond lease value (area: 1 ha)	10,000
2.	Prawn seed @ 60,000/ha @Rs. 1000/1000 Nos. with transportation cost	60,000
3.	Fertilizers and lime	6,000
4.	Supplementary feed (pellet form @ 3 t/crop @ Rs. 30/kg)	90,000
5.	Wages (One @ Rs. 3000/month for 9 months)	27,000
6.	Electricity and fuel	3,000
7.	Harvesting charges	5,000
8.	Miscellaneous expenditure	3,000
	Sub-Total	2,04,000
B.	*Total Cost*	
1.	Variable cost	2,04,000
2.	Interest on variable cost (@ 15% per annum for 6 months)	15,300
	Grand Total	2,19,300
II.	*Gross Income*	
	Sale of prawn (@ Rs. 600/kg for 1000 kg)	6,00,000
III.	***Net Income (Gross income – Total cost) (420000 - 219300)***	**2,00,700**

Economics of Polyculture of Giant Freshwater Prawn with Carps

S.No	Item	Amount (in Rs.)
I.	*Expenditure*	
A.	*Variable Cost*	
1.	Pond lease value (area: 1 ha)	10,000
2.	Fish seed [7000 no./ha (@Rs. 300/1000 nos.)] = Rs. 2100/- Prawn seed [25,000/ha (@Rs. 1000/1000 nos.)] = Rs. 25000/-	27,100
3.	Fertilizers and lime	6,000
4.	Supplementary feed (pellet form @ 3 t/crop @ Rs. 25/kg)	75,000
5.	Wages (One @ Rs. 3000/month for 10 months)	30,000
6.	Electricity and fuel	3,500
7.	Harvesting charges	5,000
8.	Miscellaneous expenditure	3,000
	Sub-Total	1,59,600

S.No	*Item*	*Amount (in Rs.)*
B.	*Total Cost*	
1.	Variable cost	1,59,600
2.	Interest on variable cost (@ 15% per annum for 10 months)	19,950
	Grand Total	1,79,550
II.	*Gross Income*	
	Sale of prawn (@ Rs. 350/kg for 500 kg)	1,75,000
	Sale of fish (@ Rs. 60/kg for 2500 kg)	1,50,000
	Grand Total	3,25,000
III.	*Net Income (Gross income– Total cost) (325000-179550)*	*1,45,450*

Conclusion

The major bottlenecks for freshwater prawn culture includes lack of knowledge to care post-larvae, non-availability of seed, nutritionally balanced feed, short rearing period and marketing. The grow-out culture technology for freshwater prawn culture is already standardized. The work on development of low-cost feed is going on. However, to popularize the farming of freshwater prawn in different regions, the State government should encourage its culture by providing subsidize seed and feed (as it costs about 60-70% of the total cultural cost), ensure quality seed, feed supply, and better marketing platform.

References

1. Gupta A. Formulation and evaluation of some alternative practical feeds for giant freshwater prawn, Macrobrachium rosenbergii (De Man). Ph.D. thesis Punjab Agricultural University, Ludhiana (Punjab), India. 2006.
2. Gupta A., Sehgal H.S., Sehgal G.K. Growth and carcass composition of giant freshwater prawn, Macrobrachium rosenbergii (De Man), fed different isonitrogenous and isocaloric diets. Aquaculture Research. 2007; 38: 1355-1363.
3. Gupta A., Sehgal H.S., Sehgal G.K. Low cost diet for monoculture of giant Macrobrachium rosenbergii. Indian Journal of Animal Nutrition. 2011; 28: 54-63.
4. Gupta A., Verma G., Gupta P. Growth performance, feed utilization, digestive enzyme activity, innate immunity and protection against Vibrio harveyi of freshwater prawn, Macrobrachium rosenbergii fed diets supplemented with Bacillus coagulans. Aquaculture International. 2016; 1-14, DOI 10.1007/ s10499-016-9996-x.
5. New M.B. Status of freshwater prawn farming: a review. Aquaculture Research. 1995; 26: 1-54. 6. New, M.B. Freshwater prawn farming: global status, recent research and glance at the future. Aquaculture Research. 2005; 36: 210-230.

Transforming Rural Areas through Veterinary Science *Pages* **103-116**
Editor: Dipanjali Konwar, Shilpa Sood, & Shahid Ahamad
Published by: **ASTRAL INTERNATIONAL PVT. LTD., NEW DELHI**

7 Commercial Layer Farming in Jammu Province

Dr. Suraj Amrutkar & Dr. Surinder K. Gupta

Introduction

Poultry eggs are important sources of high quality proteins, minerals and vitamins to balance the human diet. Commercially egg type chicken breeds are now available with an ability of high egg production and high feed conversion efficiency. Layer (for eggs) farming can be main source of family income and gainful employment to farmers throughout the year.

Scope for Layer farming and its National Importance

In the last three decades, India has made considerable progress in egg production. High quality chicks, equipments, vaccines and medicines are available easily at market. Technical and professional guidance is available to the farmers. Disease and mortality incidences are much reduced due to the management practices have improved. Many institutions are providing training to entrepreneurs. The per capita egg availability at present is 58 eggs; while as per ICMR recommendations about 182 eggs per person per year are required to balance the common vegetarian diet. Increasing assistance from the Central/State governments and poultry corporations and NABARD is being given to create infrastructural facilities so that new entrepreneurs take up this business. Layer farming has been given considerable importance in the national policy and has a good scope for further development.

Present Status of Poultry in India

Today, poultry is one of the fastest growing segments of the agricultural sector in India. Poultry industry influence by demands upon the eggs to human being. Poultry industries are the source of income and food. The National Institute of Nutrition has recommended 180 eggs per capita consumption for our country.

Poultry sector has shown a healthy increase by 12.39% over the previous census (2007) and the total poultry in the country was 729.2 million numbers in 2012. China has the 1st rank in poultry population in world. India has 5th rank in poultry population and 3rd rank in egg production.

All India Livestock Census in 2007 and 2012 (Birds in Thousands)

Species	*2007 census*	*2012 census*	*% change*
Fowl	617734	692646	12.13
Ducks	27643	23539	-14.85
Turkey and others	3452	13025	277.32
Total poultry	648829	729209	12.39

The largest producer of egg is Andhra Pradesh which produces 32% of the total egg production in the country followed by Tamilnadu that produces 17.1% of the egg production. West Bengal is the third largest egg producer state in the country which produces 6.8% of the total production. Per capita availability of egg in India is 58 eggs.

India	*Egg production (Million number)*	*Human production (million number)*	*Per capita availability (number / annum)*
2012-13	69731	1202.25	58

Present status of Poultry in Jammu & Kashmir

The Indian Livestock census is an exercise conducted every fifth year in the entire country. The 19th Livestock census was conducted with 15th October 2012. The poultry population is mainly contributed by fowls in Jammu & Kashmir with total poultry population of 8.27 million numbers in 2012. The changes in the poultry population over previous 3 census (2003, 2007 and 2012) are 5568, 6683 and 8273 (values in thousands), respectively. The total poultry population is showing increasing trend over 2003-2012. The birds have increased from 5.56 million numbers in 2003 to 8.27 million numbers in 2012. There is an increase of 23.8% in the poultry population during the inter census period (2007-2012).

The population of fowls has been increasing continuously since 2003. The fowls have increased from 5.32 million numbers in 2003 to 0.12 million numbers in 2012. The duck population has decreased by 35.98% over the previous census. The turkey and other birds have increased from 0.006 million in 2003 to 0.018 million in 2012 and registered a drastic increase during inter censuses period (2007-2012).

Recent Trends of Change in Population in J & K States of Fowl, Duck, Turkey and others (Note: Values in Thousand)

Species	*2003*	*2007*	*2012*	*% change from 2007-2012*
Fowl	5325	6487.4	8134.35	25.39
Ducks	237	190.30	121.84	-35.98
Turkey and other poultry	6	5.86	17.53	199.35
Total poultry	5568	6683	8273.71	23.8

Breeds of Layer Reared for Egg Production

Layers		
White leghorn	Cari priya	Cari sonali

Common Management Practices Recommended for Poultry Farmers

Layer bird's life cycle divide into three phases for easy management:

- Brooding stage: 0-8 weeks of age
- Grower stage: 9-20 weeks of age
- Layer stage: 21-72 weeks of age

Some of the major norms and recommended practices are given below:

Chicks

- Chicks should purchase improved strain of one day old healthy egger type chicks from a reputed hatchery. Usually 2-5% extra chicks are supplied.
- If cages are used for housing of birds ensure proper cage space *i.e.* half of the recommended floor space on deep litter.
- All equipments should clean, wash and disinfect with 0.5% malathion spray after every batch of birds is disposed off.

Brooding Management

Brooding is an art and science of rearing large number of baby chicks in the absence of a broody hen. In newly hatched chick, the thermoregulatory mechanism has not developed fully and takes about two weeks to develop this mechanism and homeostasis. Therefore, they can't maintain the body temperature properly for the first few weeks of life and may be subjected to chilling, if not properly taken care of. Hence, artificial brooding is mainly aimed at, providing the right temperature to the chicks. In addition to the temperature, adequate floor, feeder space, water space, relative humidity, ventilation and light should be provided for optimum comfort and growth of the chicks.

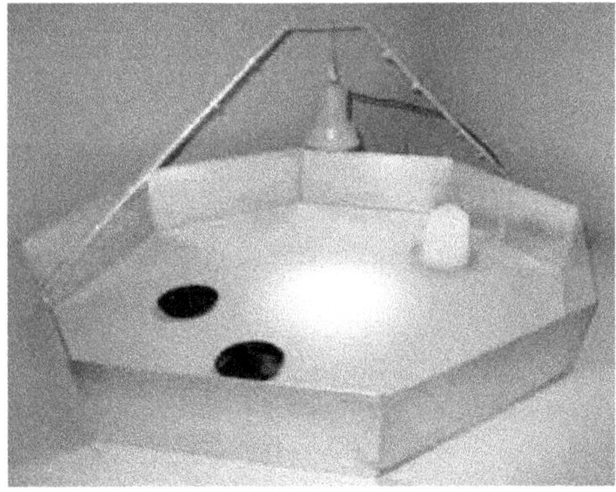

- ☆ Maintain the correct temperature, light, ventilation, space, feeding, watering etc. in brooder house
- ☆ Of these, the temperature is the most important criterion
- ☆ Room temperature of about 35°C has to be maintained during the first week of age
- ☆ Gradually reduced by about 3°C every week until the room temperature or 18-20°C is reached

Types of Brooders

- ☆ Incandescent bulbs and other types of bulbs
- ☆ Heater coil with thermostat
- ☆ Centralized heating system
- ☆ Battery brooder
- ☆ Biogas brooder
- ☆ Gas brooder
- ☆ Kerosene stove
- ☆ Charcoal stove

Behaviors of Chicks

- ☆ If they crowd under or near the source of heat, then the warmth given is not sufficient.
- ☆ If the chicks have moved to the periphery and are reluctant to come to the center under heat source, then temperature in the environment is higher than required.
- ☆ If the chicks feel comfortable at a given temperature, they walk actively throughout the area unmindful of heat provided and some take rest setting their head down on the side, the posture being given the name as "Chick comfort".

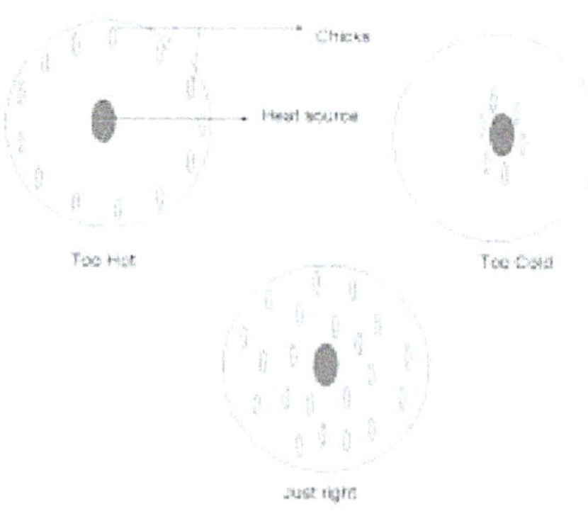

Feeding

- ☆ Feeds should be use high quality balanced. Starter feed (upto 8 weeks of age), grower feed (9 to 20 weeks of age) and layer feed (21 to 72 weeks of age) manufactured by reputed institutions/companies should be used. BIS feed formulae and specifications are available. With proper knowledge/ experience, the feed can be prepared on the farm.
- ☆ The feed should store in clean, dry, well ventilated room. A wet feed may bring fungus infection.
- ☆ Should use properly designed feeders and control the rats to avoid feed wastage
- ☆ Adequate feeding space should provide per bird. More space is required as the bird grows in age
- ☆ Keep proper records on feed consumption per bird for each batch. About 7 kg. feed upto 20 weeks and 38 kg. feed from 21 to 72 weeks of age is required. Excess consumption may be due to feed wastage, rats, low temperature of shed or poor feed quality (low energy feed).
- ☆ Too low feed consumption may be due to disease condition, low quality/ unpalatability of feed, high temperature in poultry shed.

Watering of Birds

- ☆ Always give fresh and clean drinking water
- ☆ Water should be always available at birds
- ☆ Use properly designed watering equipment
- ☆ Provide adequate watering space per bird
- ☆ Always keep water-pots clean
- ☆ Avoid birds entering inside pots
- ☆ Provide cool water during summer
- ☆ Store the water in tanks that are not exposed to hot sun in summer

Disease Prevention/Control

- ☆ Sanitary conditions of poultry sheds and equipment, balanced feed, fresh clean water, healthy chicks are essential to prevent diseases.
- ☆ Strictly avoid entry of visitors to farm, especially inside the sheds. If visitors come, ask them to dip their feet in a disinfectant solution, wash and clean hands and to wear apron/boots provided by the farm.
- ☆ Use proper vaccination schedule
- ☆ Use high quality vaccines purchased from reputed manufacturers. Keep vaccines in cool, dry conditions away from sunlight.

- Any left-over vaccine should be properly disposed off. Vaccines should not be used after their expiry date is over.
- Dead bird should be immediately removed from the shed and sent to laboratory for post-mortem examination or buried/burnt suitably away from the poultry sheds.
- The waste of farm should be suitably disposed off. Different workers should be employed in brooding and laying sheds.
- If any bird showing advanced signs of a disease, should be removed from the shed and culled. It can be sent to laboratory for diagnosis.
- If birds showing advanced signs of a disease, then it should be shown to a qualified veterinarian; and suitable medication/treatment be given as per his/drug manufacturers recommendations.
- Infected poultry manure can spread disease from one batch to another. Keep the litter dry, remove it after flock is sold and dispose the manure properly and quickly.
- Always keep the records on mortality and its causes and the treatment given to birds. Dates of vaccination for each flock should be properly recorded.
- Avoid rats because rats are important carriers of poultry disease. Use suitable rat poisons/rat traps.
- Poultry medicines can be given in drinking water. When medication is to be given, remove the waterers in poultry sheds on the previous evening. Next morning give medicine in measured quantity of water, so that entire medicine will be quickly consumed and there will be no wastage of medicines.
- Mild infection of disease may not cause mortality but it will reduce growth. Keep sample record of body weight for growers, mortality rate and egg production. Study the possible causes, if weight is low or egg production is low and take steps to improve the management of the subsequent batches. A constant vigil and analysis of records/results is necessary to keep up the efficiency in farming.

Processing/Marketing

- The market should be nearer to the farm. Ensure the constant and steady demand for eggs is available.
- The market should be study for demand of particular egg weight. Provide one nest box for every 5 birds. Collect eggs from the shed 4 times a day. Store them in a cool dry place and market them quickly.
- Birds should not be kept on the farm beyond 18 months of age, as their egg production will go down considerably and their efficiency of feed conversion will reduce progressively as they grow older.

Pointers for Higher Egg Production

Quality Birds

Choose the breed and strain that will perform best and is known to have good livability under reasonable environmental conditions. Good chicks may cost more but they will perform better and pay more too.

Housing

There should be ample fresh air, free from drafts. Air must be circulating. High levels of non-desirable gases decrease growth rate and increase flock's susceptibility to respiratory disease. Ensure that the litter is dry. A well-managed litter helps the birds in putting on feathers and improve feed conversion ratio. It also reduces coccidiosis problem.

Crowding

Overcrowding increases the mortality, stress as well as production cost.

Feeding

Always ensure adequate fresh feed. Birds that are without feed for six hours will record a drop in production and a 12 hour starvation will result in moult of wing feathers. There should be adequate feeder space for the birds. Guard against feed wastage. Maintain records of daily feed consumption. It will enable to determine feed utilization and bird's performance.

Watering

Provide plentiful and clean disinfected water. Ensure that the waterers are so placed that they are easily accessible to birds.

Lighting

During grower stage, no need to give artificial light. During laying stage, the duration of light should be 16 hours per day, but not beyond 17 hours. No advantage is obtained by exceeding this limit. The amount of light given to the flock in one day should never be less than that given the day before. A decreasing day length can prematurely cause hens to go out to production.

Vaccination

Ensure that all birds are vaccinated for Marek's Disease and Ranikhet Disease. Birds not vaccinated are highly susceptible to these diseases. Please adapt vaccination schedule.

Debeaking

Follow correct debeaking programme. Poor debeaking can adversely affect egg production.

Culling

Uneconomic and unsuitable and birds should be timely culled.

Health

Watch for early signs of disease for its timely treatment. Some of the symptoms that indicate the onset of disease problems are:

- Drop in egg production
- Feed consumption
- Increased morbidity
- Mortality
- Inactivity and lack of vigor
- Droopy ruffled appearance
- Respiratory distress.
- Look for any sudden change in egg quality

Sanitation

Sanitary measures are the most importance in poultry operation. Keep roundworms, tapeworms and caecal worms under control. External parasites are a serious farm hazard, and can reduce production if unchecked. Deworming at regular intervals should be practiced.

Egg Quality

Respiratory and intestinal diseases should be under control for the maintenance of quality of egg shells. Indiscriminate use of sulpha drugs can affect the egg shell quality.

Records

A daily record of feed consumption, egg production, mortality, income and expenditure is essential to help improve farming efficiency and pinpoint troubles and their solutions.

Routine Checking

Critical items of management should be listed on a daily, weekly or seasonal check list. Every item must be checked. It helps to locate the cause of trouble when it occurs. Routine checks are: Cleaning and refilling of waterers and feeders: cleaning the house and spraying insecticide; stirring the litter; dusting; culling of birds; egg collection, etc.

Space Requirement Data

Age	*Floor space (sq.ft./ bird)*		*Feeding space (inches)*	*Watering space (inches)*	*Height of feeders & waterers*	*Litter depth (inches)*
0-8 weeks	0.5	0.25	2.0	0.6	1.5	3
9-16 weeks	1.0	0.55	2.5	0.8	2.5	4
17-76 weeks	2.0	0.80	3.0	1.0	5.0	6

Average Growth Rate and Feed Requirement for Egg Type Chickens:

Age in weeks	*Average weight of bird (gms.)*	*Cumulative feed in kgs. Per 1,000 birds*
4	275	650
8	590	1900
12	850	3400
16	1100	5000
20	1300	7000
24	1550	10000
30	1600	14500
40	1700	22000
60	1700	37000
80	1700	52000

Recommended rations (per quintal of feed) for various age groups of layers:

Composition	*Unit*	*Chick mash (0-8 weeks of age)*	*Grower mash (9-20 weeks of age)*	*Layer mash*	
				Phase I (21-42weeks)	*Phase II (43-72weeks)*
Yellow Maize	kg.	29.0	26.0	35.0	40.0
Rice Polish	kg.	33.7	43.8	32.1	31.1
Wheat Bran	kg.	-	2.0	-	-
Groundnut cake (expeller pressed)	kg.	22.0	13.0	17.0	12.5
Fish Meal	kg.	10.0	7.0	6.0	6.0
Lucerne Meal	kg.	3.0	3.0	3.0	3.0
DL-Methionine	gm.	4.0	-	-	15
Molasses	kg.	-	3.0	-	-
Mineral Mixture	kg.	2.0	2.0	3.0	3.0
Vitamin A+B2+D3 supplement	gm.	20	20	30	30
Vitamin B12 supplement	gm.	20	20	20	20
Vitamin K	mg.	100	100	100	100
Vitamin E	mg.	200	200	200	200
Potassium Iodide	mg.	20	20	20	20
Manganese Sulphate	m.	5	3	3	3
Zinc Carbonate	gm.	8	5	3	3
Shell Grit	kg.	-	-	3.8	4.3
Antibiotic feed Supplement	gm.	50	50	50	50
Zinc Bacitracin	gm	100	100	-	-
Coccidiostats	gm	50	32	-	-

Vaccination Schedule for Layers

Proper vaccination programme in poultry is necessary to prevent mortality and losses from many dreadful poultry diseases. Vaccination programs are available against the major poultry diseases *viz*. Ranikhet, Marek's disease and Fowl pox.

Precautions

Water soluble antibiotic/electrolyte can be given in the water 4 days prior to and 5 days after the vaccination to reduce stress.

Vaccination Calendar

The vaccination schedule is a general guide. Each farm and area will require some changes in the schedule. Following table can be used as a general guideline.

Name of Vaccine	*Route*	*Age of birds*
La Sota or F vaccine Ranikhet	Intranasal drop	3 to 7 days
Marek's vaccine (in Hatchery)	Intramuscular	1 day
Infectious Bronchitis (1st dose)	Eye drops	2 - 3 weeks
La Sota Ranikhet	Drinking water	5 - 6 weeks
Fowl Pox (1st dose)	Wing Web	7 - 8 weeks
R2B Ranikhet	Sub cut or Intramuscular	9 - 10 weeks
Infectious Bronchitis	Eye drop or drinking water	16 weeks
Fowl Pox (2nd dose)	Skin Scarification	18 weeks
La Sota (if necessary) Ranikhet	Drinking Water	20 weeks
La Sota (if necessary) Ranikhet	Drinking Water	40 weeks
IBD :		
Mildly invasive vaccine	Drinking Water	0 - 3 day
Intermediately invasive vaccine	Drinking Water	15th day
Intermediately invasive vaccine	Drinking Water	28-30th day

It is necessary to keep proper records on date of vaccination and on vaccines used including type, brand, serial number, date of purchase and date of use of vaccine.

Guidelines for Integrated Biosecurity in Poultry Production

A set of recommended biosecurity practices to be adopted by the poultry farmers for minimizing the disease occurrence is given here under in brief.

1. Locational Biosecurity: Farm should be located

- ☆ Elevated and well ventilated site
- ☆ Away from any existing farms
- ☆ Away from water ways/water pools/lakes/tanks
- ☆ Away from any nearby village poultry
- ☆ Broiler and layer units should not be established in close vicinity

- ☆ Farms having more than 50000 (Layers) should have preferably separate facilities for brooding/growing
- ☆ The new poultry farms may be one kilometer away from the existing farms or complexes.

2. Structural Biosecurity

- ☆ Construct separate sheds for brooding/growing/laying operations with East-West orientation.
- ☆ A minimum distance of 150 ft. between brooding/growing sector and layer sector should be maintained. The distance between the sheds within the sector should be at least 50 ft.
- ☆ In case of farms where in brooding/growing operations are carried out along with layer operations 1:3 system of rearing may be adopted, while in case of units where brooding/growing operations are carried out at separate places, 1:1:4 or 1:1:5 system of rearing may be adopted.
- ☆ Multi-storied poultry sheds are not desirable.
- ☆ Individual farms should be provided fencing with wheel dip at main gate. Provide foot dips at every doorstep.
- ☆ The maximum width of the sheds in case of deep litter system should not exceed 30 feet and the shed should be 2 feet above ground level with pucca floor.
- ☆ A minimum overhang of 3 feet must be provided.
- ☆ The maximum width of the sheds should be 33.5 feet in case of layer houses under cage system.
- ☆ In case of cage system rows as well as tiers should not be more than three.
- ☆ The height of the plat form from the ground should not be less than 6 feet in case of cage system.
- ☆ For ideal farming 3 birds per cage with adequate water and feeding facilities should be ensured
- ☆ Provide closed disposal pit or incinerator at least 500 feet away from the active operational area.
- ☆ A store house for proper storage of litter material should be provided to avoid contamination.
- ☆ Provide proper area for used litter disposal away from the active operational area.
- ☆ Feed store/mill should be 150 feet away from the sheds and preferably near the gate.
- ☆ Office and egg store should be away from active operational area and preferably at the main gate.
- ☆ All the sheds and other structures should have rat proof arrangements.

3. Operational Biosecurity

- ✰ Procure the day old chicks, which are free from diseases from reputed hatcheries
- ✰ It is advisable to have cage system of rearing in place of deep litter system of rearing.
- ✰ As far as possible automated equipment should be considered to minimize the manual handling of feeds and water.
- ✰ Testing feed ingredients/feeds must be arranged to ensure that they are free from intection.

4. Microbial Agents or Toxins at Periodic Intervals

- ✰ Storage facilities for feed ingredients/feeds must be managed in a hygienic manner.
- ✰ Ensure the feed manufacturing area free from dust and should be equipped with appropriate screens to protect from fly problem.
- ✰ It is advisable to feed the birds with pellets for improved biosecurity.
- ✰ Sheds having infected flocks should be served with feed at the end of a delivery day.
- ✰ Always ensure the supply of clean and potable water. If necessary use appropriate sanitizers.
- ✰ Periodic inspection of wells, piping and tanks to ensure that water supplied is clean.
- ✰ An area specific vaccination schedule as recommended by hatchery doctor must be practiced with utmost care.
- ✰ Rodent control programme, where ever necessary, must be adopted by employing mechanical (traps) or chemical techniques along with strict sanitation measures.
- ✰ After selling of each crop from the sheds, thorough cleaning of sheds by removing all fixtures, equipment, litter dust, debris followed by brooming and burning. The rat holder cracks, worn out area should be packed with cement.
- ✰ Cleaning of the vegetation thoroughly six feet around the sheds and spraying of bleaching powder (1 parts) with lime (3 parts) around the sheds a minimum of 3 feet.
- ✰ Avoid use of litter as manure around the farms.
- ✰ Well cleaning of sheds and equipment with water and appropriate detergent.
- ✰ A thorough disinfection of sheds, equipments as well as farm surroundings by formalin spray at recommended concentration.
- ✰ Foot baths should be always filled with disinfectant.

- ☆ Vehicles visiting the farms should be thoroughly disinfected by appropriate disinfectant spray.
- ☆ Personnel working in laying sectors should not be allowed into brooding/ growing sector or feed manufacturing facilities. All visitors must be ensured to walk through foot baths.
- ☆ Disposal of dead birds in hygienic manner either by using incinerator or by pit method is very essential.

Financial Assistance Available from Banks/NABARD

NABARD is an apex institution for all matters relating to policy, planning and operations in the field of agricultural credit. It serves as an apex refinancing agency for the institutions providing investment and production credit. Loan from banks with refinance facility from NABARD is available for starting poultry farming. For obtaining bank loan the farmers should apply to the nearest branch of a Commercial or Cooperative or Regional Rural Banks in their area in the prescribed application forms which is available in the branches of financing banks. The technical officers attached to or the manager of the bank can help/give guidance to the farmers in preparing the project report to obtain bank loan. Banks provide financial assistance for the following purposes:

- ☆ For construction of brooder/grower and layer sheds, feed store, quarters etc.
- ☆ For purchase of poultry equipment such as feeders, waterers, brooders etc.
- ☆ For creating infrastructure items for supply of electricity, feed, water etc.
- ☆ For purchase of day old chicks or ready to lay pullets.
- ☆ For meeting working capital requirement in respect of feed, medicines and veterinary aid etc. for the first 5 to 6 months (i.e. till the stage of income generation).

The Cost of land is not considered for loan. However, if land is purchased for establishing a poultry farm, land cost can be treated as party's margin upto a maximum of 10% of total cost of project.

Transforming Rural Areas through Veterinary Science *Pages* **117-128**
Editor: Dipanjali Konwar, Shilpa Sood & Shahid Ahamad
Published by: **ASTRAL INTERNATIONAL PVT. LTD., NEW DELHI**

8 Employment Generation Through Poultry Entrepreneurship

Dr. Amandeep Singh & Dr. Pranav Kumar

Introduction

Over the last two decades South Asian economies have been growing at an average rate of over 6 percent per year, with gains in real per capita income ranging from 2.5 to 5 percent per annum. While structural transformations have led to the industry and service sectors now contributing the most to gross domestic production, agriculture remains a critical component, accounting for about 20 percent of the GDP. The largest majority of poor households continue to depend on agriculture for their livelihoods, directly or indirectly and investments in agriculture are recognized as an effective strategy for poverty reduction. The capacity of agriculture especially animal husbandry to contribute to poverty reduction and nutritional security does not only depend on the overall rate of growth, but also on the ability of poor households to participate in that growth, *i.e.* on the quality or inclusiveness of the growth process. In India, it is estimated that over 50 percent of landless and marginal farmers depend on poultry and small ruminant rearing and with the increasing demand for meat and eggs; the poultry sector provides direct employment to over two million people.

Poultry entrepreneur is a person who undertakes poultry based activities such as poultry rearing, production of poultry/ poultry products, processing and other inputs of poultry business. He finds ways and means to create and develop a profitable poultry business. Poultry entrepreneurs see their farming as a business and as a means of earning profits. So they are willing to take calculated risks to make profits and to grow their businesses. They are also motivated to improve poultry production through mechanization and application of technologies in the field of poultry and allied enterprises.

Qualities and Skills Required by Average Farmer to Become Poultry Entrepreneur

Technical Skills Required by a Poultry Entrepreneur

Technical competencies are needed particularly in these areas

1. Managing inputs
2. Managing production
3. Managing marketing
4. Financial Management
5. Labor Management

1. Managing Inputs

The entrepreneur is good at identifying, sourcing and acquiring inputs for the farm. For effective management of inputs, the farmers should know the requirement of inputs for the farm, where to get them and how to use them. The entrepreneur should look for good quality input at low prices.

2. Managing Production

The entrepreneurial farmer knows the most profitable and sustainable way to produce. Every good farmer will have all the production skills needed to produce a good crop *viz.* ploughing, planting, pest control, weed control, harvesting. Similarly for poultry farming: rearing, feeding, watering, disease control, correct record keeping for all production activities is mandatory. The entrepreneurial farmer is aware of time – doing things now rather than later. The entrepreneurial farmer is also ready to experiment with alternative production systems. Managing production involves poultry production skills as well as ability to make most of the modern technologies which can help poultry farmers to improve their production processes.

Managing Marketing

In order to make profits, produce has to be marketed and sold. Poultry-entrepreneurs know where the most profitable market is for each product. They are good at negotiating contracts. Keep records of transactions. They look for more profitable markets. Adapt quickly to market changes and market opportunities Large scale poultry businesses require marketing management skills, market and customer orientation, identifying market opportunities, sales management, customer management; assessing customer needs through dialogue and feedback.

Financial Management

This involves accountancy and financial skills. It is important for the assessment of profits and losses.

Labor Management

This is important for production management, as well as for risk management. Hiring the wrong laborer can quickly change profits into losses This involves determination of job requirements of different types of work, determine cost of labor, recruitment, selection, orientation and training, working with employees, motivating employees and evaluating employees.

Avenues of Poultry Entrepreneurship

Poultry Farms

The poultry farmers can start their own poultry farms with their vast technical knowledge; they can infuse scientific management techniques in their own farms. In the WTO (World Trade Organization) era, GMP (Good Manufacturing Practices) and SPS (Sanitary and Phytosanitary) measures are of great importance for export of poultry commodities, as the emphasis in international trade is on quality and food safety. Further, the veterinarians can extend need based knowledge to the interested poultry farmers for poultry farming.

Feed Manufacturing

The interested persons can start their own feed mill units for various poultry species. Commercial feed availability for various unconventional poultry species such as Quail, Emu, Ostrich, etc. are far less than the demand. Manufacturing feed for these species is a niche business as their energy requirement is different from the existing commercially available broiler or layer feed.

Poultry Feed Supplements

The main constraint which hampers the growth of poultry production is the inadequacy of nutritious and balanced feed. To overcome such deficiency in the feed sector, feed supplements like mineral mixtures, vitamin supplements, feed additives, growth promoters, etc. can be effectively used. The enterprises related to manufacturing of such supplements are very inviting and profitable and the poultry entrepreneurs can increase the scale of their income.

Farm Equipment Manufacturer/Dealer

Numbers of farm equipment are needed for poultry farms. Poultry farmers need debeaker, vaccinator, automatic feeder, waterer, egg candler, weighing scale, etc. Demand for farm equipment increases with the wide adoption of intensive poultry and poultry farming system. The poultry entrepreneurs can either start their own business or they can act as dealer for these equipment.

Hatchery

Though starting a hatchery requires higher investment, it offers good return.

Value Addition of Poultry Meat

Value addition to the poultry products such as egg and meat has huge profit potential. Value of the products get increased many folds during processing, and thereby provide excellent returns. Interested entrepreneurs can start their own outlets and food corners where they can sale value added chicken meat products like sandwiches, patties, popcorns, soups, burgers, etc. Marketing of such value added products could be done in their own brand name and they can start chain of hotels later.

Dealer/Manufacturer of Equipment Required for Value Addition of Poultry Meat

The various equipment required for the value addition of poultry meat are meat mincer, bowl chopper, ovens, texture analyzer for quality check, etc. The persons interested in poultry entrepreneurship can either start their own manufacturing units for production of such equipment or can become dealers for different enterprises dealing with such equipment.

Farm Consultant

Poultry farm consultant is a lucrative avenue. Veterinarians or experienced poultry entrepreneurs with skill and knowledge can earn well in specialized poultry farms, hatchery units, poultry breeding farms, processing units, and can act as feed and poultry healthcare experts. After some years of experience in managing the farms, they can start their own farms independently or with partnerships.

Contract Farming

Contract farming is emerging system where the poultry farmers are given all the inputs such as chicks; feed, medicines, technical inputs. Farmers have to rear the chicks and the integrator will take care of the marketing activities. Veterinarians can join together and venture into contract farming. Being technical savvy would help them in getting loans, maintaining farm business and marketing the products.

Agents for By Products Utilization

The poultry feed manufacturers and pharmaceuticals require several ingredients such as bone meal, fish meal, blood meal which they are getting from the agents at contract basis. Here, veterinarians can make interventions. They can make a tie-up and could meet the requirements of feed manufacturers at a reasonable price and also can earn money.

Veterinary Pharmaceutical Industry

It is also a lucrative opportunity but needs huge investment. After working some years in the pharmaceutical industry and learning experience, veterinarians can initially start a small one with fewer drugs which can be expanded later to the needs of local farmers. From thereon, they can grow slowly.

Private Service Provider

Development of poultry farming can open up avenues for mobile poultry breeding and extension services. Poultry breeding (AI), vaccinations, health care, detection of health problems, providing first aid and management of poultry are the services required by farmers at their doorstep. Veterinarians, experienced poultry entrepreneurs as well para-veterinary staff/poultry health workers have huge self-employment opportunities to provide these services.

Commercial Broiler Farming or Poultry Enterprise

Broilers are those birds which are reared for meat purposes, therefore due to their short generation interval; they are suitable for commercial poultry production or for establishing poultry enterprise. Broiler farming has several advantages: firstly the initial investment is low, and there is a faster return from the investment. Layers start laying at the age of 6-21 weeks. Broilers start paying within 4 to 5 weeks. Since broilers have high feed conversion efficiency, only a minimum amount of feed is required for unit body weight gain in comparison to other livestock. The demand of poultry meat is always increasing and is even **than** the demand for mutton/ chevon. A large section of people are engaged in producing essential inputs required for poultry farming such as high yielding breeding stock, specialized equipment for hatchery and farm automation, poultry feed etc. The total cost of production constitutes good quality Day old chicks (DOC's) and feed; hence, availability of these two is a very important factor. To develop poultry sector in a competitive way creation of basic facilities and infrastructure relating to hatching and feed mixing centers are essential. Strict sanitary precautions, intelligent use of antibiotics and vaccines are necessary for satisfactory disease control.

Benefits of Rearing Broilers for Rural People

1. The broilers grow to 1.5kg of weight in just 28 days with proper managemental conditions, so the profit can be obtained in a month's time.
2. The deep litter so formed by them consists of 3% nitrogen, 2% potassium and 2% phosphorous which serves as an excellent fertilizer for crops.
3. The year round employment can be generated by the unemployed villagers by adopting broiler farming.
4. Along with income, broiler farming serves as boost to nutritional security.
5. With a slight knowledge, even children of the family and women can uptake the work of rearing broilers.
6. Social and economic empowerment can be brought about by the clubbing the agriculture farming with broiler farming.

Financing the Poultry Enterprise

Poultry rearing provides triple benefits of income, employment and nutritional security to the society and is important source of subsidiary income to small/ marginal farmers and agricultural laborers. Finance is a prerequisite and of paramount importance for setting up of a poultry enterprise whether poultry farm, breeder farm, feed mill, equipment manufacturing unit, processing plant. Decisions about credit are often most important judgments that people in the poultry industry must make. These decisions often determine whether individuals operating in input, production, processing, and services based poultry enterprise would succeed in making profit.

Importance of Credit in Poultry Entrepreneurship

Credit helps to overcome shortage of equity capital in poultry enterprise. Restricted credit, changing interest rates, lack of credit information are most common problems faced by a poultry entrepreneur.

Credit serves many purpose of an entrepreneur such as

1. Start up and increase production
2. Improvement in quality of what is being produced
3. Revise operations to make them more profitable

The money borrowed must generate enough additional income to pay for the cost of the borrowed money (interest) and to ensure that principle is repaid according to specified terms of the loan. Credit is normally needed in three broad expenses in an enterprise: Fixed expense, operating expenses and start-up expenses.

Fixed expenses are items which can be used over and over for a long period of time incurring the same price (expense) each year. Examples are land, buildings, equipment, tools and machinery.

Operating expenses are needed to run an enterprise production entrepreneur would need money to buy feed, manpower expenses to run his poultry enterprise. In poultry sales enterprise operating expenses would need communication, transportation, fuel, advertising expenses.

Start-up expenses are before the business begins operation. It may include cost of construction of farm housing, fees to architects and construction work.

Type of Credit Requirement in Poultry Enterprise

The financial credit needs of poultry farmers according to length of the loan period can be classified into three parts:

1. Short Term Credit: Short term credit is required for a period of six to 12 months. This type of credit is needed for maintenance of expenses as well as to purchase items like feed, feed additives, and medicines for poultry. Short term credit is important for survival of poultry enterprise as it finances everyday operations of the firm which generate the cash flow in the business. Such type of credit is taken from money lenders, relatives, friends and the co-operative societies. To maintain good flow of credit these loans should be repaid upon receipt of money at harvest or auction time.

2. Medium Term Credit: These loans are needed from 1 to 10 years. These types of loans are needed by poultry farmers to repair and construction of housing systems, fencing, sophistication in poultry enterprise, purchase of poultry equipment such as waterers, feeders, automatic vaccinators, debeakers, lightning systems, brooders. Such type of credit is taken from money lenders and the commercial banks or lender may require collateral when considering a loan application.

3. Long term Credit: Loans that extend over 10 years are long term credit. Long term credit is especially important when starting a poultry enterprise. The entrepreneur has to determine how much land and what type of building are suitable to the scale of operations. In fact start up of poultry venture depends on whether a lender is willing to extend this credit. Loan repayment of long term credit depends on funds left over after deductions of all exenses for the year. Net income are examples of sources of repayment for long term loans.

Sources of Farm Credit

The different sources for poultry start-ups can be obtained from formal and informal sources.

a. Formal sources include Credit co-operatives, commercial banks, government, Regional Rural Banks.

b. Informal sources include money lender, friends and relatives, traders and landlords.

Government Sponsored Subsidy Schemes for Poultry Rearing

1. Under NABARD;

a. Centrally sponsored scheme for establishing "poultry estates" and mother units for rural poultry.

b. Scheme for development/ strengthening of agriculture marketing infrastructure, grading and standardization.

2. Under Department of Animal Husbandry & Dairying

a. Assistance to State Poultry or Duck farms

b. National Project for improvement of Poultry and Small Animals

c. Assistance to Dairy Cooperatives/Poultry Venture Capital Fund Schemes

d. Central Poultry Development Organization

3. Poultry Development Scheme; (by Centralized Banks of India)

Bank Support Schemes for Poultry Entrepreneurship in India

Two major schemes for poultry entrepreneurship in India are:

a. Poultry Venture Capital Fund Scheme

b. Poultry Development Scheme

Poultry Venture Capital Fund Scheme (PVCFS)

This scheme is implemented by NABARD through various commercial banks, co-operative banks, regional rural banks and other agencies. All individual entrepreneurs, farmers, Non Govt. Organizations, Companies, groups of organized and unorganized sector are eligible for this scheme. The objectives are to establish the poultry breeding farms with low input technology birds and also for creating the necessary infrastructure facilities such as feed godown, feed mixing unit, egg grading, packing and storage for export, retail poultry dressing units.

Features of the Scheme

This scheme provides financial assistance to open breeding units for low input technology birds and turkey, ducks and other poultry species. Assistance up to Rs. 30 lakh is available. Similarly poultry feed unit, feed godown or analytical lab can also be established for which assistance of Rs. 16 Lakh is available. Similarly retail poultry dressing units, egg grading, packing and storage for export purpose, transport vehicle and cold room egg/broiler carts, central grower units can be established for which financial assistance is available.

PoultryBased Entrepreneurships can be Covered Under Following Activities

Component	*Unit cost in Rupees*
Hybrid Broiler (chicken) Units – upto 5000 birds. Can be weekly, fortnightly, monthly, all in all-out batches. Bird strength at any point of time should not exceed 5000 birds	Rs. 2.24 lakh for a batch of 1000 broilers- Varies with unit size
Transport Vehicles – open cage	Rs. 8.00 lakh
Retail outlets –Dressing unit	Rs. 6.00 lakh
Retail outlets –marketing units	Rs. 6.00 lakh
Mobile marketing units	Rs. 8.00 lakh
Egg / Broiler Carts	Rs. 10,000/-
Breeding Farms for Low Input Technology Birds like turkey, ducks, Japanese quails, emu etc.	Rs. 30.00lakh
Central Grower Units (CGU) – upto 16000 layer chicks per batch.	Rs. 40 .00 lakh for a unit of 16000 layer chicks per batch (three batches a year) – varies with size.
Rearing other species of Poultry (Other than commercial layer and broiler chicken)	Rs. 10.00 lakh- Varies with the species and unit size

Eligibility

1. Farmers, individual entrepreneurs, NGOs, companies, cooperatives, groups of unorganized and organized sector which include Self Help Groups (SHGs), Joint Liability Groups (JLGs).
2. An individual will be eligible to avail assistance for all the components under the scheme but only once for each component.
3. When more than one member of a family is assisted under the scheme, the units set up by each member should be with separate infrastructure at different locations with distinct identity. The distance between the boundaries of two adjacent farms should be at least 500m.
4. Biosecurity norms should be kept in view while locating the units.

Funding Pattern

- ✰ Entrepreneur contribution (margin money) - For loans upto Rs one lac, banks may not insist on margin as per RBI guidelines. For loans above Rs 1.00 lac : 10% (minimum)

- ☆ Back ended capital subsidy –25% for general and 33% for SC/ST.
- ☆ Effective Bank Loan (excluding eligible subsidy as above) – Balance portion, Minimum 40% of the outlay.

Repayment

- ☆ Repayment Period will depend on the nature of activity and cash flow and will vary between 5- 9 years. Grace period from 6 months to 1 year.

How to Apply

Approach the nearest Veterinary Assistant Surgeon, Block Veterinary Officer or the Chief Animal Husbandry Officer of the concerned District along with:

- ☆ Affidavit of being unemployed and not a defaulter of any bank or financial institutions
- ☆ Photocopy of Ration card/State Subject
- ☆ Land papers for mortgage if loan amount exceeds Rs.1.00 lac.
- ☆ Photocopy of category certificate if any
- ☆ Three passport size photographs
- ☆ Copy of driving license if the unit is Transport vehicle

Poultry Development Scheme (PDS)

By centralized banks of India

Objective

The main objective of financing poultry is to increase egg/meat production by meeting financial requirement of the proponents who are willing to undertake poultry as a subsidiary or main occupation.

Purpose

1. Financing can be considered for the following types of poultry schemes.
2. Establishment of small poultry (layer or broiler) units of 200 to 500 birds as subsidiary occupation by the farmers and agricultural labourers. Individual registered partnership firms limited companies and registered co-operative societies having necessary trained and technical personnel and management experts for running following commercial poultry units.
3. Establishment/expansion of layer farm
4. Establishment/expansion of broiler farm
5. Establishment /expansion of hatchery farm
6. Establishment / expansion of production –cum-processing units

The Following Items are Eligible for Finance Under Different Poultry Schemes

a. Construction of brooder/grower houses, feed godowns, acquisition of electricity and water supply, purchase of cages, purchase of feeders, waterers, feed/egg, trolleys, vaccination equipment.

b. Poultry co-operative may require finance for purchase of feed mixing plant, feed ingredients and for stocking of feeds for their members.

c. Integrated layer units will also require finance for construction of broiler houses, purchase of machinery/equipment for dressing of bird, refrigerated storage facilities for dressed birds and refrigerated van for their transport.

d. Hatchery units will require finance for egg rooms fumigation room, egg cooling room, room for egg incubators, room for chick sexing as well as vaccination and packing room.

e. Larger poultry units may also require finance for purchase of air conditioners, stand-by generator.

Eligibility

Individual farmers/agricultural laborers who are experienced/trained in poultry management are taking up poultry farming as a subsidiary occupation. Individual registered partnership firms, limited companies are eligible for bank credit for large poultry units. These units should have trained/ technically qualified personnel for running the unit.

Technical Feasibility

The following aspects should be taken into account while assessing the technical feasibility for a poultry project

a. Sustainability of climate

b. Availability of day old chicks, feed

c. Requirement of housing and equipments

d. Availability of electric power

e. Veterinary care

f. Marketing arrangements

g. Experience of the proponent/availability of the trained/technically qualified personnel for running the unit.

Financial Viability

The assessment of financial viability of poultry units should include reasonableness of cost of various items of the scheme. Cost benefits analysis of the scheme should be worked out over the scheme period to find out net income generation **vis-à-vis** servicing of the debt apart from the entrepreneur getting a fair amount of return on the investment. Subsidies available to small/marginal farmers, agricultural labourers, scheduled casts and scheduled tribes under various programmes should be taken into account while studying the financial viability of the scheme.

Quantum of Finance

The amount of finance will depend upon the type and size of the poultry unit and the fixed costs and the working capital requirement during the gestation period. Working capital for the first 5 to 6 months in case of layer farms, 1 to 1.5 months in case of broiler farms and normally 7 to 8 months for hatcheries should be capitalized and included in the project cost.

Margin

- ✰ For marginal/small farmers, agricultural laborers and scheduled castes/scheduled tribes and other weaker sections, subsidy available from various sources to be treated as margin.
- ✰ For others, 15 to 25% depending upon the financial capability of the proponent and size of the project.

Type of Facility

Term loan

Security

Demand Promissory Note (L-434), Composite Agreement for Hypothecation (CHA-1/CHA-2), Borrower's loan application should clearly state the purpose for which the advance is sought and being an integral part of the documents, a copy of such application must be attached to the Agreement for Hypothecation. L-515 declaration as to relationship with Director/Officials, L-516 or Annex the clauses on non-diversion of funds and securitization enclosed to Br. Cir.No.97/186 dated 08.03.2004 with CH I/CHA-II/CHA-IV Equitable or legal mortgage or deed of declaration of land/superstructure, as appropriate where the limit exceeds Rs.50000/- (legal mortgage of land is to be taken in form CHA-4), Letter of Guarantee from a guarantor wherever considered necessary in the limit above Rs.50000/- (CHA-3).

Insurance

Comprehensive insurance of birds covering diseases to be obtained for poultry development under all government sponsored schemes, small and medium poultry farms having bird strength upto 10,000. In respect of commercial farms and hatchery units having fully automated management system or environmentally controlled management, obtention of comprehensive insurance of birds covering diseases be waived, irrespective of its size. Comprehensive insurance of poultry birds covering diseases may not be insisted upon in respect of large poultry farms and hatchery farms with strength of birds above ten thousand, obtention of such insurance be left to the discretion of the borrowers. Obtention of regular fire and strikes, riots, civil commotion (SRCC) comprehensive insurance policy for poultry structure, hatchery building, other civil work, machinery, equipment, feed mill, stock of feeds, medicines, vehicles. financed under poultry development schemes.

Disbursement

The execution of the scheme should be planned in a phased manner. Disbursement should be in accordance with the progress made in execution of different items of the scheme. At every stage of disbursement, the progress of the work should be verified by conducting post-disbursement inspections. As far as possible the loan amount should be disbursed directly to the concerned contractor/dealer/supplier/agency against proper bills/receipt and statement of completion from the borrower.

Repayment

- **Layer Farms:** Monthly installments after a gestation period of 5-6 months after purchase of day old chicks.
- **Broiler Farms:** Monthly or quarterly depending upon the size of the unit and income generation pattern after a gestation period of 3 months after purchase of day old chicks.
- **Hatchery Units:** Monthly installments to start 7 to 8 months after the first purchase of parent stock as day old chicks.

Conclusion

Poultry industry has been a dynamic industry in terms of both growth and policies. The growth is ever increasing and the policies related to poultry farming have also seen a surge during past few decades. This sector shows a potential opportunity for the unemployed youth of the country to start a business and earn their livelihood. One can start the enterprise by taking credit from the government at subsidized interest rates. Many villagers from past many years are rearing backyard poultry primarily for entertainment and secondarily for livelihood generation. There is a strong need for capacity building of such villagers and transforming them into successful poultry entrepreneurs by giving them proper training and guidance. Poultry entrepreneurship will not only help to improve the economy of the rural areas but also provide nutritional security to the deprived masses.

Transforming Rural Areas through Veterinary Science Pages 129-144
Editor: Dipanjali Konwar, Shilpa Sood & Shahid Ahamad
Published by: ASTRAL INTERNATIONAL PVT. LTD., NEW DELHI

9 Transformation of Rural Livelihood through Recent Advances and Approaches in Aquaculture

Dr. Prem Kumar, Dr. Amit Mandal & Dr. Shiv Kumar Sharma

Introduction

Aquaculture, an important component of agriculture and farming systems is contributing to the alleviation of food insecurity, malnutrition, and poverty by providing high-quality protein-rich food of high value. It is helping in generating employment and income to the needy farmers by the use of baron and saline lands for fish and shrimp culture. Aquaculture in India has received its due attention in recent years after proving its worth in generating foreign income, nutritional security, reducing inequality and employment generation, both in the sector itself as well as in support services. Knowing the importance, Prime Minister has given the vision of Neel Kranti Mission-2016 (NKM 16) which will have a multi-dimensional approach to all activities concerned with the development of the fisheries sector. The government of India has kept the target of 15 million metric tonnes (MMT) of fish production by the year 2020.

All over the world, more than 30 million fishers and fish farmers and their families gain their livelihoods from fisheries. Globally, fish provide about 16 percent of the animal protein consumed by humans and are a valuable source of minerals and essential fatty acids. Global fish production has grown steadily in the last five decades with food fish supply increasing at an average annual rate of 3.2 percent, outpacing world population growth at 1.6 percent. According to the State of World Fisheries and Aquaculture (SOFIA) 2018, total world fisheries and aquaculture production have reached to 170.9 million metric ton (mt) collectively including 90.0 mt from capture fisheries and 80.0 mt from aquaculture during 2016. Although wild fishery resources are contributing more in production if they are overexploited, production declines and may even collapse. What made possible the continuing rise in overall fish production is the rapid growth of aquaculture. Aquaculture farmed food fish production included 54.1 mt of finfish (USD 138.5 billion), 17.1 mt of molluscs (USD 29.2 billion), 7.9 mt of crustaceans (USD 57.1 billion) and 0.94 tonnes of other aquatic animals (USD 6.8 billion) which includes edible jellyfish, sea urchins, turtles, frogs, and sea cucumbers. Finfish farming still dominates inland aquaculture, accounting 92.5 % (47.5 mt) of total production, besides strong growth production of other species groups, particularly crustaceans including shrimps, crayfish and crabs in inland aquaculture in Asia. Total fish production of India during 2016-17 was projected 11.41 million metric tonnes (MMT) which included 3.64 MMT from capture fishery and 7.77 MMT from aquaculture (http://dahd.nic.in/reports/annual-report-2017-18). Aquaculture contributed 68.1% of the total fish production of the country in which three Indian major carps species hold a lion's share. Composite fish farming of Indian major carps in combination with exotic carps is the main reason behind higher contribution and it is most popular among small and medium fish farmers who usually adopt extensive or semi-intensive low-cost production technology appropriate to their resource base. Increase in inland aquaculture production can be accomplished either by increasing the area devoted to aquaculture or by intensifying production in existing aquaculture areas to harness the full production potential and enhance productivity substantially. It will ensure doubling the income of the fishers and fish farmers with the inclusive participation of the socio-economically weaker sections and ensure sustainability with environment and biosecurity (DADF, 2016).

Aquaculture becomes an attractive and important component of rural livelihoods due to increasing population pressures, environmental degradation or loss of access, limit catches from wild fisheries (IIRR *et al.*, 2001).

Prospects for an Increased Contribution by Aquaculture

Due to increased awareness, market price and different Government schemes related to Aquaculture, the numbers of fish culture ponds have been increasing rapidly in recent past and fish farming is becoming popular among the farmers. However, till now fish farming is practiced at the level of extensive and semi-intensive while aquaculture has huge potential for expansion and intensification. The average productivity from ponds on the national level is around 2,500 kg/ha/year, though in Bihar and UP it is anywhere between 1,500 and 2,500 kg/ha/year, while some other states like Andhra Pradesh and Haryana it is more than 5,000 kg/ha/year (jpn-virtualvarsity.org). Thus, there is potential for an increase in production to 5000 kg/ha/year and has huge potential for both vertical and horizontal expansion in the coming years.

The foremost reasons for low productivity are poor knowledge of advance technologies of fish farming so non-adoption of recent technology at the village level, lack of understanding about the dynamics of pond production, poor or lack of technical knowledge especially in rural areas and insufficient resources. With this background, the current chapter aimed at providing knowledge of recent scientific technologies for adoption in fish farming systems.

Intensification in Aquaculture

The current trend of increased production can be maintained, either through intensification or expansion of areas under aquaculture production. Generic technologies for intensification of existing production systems are in place, and it is mainly socio-economic and institutional issues that will be the most important constraints for a greater contribution by aquaculture to rural development. The expansion of land-based culture systems in inland areas has the greatest potential because aquaculture can be integrated with agriculture on current agricultural land in smallholder and commercial farms (Edwards, 1999). The considerable potential lies in the integration of aquaculture and irrigation systems (Fernando and Halwart, 2000; Moehl *et al.*, 2001) and aquaculture can make also use of land that is unsuitable for agriculture, such as swamps or saline marsh areas in the form of shrimp farming.

In addition, there's a large diversity of midland and coastal aquatic resources as well as rivers, floodplains, lakes, reservoirs, rice fields, estuaries, lagoons, coral reefs, mangroves, and mudflats that give opportunity for the integration of well-controlled, sustainable aquaculture, enhancement or other form of aquatic animal management, into rural development (IIRR, 2001). Increasing yields through intensified production require increased use of feeds and/or fertilizers, which may be derived from on- or off-farm sources, or a combination of the two. As mentioned previously, many of the technical aspects of aquaculture are relatively well developed, however, there is a knowledge gap between what is known globally and what is available to farmers. Weak rural extension systems and a lack of local examples of intensified aquaculture limit farmers' ability and willingness to risk intensification (Halwart et al., 2003).

Genetic and Reproduction Technologies

In recent decades there has been a revolution in the application of genomics and gene-related biotechnology in agriculture and aquaculture (Foresti, 2000, Hew and Fletcher, 2001, Melamed *et al.*, 2002). Biotechnological advancement in genetics helps to extend production and cut back prices particularly through the manipulation of the genes and chromosomes of cultivated species. Equally, biotechnology is also applied to wild fisheries resources to improve their management, for example, DNA is being used to differentiate populations and to manage captive breeding programs for stock enhancement/replenishment.

Improved Jayanti Rohu is the first genetically improved fish variety in India. Jayanti Rohu has higher growth percentage (17%) over traditional rohu. The inbreeding factor also less in Jayanti as compare to conventional rohu. In order to capitalize on the effort made for the development of Jayanti Rohu, its dissemination to farmers must be effective. Another fish is Amur Carp, Superior common carp breed released by KVAFSU, Bidar. Amur carp is having a fast growth rate and late maturity in comparison to common carp, a victim of inbreeding. Farmers will get the maximum benefit offered by the improved seed, but this will require adequate quality training, education, and technical support.

Transgenic Fishes

Organisms into which heterologous DNA (transgene) has been artificially introduced and integrated into their genomes are called transgenic. Transgenic technology has been developed in a number of fishes for achieving genetic change for fast growth, disease resistance, resistant to freezing temperature and tolerance to low-level oxygen in the water. Transgenic fish with remarkable growth rates have been obtained by micro-infecting into freshly fertilized eggs a fish- growth hormone gene, linked to a suitable fish promoter. In order to grow fishes that are longer and heavier, one method in use is to dip the fish in a solution, containing the desired growth hormone. However, there are some problems with this technique. Firstly, it may be difficult to determine if the fish is getting the right amount of growth hormone. Therefore, the current research focus is to develop new strains or transgenic fish which naturally produce just the right amount of growth hormone to speed their growth. The two main techniques which researchers use to transfer genetic materials in fish as microinjection explained above; and electroporation that involves transferring the genetic material or DNA into fish embryos through the use of an electric current. Research is being pursued to produce transgenic fish carrying genes that encode antimicrobial peptides such as lysozyme. This is one approach to obtain disease resistance in fish. Other approaches to enhance disease resistance in fish including using antisense and ribozyme technologies against viral RNA.

Mono-Sex Culture

Mono-sex culture is the culture of fish belonging to single-sex either males or females depending upon the sex which have better food conversion ratio and growth rate. Sex of fish is genetically determined by the sex chromosomes (X, Y, Z, or W). The M gene responsible for male sex is present on any of the three X, Y and W. Some species have ZZ female and ZW male. Platy fish has 3 sex chromosomes – X, Y and W which make different combinations like XX, WX, and WY.

Treatment with sex hormones is the easiest way when male sex hormone methyl testosterone is administered through feeding in early developmental stages of female fish. The genotype female (XX) then transferred to phenotype male (XX). When this phenotypic male is crossed with a normal female, 100% female progeny occurs. The gonads of fish (teleost) are undifferentiated at early stages of maturity so sex hormones may be used to produce male or female gonads by that process.

Considering the suspected harmful effect of sex hormones on human, the hormone-treated sex-reversed male may not be used for human consumption but the next generation, normal female offspring is completely suitable for human consumption. The production of all female by this technique has been carried in salmon and trout. Oral administration of 17-ß estradiol at 20 mg/kg of food is given to the juvenile trout and salmon up to 60 days resulted in sex reversal of males to females. In the case of Tilapia, the little amount of methyl testosterone (@15-60 mg/kg of food) is administered for 30-50 days of life, during which gonadal differentiation takes place. The uses of estrogenic steroids are not successful in tilapia. In Pacific salmon (*Oncorhynchus* spp.), immersion of young fish in drug and feeding the drug simultaneously was found necessary for sex reversal.

Tilapia fish has a great demand and value in the local and international market due to which its culture areas are expanding. It is having a high ability to take a natural feed from the pond, proper utilization of supplementary feed, surviving capacity in adverse weather and they have high diseases resistance power. But male monosex tilapia is the most preferred culture method due to some important reasons. Female fish attain maturity early and belongs to prolific breeder community so it invests most of the energy in breeding in place of growth.

Alternate Carp Species for Diversification

Indian water contains about 3035 species which includes 1016 freshwater species, 113 brackish water, and 1906 marine species which shows the ample scope of diversification. Carp culture in India originated traditionally as the polyculture of Indian major carp catla (*Catla catla*), rohu (*Labeo rohita*), and mrigal (*Cirrhinus mrigala*). Polyculture implies incorporation of more than one species with different feeding habits and different habitat preferences. In the late 1950s, the composite fish culture was adopted in India using the Bangkok strain of common carp (*Cyprinus carpio*) and Chinese carp like silver carp (*Hypopthalmichthys molitrix*) and grass carp (*Ctenopharyngodon idella*) with the three Indian major carp. In composite fish culture, different niches of a pond are effectively utilized and the productivity of per unit water spread area also gets multiplied as the fishes have different feeding habits. Adoption of techniques in a polyculture of carp and composite fish culture has been with several modifications depending on the market demand and resource availability. Indian aquaculture is completely dominated by carp species but due to arise of certain problems like disease, inbreeding depression, the pressure to increase production by complete use of niche and increasing demand of other fishes, diversification of cultivable species is receiving utmost importance. Many of the carp species like minor barbs and minnows are not economical from the commercial culture point of view but at least 15-20 varieties of minor and medium carps have a high potential for freshwater aquaculture, which has yet to be exploited. These carp species can be considered as alternatives to the major cultured carp species, for diversification in freshwater aquaculture. The country possesses many endemic potential and cultivable medium and minor carp species having regional demand, such as, *Labeo calbasu*, *L. fimbriatus*, *L.gonius*, *L.dussumieri*, *L. bata*, *Cirrihinus cirrhosa*, *C. reba*, *Puntius sarana*, *P. jerdoni*.

In India, shrimp farming has been traditionally practiced in the coastal states of West Bengal and Kerala. The traditional trap and culture system was characterized by low production levels of mixed species of fin and shellfishes. The shrimp farming areas are mainly located in the coastal states of Andhra Pradesh, West Bengal, Kerala, Orissa, Tamil Nadu, Karnataka, Maharashtra, Gujarat, and Goa. The major importers of Indian shrimp are Japan, Western Europe, and the USA. There were 33 numbers of feed mills in the country in 2005 with a total installed capacity of 1,50,000 t/year to cater to the shrimp industry (Rukmani *et al.*, 2007). Catfish (*Pangasius* sp.) introduced as an alternative species in the brackish water shrimp ponds due to its survival and fast-growing nature in the harsh pond environmental conditions.

Intensive Cage Fish Culture

The development of intensive inland and coastal cage aquaculture of high-value fishes has been encouraged and supported by different governments, as an opportunity for developing remote rural areas. Many fishermen without any land ownership changed into the fish farmer by setting the cage. Intensive aquaculture industries are also emerging for high-value warm water piscivorous fish, such as groupers and barramundi (in Hong Kong, Malaysia, Thailand, Indonesia, the Philippines, Taiwan Province of China, Singapore and Australia). In India, cage culture is still in its infant stage and developing fast to culture tilapia in freshwater and cobia in seawater. In tilapia cage culture, fry from the reproduction ponds is passed through a 3.1 mm mesh grader to remove fry larger than 14 mm. The smaller fry is stocked in cages of mesh size 1.5 mm and stocked at stocking densities of approximately 2-3,000 per square meter.

Recirculatory Aquaculture System

Recirculating Aquaculture Systems (RAS) reprocess the water repeatedly, passing the water through treatment processes to get rid of waste and to revive water quality. It could be a technique for raising water-borne animals in a very closed (usually indoor) system that minimizes water consumption, allow to control environment, and reduces the risk of exposure to parasites, disease, and predators. The technology relies on the employment of mechanical and biological filters, and therefore it can be used for any species like fish, shrimps, clams, etc. Also, the restricted use of water makes it a lot of easier and cheaper to get rid of the nutrients excreted from the fish because the volume of discharged water is far lower than that discharged from a traditional fish farm. The nutrients from the farmed fish are used as fertilizer on agricultural farming land or as a basis for biogas production.

Traditional fish farming completely depends on external conditions like the water temperature of the water resource, cleanliness of the water, oxygen levels, or weed and leaves drifting downstream and blocking the inlet screens, etc. In a recirculated system these external factors are eliminated either fully or partially, looking on the degree of recirculation and therefore the construction of the plant. (Jacob, 2015).

Multiple Breeding in Carps

Carp seed production isn't any more confined to monsoon months. Nowadays carps have been domesticated to breed multiple times i.e. much before monsoon and post-monsoon months, making certain the seed throughout pre and post-monsoon periods. Such brooders are called professional brood.

a. Pre-monsoon Breeding: Success in Pre-monsoon breeding depends on pre gonad maturity. This can be achieved by simple brood stock management practices. Pre-monsoon breeding commences as early as March. The yield is 0.5 – 0.6 lakh spawn/kg body weight of fish. Second spawning of same fish is achieved within 40 – 45 days again with a production rate of 1.0 – 1.5 lakh spawn/kg body weight. Both the spawning are completed between March and May.

b. Monsoon Spawning: A time-lapse of another 40-45 days following the second spawning brings the 3rd crop (June-July) and yield increases to 1.5 – 2.0 lakh spawn/kg of body weight due to a favorable condition.

c. Late Monsoon Spawning: Quality of mature eggs can't be maintained in situ for an indefinite period. Therefore, monsoon-dependent old broods may not be useful for late monsoon breeding. Only the chosen brooders fish may be used repeatedly with an optimum time interval between two successive spawning. The fish has already spawned twice or thrice in a season expected to come for late monsoon breeding i.e. between August & September. However, the yield of spawn declines in comparison to monsoon breeding.

The principle of Multiple Spawning: The fishes are bred by adopting the routine hypophysation technique. Further re-maturation rate declines 30 – 50% which may need some more management manipulation for the purpose (fisheryscience. blogspot).

Central Institute of Freshwater Aquaculture, ICAR, Bhubaneswar developed feed for brooders with name CIFABROOD™ for early maturation of carps.

FRP Hatchery

The fiberglass reinforced plastic hatchery, is an alternative to the concrete hatchery, for production of healthy carp seed. The system consists of one breeding pool; one hatching pool; and egg collection chamber and an overhead storage tank. It can produce 10 lakh carp spawn per operation.

Stunted Yearling Stocking

Since carps are known to grow faster during their second year, nowadays ponds are stocked with 8-12 month-old stunted fishes of 100 -150g, instead of fry or fingerlings as practiced in the traditional system.

Biofloc Technology

Biofloc technology help in enhancing water quality in aquaculture through reconciliation carbon and nitrogen within the system. The technology has recently gained attention due to control over water quality, with the added value of producing protein-rich feed *in-situ*. The environmental friendly aquaculture system called "Biofloc Technology (BFT)" is considered as an efficient alternative system since nutrients could be continuously recycled and reused (Emerenciano, 2013). The principle of biofloc system is based on the growth of a microorganism in the culture medium, benefited by the minimum or zero water exchange. These microorganisms (biofloc) has two major roles:

a. maintenance of water quality by the uptake of nitrogen compounds generating "*in-situ*" microbial protein

b. increasing culture feasibility by reducing feed costs due to lower feed conversion ratio

Probiotics

Probiotics and prebiotics have emerged as exciting feed additives due to their potential benefits for aquatic animal health and performance. Probiotics and prebiotics are now commonly incorporated into farm-made feeds and private companies' aqua feed formulations. The common organisms in probiotic products are bacteria *Lactobacillus acidophilus, L. bulgaricus, L. plantarum, Bifidobacterium bifidium, Streptococcus lactis, Saccharomyces cerevisiae etc.* and fungus *Aspergillus oryzae.* These cultures may be administered through water or incorporated within the feed.

The most significant parameter of probiotics is its capacity to multiply in the gut and suppress the growth of harmful bacteria. Genetic engineering would facilitate in developing probiotics with special properties like secreting enzymes and vitamins in good quantities. These genetically engineered products would be the next generation of feed additives. The mechanism of action is

a. Competition for binding sites: also known as "competitive exclusion", where probiotics bacteria bind with the binding sites in the intestinal mucosa, forming a physical barrier, preventing the connection by pathogenic bacteria

b. Production of antibacterial substances: probiotic bacteria synthesize compounds like hydrogen peroxide and bacteriocins, which have antibacterial action, mainly in relation to pathogenic bacteria. They also produce organic acids that lower the environment's pH of the gastrointestinal tract, preventing the growth of various pathogens and development of certain species of *Lactobacillus*

c. Competition for nutrients: the lack of nutrients available that may be used by pathogenic bacteria is a limiting factor for their maintenance

d. Stimulation of the immune system: some probiotics bacteria are directly linked to the stimulation of the immune response, by increasing the production of antibodies, activation of macrophages, T-cell proliferation and production of interferon.

Other than improving gut micro-biome, some probiotics are also used in the pond as cleaners. Probiotic bacteria directly uptake or decompose the organic matter or toxic material and improve the quality of water. The microbial cultures produce a variety of enzymes like amylase, protease, lipase, xylanase, and cellulase in high concentrations than the native bacteria, which help in degrading waste. These bacteria have a wide range of tolerance for salinity, temperature, pH which usually exists in aquaculture operations.

Disease Management

Specific pathogen free (SPF) and Specific pathogen resistant (SPR) stocks are very much in use in shrimp farming to combat the most prevailing diseases and these stocks are developed through shrimp broodstock management programmes. The specific pathogens for these programs are those listed as 'notifiable' by the OIE, representing direct trade concerns, as well as, significant threats to optimal production (OIE, 2000, 2001). SPF shrimp are produced from brood stocks which are free from specific pathogens and raise their offspring under strictly controlled sanitary conditions. SPF shrimp are important for trade to countries or areas that are free of the particular disease, or for restocking ponds following a disease outbreak and disinfection.

SPR shrimp are developed through selective breeding of individuals that have survived challenges/infections by specific pathogens. therefore, These have great potential to enhance production in waters endemic for the specific diseases, but are inappropriate for use in non-endemic waters, as they may carry sub-clinical infections of the pathogen in question. These specific pathogen approaches are now being applied to shrimp stocking in different countries including India for *P. vannamei*. Both approaches produce 'high health' (HH), however, many SPF stocks perform poorly when challenged by other pathogens, since their production under sterile conditions impedes the development of acquired resistance to common, but normally less significant, pathogens (Browdy, 1998). The inheritable immune or physiological traits of SPR may have the potential to confer significant performance improvement at the farm level. Taking this technology beyond specific pathogens, there is exciting potential for this approach to be adapted to the selection of lines with high non-specific immunity or high tolerance of physiological stresses that facilitate opportunistic infections or other pathology (Bedier, *et.al.*, 1998).

Feed Technologies

The use of fishmeal and other animal proteins in aquafeeds is the topic of concern and replacement is needed for aquaculture development (Naylor *et al.*, 2000). Although fishmeal is used for its high-quality protein content, it has several disadvantages too, including high cost and instability of supply. Capture fisheries are not sustainable and a lot of fishes are under overexploitation and there are increasing environmental concerns, ethical concerns over feeding fish to non-piscivorous fish, and social considerations over feeding aquatic protein to fish that might be used for human nutrition (especially in nutritionally-deficient areas of the world). Biotechnology offers opportunities for the development of alternatives to fishmeal, especially plant-based protein sources, by enhancing production and processing techniques.

Plant protein has significant potential for addressing the problem of phosphorus pollution since plants do not contain the high levels of phosphorus found in animal protein. The use of plant protein in aquafeeds also helps reduce pressure on wild fish stocks. A lot of research is going on various plant species and plant-animal protein mixes, as new sources for protein for aquafeeds for shrimp (Mendoza et *al.*, 2001); molluscs (Shipton and Britz, 2000) and finfish (Ogunji and Wirth, 2001). Other technologies offer the potential for reducing the cost of feed by use of local ingredients in fish feeds and preparation of pelleted feeds at the farm.

Although dietary requirements of most fish and shellfish species are known, large-scale hatchery production of most aquatic species still depends on live feeds, such as selected species of the brine shrimp *Artemia*, the rotifer *Brachionus* and microalgae. This has created a whole new area of biotechnological research aimed at finding cost-effective and efficient supplements to live microalgae, commercial production of freeze-dried algae, microencapsulated diets, and manipulated yeasts. Results of much of this work have shown significant success (Oliva-Teles and Goncalves, 2001).

Enrichment of *Artemia* through bio-encapsulation to improve the nutritional value, particularly with highly unsaturated fatty acids and vitamins, has improved larviculture outputs in terms of quality, survival, growth, and stress resistance (Merchie *et al.*, 1995). Bioencapsulation has also been applied for oral delivery of vaccines, vitamins, and chemo therapeutants notably for hatchery developmental stages of finfish and shrimp.

Bag Feeding

The mixture of uncooked defatted rice bran and oil cakes are suspended in perforated polyethylene bags on poles at various locations in the pond. About 20 to 25 feed bag poles are deployed per hectare. Fish browse on the feed through the perforations and within 2-3 hours most of the feed in the bag is utilized. This technique ends up in minimum wastage of feed and permits for stress-free application of medication.

Mobile Apps

Mobile communication technology has quickly become the world's easiest way of sending voice, data, and services in the developing world. Mobile applications for aquaculture hold significant potential for advancing development. They could provide the most affordable ways for millions of people to culture information, fish markets, finance, and government schemes previously unavailable to them. Mobile phones have several key advantages: affordability, wide ownership, voice communications, and instant and convenient service delivery. As a result, there has been a global explosion in the number of m-apps, facilitated by the rapid evolution of mobile networks and by the increasing functions and falling prices of mobile handsets (Qiang *et al* 2011). Some aquaculture apps are Vanami Shrimp app, m-Krishi, Aquaculture techniques, Aquabrahma, Blue aqua *etc.*

Integrated Farming Approach

Integrated Aqua farming is a diversified and co-ordinated way of farming of producing agricultural items in fish farms as the main product. The items produced are to be used either as a source of feeds and fertilizers, the source of additional income, or both. The principle of integrated fish farming involves the farming of fish along with livestock or/and agricultural crops. Generally, integrated farming means the production or culture of two or more farming practices but when fish becomes its major component it is called as integrated fish farming. Advantages of this system are-

- An artificial ecosystem with no waste
- Efficient recycling of organic material (waste)
- Assured profitable production of fish
- Reduction in cost of fish production
- Diversification of products
- Increase in overall productivity
- Effective utilization of available resources
- Abatement of environmental pollution
- Enhancement of income
- Sustainable system

Integrated fish farming can be broadly classified into two, namely:

- **Agriculture-Fish**- Agri-based systems include rice-fish integration, vegetable-horticulture-fish system, mushroom-fish system, seri-fish system etc.
- **Livestock-Fish Systems-** Livestock-fish system includes cattle-fish system, pig-fish system, poultry-fish system, duck-fish system, goat-fish system, rabbit-fish system.

Cultivation of Vegetables

- The vegetables like Brinjal, Tomato, Cucumber, Gourds, Chilli, Carrot, Radish, Turnip, Spinach, Peas, Cabbage, Cauliflower, Ladies finger can be grown according to their season throughout the year. The flower plantation like Rose, Jasmine, Gladiolus, Marigold and Chrysanthemum *etc.* on the embankment is also useful and it provides additional income of 20-25% in comparison to aquaculture alone.

Horticulture Crops on Pond Bunds

- The plant should be dwarf, seasonal, evergreen, remunerative and less shady. The fruit crops which can be used are Mango, Banana, Papaya, Coconut, Lime *etc.*

Rearing of Cattle and Poultry – It may be Adopted in Different Combinations Like

- Fish-cattle
- Fish-duck
- Fish-poultry
- Fish-pig

- Fish-goat or –sheep
- Combination of fish with two or more types of livestock(*e.g.*, poultry, pig and fish)

Cluster Farming

In a cluster model, some farmers may ultimately choose to specialize in one aspect of the fish farming chain, such as in hatchery production, fingerling nursery, or feed manufacture. Other farmers, doing the same vocation then cluster around these centers of aquaculture services and are able to concentrate their own efforts strictly on fish grow-out.

Example: Ornamental Fish Village

The ornamental Fish village was established under the guidance of Central Institute of Freshwater Aquaculture (CIFA) which played an instrumental role in developing two ornamental fish villages in 2011 (Nath *et al.*, 2012). The local fishery officer initiated this new way of income generation among the women. The Agricultural Technology Management Agency (ATMA) also pitched in by providing financial assistance for construction of rearing tanks. Capacity building training and exposure was provided by the CIFA, Bhubaneswar. The scientists of Krishi Vigyan Kendra, Deogarh popularised the new vocation in the village by organizing awareness camps. With all the families engaged in rearing ornamental fish, the village came to be known as 'ornamental fish village' (De *et al.*, 2012). Another ornamental fish village has also been developed recently at Sarouli in the same district with the partnership of CIFA, ATMA, and State Fisheries Department to promote livelihood development of women SHGs (De and Panday, 2014).

Women Empowerment through Aquaculture

Diversification is believed to be very important in maintaining ecosystem resilience and building social systems resilience. Integrated agriculture-aquaculture (IAA) farming systems, considered among the promising options for small-scale farming households in China and Vietnam, are likely relevant in the context of mixed crop-livestock farming systems else where as well. Aquaculture as a sub-system complemented well with the present mixed crop-livestock systems by virtue of better synergistic relationships among the three sub-systems. Food and nutrition security of the participating households increased to a notable rise in quantity and frequency of fish consumption. Development of Community Fish Production and Marketing Cooperatives exclusively owned and managed by the women themselves helped in women's empowerment through their improved access to and control over resources and increased roles in decision-making at both household and community levels (Pant *et al.*, 2009).

Involvement of rural women in aquaculture production activities including composite carp culture, seed rearing, and integrated fish farming has been advocated for their socio-economic upliftment (Bhanot *et al.*, 1999) and generation of self-employment (Sharma *et al.*, 1988, Thakur *et al.*, 1988). However, lack of focus coupled with cultural and social constraints limit the participation of women in training and empowerment. Women are in subsistence aquaculture in India, taking care of fish after stocking (Nandeesha, 2007). Appropriate methods in aquaculture extension coupled with appropriate technologies can draw rural women towards aquaculture practice in a sustainable way. Women can easily manage small backyard ponds (0.01 – 0.1 ha) for raising of fish seed within a short period (Goswami and Ojha, 1997; Radheyshyam, 2002). Besides, they can undertake common carp breeding including a collection of brood fish, breeder maintenance and egg hatching for production of fish seed and also their nursing (Radheyshyam *et al.*, 1999; De *et al.*, 2005). Aquaculture is increasingly being recognized as a tool for empowering women even in most difficult areas. The initiatives by the government as well as non-government also helped to bring them closer to Govt. establishments, Banks *etc.* Office bearers of SHGs have to deal with management and financial aspects of pond management *viz.*, purchase of inputs – fingerling, lime, feed, fertilizers *etc.* and selling table fish. Additional income accruing from fish culture has also resulted in the improved social status of women.

Conclusions

Aquaculture has the potential to create new jobs and improve food security among poor households. A rural aquaculture is a good option for rural development, making an important contribution to farm income with a high adoption rate among poor farmers. Fish farmers have gained an increased level of satisfaction by means of fish culture production growth along with corresponding economic gain. Aquaculture in combination with another farm enterprise in the coastal regions of the country significantly contributes to the livelihood security of farm families in a system's perspective. Biotechnological involvement in Aquaculture to develop better quality seed, feed and disease management, and other technological innovations are showing a positive impact on aquaculture diversification success, investment potential, and international technology exchange. The development of biotechnology in aquaculture may provide a means of producing healthy and fast-growing animals, through environmentally friendly means. However, this development will largely depend on the desire and willingness of the producers to work hand-in-hand with scientists in related research, capacity building, and infrastructure development. The advancement and new proven technologies will undoubtedly help the aquaculture sector to further develop with the view to increasing sustainable aquatic animal production globally.

References

Bedier, E., Cochard, J. C., Le Moullac, G., Patrois, J. and Aquacop. 1998. Selective breeding and pathology in penaeid shrimp culture: the genetic approach to pathogen resistance. World Aquacult. 29 (2): 46-51 pp.

Bhanot, K. K., Safui, L., Jena, J. K., Mohanty, S. N. and Ayyappan, S. 1999. Fisheries technologies for women. Indian Farming 48(7):46-48 pp.

Browdy, C. L. 1998. Recent developments in penaeid broodstock and seed production technologies: improving the outlook fo superior captive stocks. Aquaculture, 164: 3-21 pp.

DADF (Department of Animal Husbandry, Dairying & Fisheries), 2016. Annual report-2016. 162 pp.

Edwards P. 1999. Towards increased impact of rural aquaculture. A discussion paper prepared for the first meeting of the APFIC Ad Hoc Working Group of Experts on Rural Aquaculture, FAO Regional Office for Asia and the Pacific, Bangkok, Thailand, 20–22 October 1999.

Emerenciano, M., Gabriela, G., and Gerard, C. 2013. Biofloc technology (BFT): a review for aquaculture application and animal food industry. Biomass Now: Cultivation and Utilization. Rijeka, Croatia: In Tech, 301-328 pp.

FAO, 2016. The State of World Fisheries and Aquaculture- contributing to food security and nutrition for all. ISBN 978-92-5-109185-2. 204 pp.

FAO. 2000a. Small ponds make a big difference. Integrating fish with crop and livestock farming. Food and Agriculture Organization of the United Nations, Rome, Italy, 30 pp.

Fernando, C.H and M. Halwart 2000. Possibilities for the integration of fish farming into irrigation systems. Fish. Manag. Ecol. 7: 45-54.

Goswami, M. and Ojha S.N. 1997. Focus on women of Assam: their role in fisheries. Aquaculture Asia 2: 41 p.

Halwart, M., Funge-Smith, S. and Moehl, J. 2003. The role of aquaculture in rural development. In FAO Inland Water Resources and Aquaculture Service. Review of the state of world aquaculture. FAO Fisheries Circular 886 (Rev. 2). Rome, FAO, pp. 47–58 (http://www.fao.org/3/a-y4490e/y4490e04.pdf).

http://eands.dacnet.nic.in/PDF/State_of_Indian_Agriculture, 2015-16.pdf

http://fisheryscience.blogspot.in/2008/11/multiple-breeding.html

https://www.researchgate.net/publication/259785868_Applications_of_nutritional_biotechnology_in_Aquaculture [accessed May 10, 2017].

IIRR, IDRC, FAO, NACA and ICLARM, 2001. Utilizing Different Aquatic Resources for Livelihoods in Asia: a Resource Book. International Institute of Rural Reconstruction, International Development Research Centre, Food and Agriculture Organization of the United Nations, Network of Aquaculture Centers in Asia-Pacific, and International Center for Living Aquatic Resources Management, 416 pp

Jacob Bregnballe 2015. A Guide to Recirculation Aquaculture: An introduction to the new environmentally friendly and highly productive closed fish farming systems. Published by FAO and EUROFISH International Organization, 2015 edition.

Mendoza, R., De Dios, A., Vasquez, C., Cruz, E., Ricque, D., Aguilera, C. and Montemayor, J. 2001. Fish meal replacement with feather-enzyme hydrolysates co-extruded with soya-bean meal in practical diets for the Pacific white shrimp (Litopenaeus vannamei). Aquacult. Nutr. 7 (3): 143-151.

Merchie, G., Lavens P., Dhert P., Dehasque M., Nelis H., DeLeenheer A. and Sorgeloos P. 1995. Variation in ascorbic acid content in different live food organisms. Aquaculture, 134 (3-4): 325-337.

Moehl, J.F., I. Beernaerts, A.G. Coche, M. Halwart and V.O. Sagua 2001. Proposal for an African network on integrated irrigation and aquaculture. Proceedings of a Workshop held in Accra, Ghana, 20-21 September 1999. FAO, 75 pp.

Nandeesha, M.C. 2007. Asian experience on farmer's innovation in freshwater fish seed production and nursing and the role of women.In: Assessment of freshwater fish seed resources for sustainable aquaculture (ed. M.G. Bondad-Reantaso), pp. 581602. FAO Fisheries Technical Paper.No.501. Rome.

Nath, S. K., Sahu, P., and Sar, B. K. 2012. Institutional linkage helping rural women of an under developed district to become self-employed. Aquaculture Asia 17(2): 34 p.

Naylor, R. L., Goldburg, R. J., Primavera, J. H., Kautsky, N., Beveridge, M. C. M., Clay, J., Folke, C., Lubchenko, J., Mooney, H. and Troell, C. 2000. Effect of aquaculture on world fish supplies. Nature, 405 (6790): 1017-1024 pp.

Ogunji, J. O. and Wirth, M. 2001. Alternative protein sources as substitutes for fish meal in the diet for young tilapia Oreochromis niloticus(Linn.). Isr. J. Aquacult. 53 (1): 34-43 pp.

OIE, 2000. Diagnostic manual for Aquatic Animal Disease. 3rd Edition. Office International des Epizootics, Paris, France, 237 pp.

OIE, 2001. International Aquatic Health Code. 4th Edition. Office International des Epizootics, Paris, France, 155 pp.

Oliva-Teles A. and Goncalves P. 2001. Partial replacement of fishmeal by brewers yeast (Saccharomyces cerevisiae) in diets for sea bass (Dicentrarchus labrax) juveniles. Aquaculture, 202 (3-4):269-278p.

Pant, J., Shrestha, M. K. and Bhujel, R. C. "Aquaculture and resilience: Women in aquaculture in Nepal." Small-scale Aquaculture for Rural Livelihoods: 19 p.

Prein, M. and M. Ahmed, 2000. Integration of aquaculture into smallholder farming systems for improved food security and household nutrition. Food Nutr. Bull. 21: 466-471.

Qiang C. Z., Kuek S.C., Dymond A. and Esselaar S. 2011. Mobile Applications for Agriculture and Rural Development. ICT Sector Unit, World Bank December 2011.

Radheyshyam, 2002. Carp seed production for rural aquaculture at Sarakana Village in Orissa: a case study. In: Edwards, P., Little, D. C. and Demaine, H. (eds), Rural Aquaculture. CABI Publishing, UK. pp 167-184.

Radheyshyam, Safui, L., Sahu, B. B. and Ayyappan, S. 1999. Rural women in common carp seed breeding (in Hindi), CIFA,Publication, 1-20 pp.

Rukmani, R., Senthilkumar, V. and Thenmathi, N. 2007. Measures of Impact of Science and Technology in India: Agriculture and Rural Development (Measures of Progress of Science and Technology in India - Part III). ISBN No. 81-88355-05-4. 279 pp.

Sharma, B. K., Thakur, N. K., Sarkar, S. K., Safui, L., Radheshyam, Dutta B. R. and Sarengi, N. 1988. Involvement of rural womenfolk in aquaculture under S &T programme at KVK/TTC, Kausalyaganga. Proceedings All India workshop on gainful employment for women in the Fisheries Field. CIFT, Cochin. 54-71 pp.

Shipton, T. A., and Britz, P. J. 2000. Partial and total substitution of fish meal with plant protein concentrates in formulated diets for the South African Abalone, Haliotis midae. J. Shellfish Res. 19 (1): 534 p.

Subasinghe, R. P., Barg, U., Phillips, M. J., Bartley, D. and Tacon, A. 1998. Aquatic Animal Health Management. Investment Opportunities within Developing Countries. J. Appl. Ichthyol. 14 (3-4): 123-129 pp.

Thakur, N.K., Sarkar, S.K., Sarengi, N. and Sharma, B. K. 1988. Self-employment of rural womenfolk through "successional" aquaculture in backyard ponds. Proceedings All India workshop on gainful employment for women in the Fisheries Field. CIFT, Cochin. 72-81 pp

Transforming Rural Areas through Veterinary Science *Pages* **145-154**
Editor: Dipanjali Konwar, Shilpa Sood & Shahid Ahamad
Published by: **ASTRAL INTERNATIONAL PVT. LTD., NEW DELHI**

10 Utilisation of Animal By-Products as Feed for the Animals

Dr. Dipanjali Konwar, Dr. Shilpa Sood & Dr. Shahid Ahamad

Introduction

Agriculture is the main stay of the Indian economy and contributes nearly 14.1 per cent of GDP (Economic survey, GOI 2012-13 base year 2004-05), as about 65-70 per cent of the population is dependent on agriculture for their livelihood. Livestock production is backbone of Indian agriculture contributing 4.11 % to national GDP and source of employment and ultimate livelihood for 70% population in rural areas. This contribution would have been much greater had the animal by-products been also efficiently utilized. India ranks topmost in the world in livestock holding and has the potential to utilize slaughter house by products to partly meet the growing requirement of animal feeds. These by-products which are also the better source of proteins and minerals can be processed into animal feed to solve the problem of nutritional needs of animals.

Animal By-Product: Animal by-product may be defined as a part of slaughtered animal that is not directly consumed by human. By-products of dairy industry and tannery by-products also fall in this group. Animal by-products are divided into two main categories viz., edible and inedible (Figure 1). Edible byproducts are those by-products that can be consumed as a food by human beings and generally include liver, kidney, heart, brain, intestine, tongue, spleen etc. They are also called as variety meats. On the other hand, those by-products which cannot be consumed as food by human beings are called inedible by-products e.g. hides, skins, ear, snout, gallbladder, foetus, hoofs, horns, hair, bristles etc. All parts of dead animal or condemned meat and organs also come in this category. The basic criterion of division between edible and inedible by-products depends upon the purchasing power, custom, tradition, food habits, religious outlook etc.

The yield of animal by-products ranges between 50-60% of the live weight. By-products (including organs, fat or lard, skin, feet, abdominal and intestinal contents, bone and blood) of cattle, pigs, and lambs represent 66.0%, 52.0%, and 68.0% of the live weight, respectively.

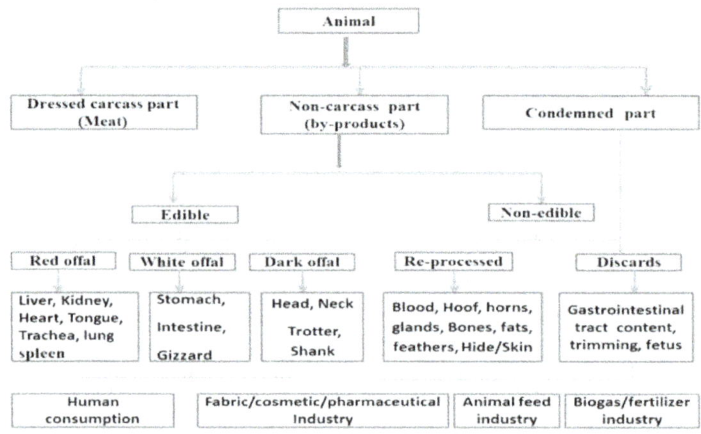

Figure 1: Classification of Animal By-Product

Importance of utilisation of by-products as animal feed: Feed constitutes the largest single factor in the cost of production of animals of all kinds. In order to achieve a successful feeding program, one should be able to provide proper nutrients at the least cost. Presently in India, live stock feed production is more of cereal based and less of animal by-product based. This results in livestock, especially poultry, pig and fish competing with humans for grains and cereals which can easily be replaced with slaughterhouse waste. According to FAO (2008) and GOI (2007) estimates 107 million livestock and more than 650 million poultry birds were slaughtered annually in India leading to production of 6.3 million tonnes meat. It leaves huge loads of by-products. The load is further increased by dead and fallen animals. Thus, India has rich resources of slaughterhouse by products which are also the better source of proteins and minerals but most of it going waste. On the other hand, at present, the country faces a net deficit of 35.6% green fodder, 10.95% dry crop residues and 44% concentrate feed ingredients. In terms of digestible crude protein and total digestible nutrients, the shortfall is about 34 percent and 37 percent, respectively. The demand of green and dry fodder for livestock will reach to 1012 and 631 million tonnes of by the year 2050. At the current level of growth in forage resources, there will be 18.4 % deficit in green fodder and 13.2% deficit in dry fodder in the year 2050. The nutrient requirements of most of the animals including poultry are well known; it is a matter of matching the ingredients to supply the required nutrients in correct proportion. India has the potential to utilise slaughter house waste to replace 13 million tonnes of animal feed annually which in turn will not only reduce the consumption of grains but will also increase the nutritive value of feedstuff and economically benefit the slaughter house and help in maintaining the environment. Efficient utilization of by-products has direct impact on the economy and environmental pollution of the country. Non-utilization or under utilization of by-products not only lead to loss of potential revenues but also lead to the added and increasing cost of disposal of these products and may create major aesthetic and catastrophic health problems.

Nutritive Value of Animal By-Product- Animal by-products have higher content of good quality protein, essential amino acids, a high energy value and is devoid of crude fibre and anti nutritional factors in comparison to product of plant origin. Some are used as medicines because they contain special nutrients such as amino acids, hormones, minerals, vitamin and fatty acids. Not only blood, but several other meat byproducts, have a higher level of moisture than meat. Some examples are lung, kidney, brains, spleen, and tripe. Some organ meat, including liver and kidney, contains a higher level of carbohydrate than other meat materials. Pork tail has the highest fat content and the lowest moisture content of all meat by-products. The liver, tail, ears and feet of cattle have a protein level which is close to that of lean meat tissue, but a large amount of collagen is found in the ears and feet. The lowest protein level is found in the brain, chitterlings and fatty tissue. The amino acid composition of meat by-products is different from that of lean tissue, because of the large amount of connective tissue. As a result, by-products such as ears, feet, lungs, stomach and tripe contain a larger amount of proline, hydroxyproline and glycine, and a lower level of tryptophan and tyrosine. The vitamin content of organ meats is usually higher than that of lean meat issue. Kidney and liver contain the largest amount of riboflavin (1.697– 3.630 mg/100 g), and have 5–10 times more than lean meat. Liver is the best source of niacin, vitamin B_{12}, B_6, folacin, ascorbic acid and vitamin A. Kidney is also a good source of vitamin B_6, B_{12}, and folacin. A 100 g serving of liver from pork or beef contributes 450%–1,100% of the RDA of vitamin A, 65% of the RDA of vitamin B_6, 3,700% of the RDA of vitamin B_{12} and 37% of the RDA of ascorbic acid. Lamb kidneys, pork, liver, lungs, and spleen are an excellent source of iron, as well as vitamins. The copper content is highest in the livers of beef, lamb and veal. They contribute 90–350% of the RDA of copper (2 mg/day). Livers also contain the highest amount of manganese (0.128–0.344 mg/100 g). However, the highest level of phosphorus (393–558 mg/100 g) and potassium (360–433 mg/100 g) in meat by-products is found in the thymus and sweetbreads. With the exception of brain, kidney, lungs, spleen and ears, most other by-products contain sodium at or below the levels found in lean tissue. Mechanically deboned meat has the highest calcium content (315–485 mg/100 g). Many organ meats contain more polyunsaturated fatty acids than lean tissue. Brain, chitterlings, heart, kidney, liver and lungs have the lowest level of monounsaturated fatty acids and the highest level of polyunsaturated fatty acids. There is three to five times more cholesterol (260–410 mg/100 g) in organ meats than in lean meat, and large quantities of phospholipids. Brain has the highest level of cholesterol (1,352–2,195 mg/100 g) and also has the highest amount of phospholipids compared to other meat by-products.

Animal By-Product as Livestock Feed

Blood Meal: Blood meal is a by-product of the slaughter house and is used as a protein source in the diets of livestock. Blood meal is prepared by collecting blood after slaughter which is then heated to induce coagulation of protein after which excess water is passed off, dried and powdered. Blood meal contains mostly protein (about 90-95 % DM) and small amounts of fat (less than 1% DM) and ash (less than 5% DM). Unlike other animal protein sources, blood meal has a poor amino acid balance. Its lysine content is relatively high (7-10 % DM) which makes it an excellent supplementary protein to use with plant-derived feed ingredients that are low in lysine. However, its isoleucine content is very low (about 1 % DM), so diets for monogastric animals must be formulated to contain enough isoleucine for the level of performance desired. Pepsin digestibility has been shown to be a good test for assessing the availability of the protein fraction of blood meal. Blood meal is rich in iron (more than 1500 mg/kg DM). Blood meal can be used upto 25% level in the diet of poultry and swine and as a substitute in calf feeding it can be used upto 40-50%. For safety reasons, blood must be heated to be used in animal feeding: a minimal temperature of 100°C for 15 min is necessary in order to destroy potentials pathogens (salmonella, mycotoxins, prions). It is recommended to avoid feeding a species with blood meal from the same species.

Meat Meal: Meat meal is the major secondary by-products of the slaughtering industry and is an important components of stock feeds for pigs and poultry. It can be prepared from the carcass trimmings, condemned carcasses, condemned livers, inedible offal, and also from the rendering of dead animals. It is used as a supplement for feeding of livestock as it is a good source of high quality proteins (well-balanced amino acid profile), energy, vitamin B and minerals. Addition of about 10% meat meal helps to satisfy the animal requirement for essential amino acids like lysine, methionine, theronine and tryptophan. Besides that meat meal also acts as a good source for vitamin B, particularly thiamine. Meat meals can be included in the diets for pigs and poultry of all ages.

Meat and Bone Meal:. When bones are added to meat meal, it becomes a product known as meat and bone meal (MBM). MBM is an excellent source of protein, calcium, phosphorous, vitamin B_{12} and numerous other minerals that are necessary to an animal's health. Normally hair, hooves and blood are not included. There can be a wide variation between plants and batches in what goes into the meat and bone meal that is being prepared. If the ash content is high, this indicates that it contains a higher amount of bones and is referred to as meat and bone meal. If the ash content is lower it is referred to as meat meal. Typically when the phosphorus content is above 4.5 %, then it is called meat and bone meal and when it is below that level it is referred to as meat meal or some other term.

Meat and bone is an excellent source of supplemental protein and has a well:balanced amino acid profile. Digestibility of the protein fraction is normally quite high, ranging from 81 to 87%. It is well suited for use in feeding monogastric and provides not only a well-balanced protein source, but also a highly available source of calcium and phosphorus and some other minerals (K, Mg, Na, *etc.*). The ash content of the meat and bone meal normally ranges from 28 to 36 %; calcium is 7 to 10 % and phosphorus 4.5 to 6 %. When using meat and bone meal as the primary supplemental protein source the mineral levels may limit its use in some diet formulations.

Meat and bone meal and other processed animal proteins were the vector of the bovine spongiform encephalopathy (BSE) epidemy in Western Europe in the 1980-1990s. For that reason, many countries have restricted the feeding of meat and bone meal and some only allow meat and bone meal derived from monogastric animals to be fed to ruminant animals and vice versa. In areas where meat and bone meal is authorized for livestock feeding, the use of proper heat treatment is required to control the spread of BSE and other disease agents such as salmonella.

Bone Meal- Bone meal is a mixture of finely and coarsely ground slaughterhouse waste products. The most common sources of these waste by-products are beef, pork, sheep and poultry. This mixture can be used as a nutritional supplement for livestock and other animals.

Bone meal, meat meal and blood meal are produced in a process known as rendering. In this process, the raw material is heated to remove moisture and release fat. The dry rendering process often begins with crushing and grinding the material, followed by heat treatment to reduce moisture content and eliminate any microorganisms. The melted fat is then separated from the solid protein through draining and pressing, and the solid material is grounded into powder, such as meat meal, meat and bone meal, feather meal and blood meal.

Animal Fat- Animal fats are produced by rendering. Animal fat is added in compound feed production as a source of energy. There are three methods of rendering viz. wet rendering, dry rendering and low temperature rendering. Heat is applied to melt down the fat and then purified by gravity. Care must be taken to prevent breakdown of fat by the action of lipase at temperature 40-60^{0}C. Animal fat is used in the range of 2-4% and sometimes as high as 7-8% when high energy feed is formulated for high producing livestock.

Dried Rumen Digesta - Rumen contents, which are commonly known as "digesta", are considered as waste, but when re-processed or utilised, can become a product of high significance and economic value for the livestock industry. The recovery of rumen digesta from ruminant animals in abattoirs offers a great opportunity as an alternate source of nutrients to complement the prevailing limited feed resources. However, many studies do not encourage rumen digesta to be fed alone to livestock but rather to be supplemented with other feed ingredients at a recommended rate during feed formulation. The chemical composition of dried rumen digesta, has drawn the interest of nutritionists to use them as cheaper feedstuff. On the other hand, rumen content are environmentally unfavourable to life, causing air pollution, ground water pollution and eutrophication if not handled properly. Conversion of these inedible by-products into livestock feed can enhance the flexibility of feed formulation and lessen environmental pollution. It was pointed out that the use of dried rumen digesta as feed ingredients has no harmful effect on growth performance of the animals. Rumen digesta are usually processed by applying light heat or sun-drying before utilisation in feed formulation. Dried rumen digesta may vary in their proximate composition because of the different chemical composition of preferred pastures consumed by different animal species. The dry matter (DM) of dried rumen digesta ranges from 13.36 to 98.4%, crude protein (CP) 11.38 to 19.6% and crude fibre (CF) 15.3 to 41.84%. Supplementation of DRC in concentrate diets resulted in improved in vitro dry matter and organic matter digestibility in buffalo rumen fluid. Diets containing DRC up to 10% improved growth performance in lamb without any adverse effect on nutrient digestibility or animal health.

Poultry By-Product Meal: Poultry by-product meal consist of ground rendered part of carcass of slaughtered poultry such as head, feet, under developed eggs and intestines exclusive of feather. The parts or organs are chopped, cooked, dried and then made into meal. Feeding trial indicate that this feed is good as meat meal. Poultry by-product meal contain 93% DM, 56.4% CP, 17.8% fat, 0.9% CF and 17.3% ash. The quality of the meal is influenced by the quality and composition of raw material used in manufacturing as well as rendering and drying process. Poultry by-product meal can be incorporated upto 5% in animal feed formulation.

Poultry Faecal Waste: A considerable amount of poultry faecal waste contains undigested material as well as non-protein nitrogen(NPN) that can be utilised in ruminant fermentative digestion. Dehydrated poultry waste contains about 95.5% DM, 24.3%CP, 4.1% fat, 10.1% fibre and 35.8% ash. In many countries poultry waste is used as valuable feed stuff for all type of livestock including poultry although predominantly to ruminant species. Because of the presence of uric acid it would appear logical to feed poultry faecal material to the ruminant, which have rumen micro organism capable of utilising this nutrient. In some case the material has been fed without any processing and in other it has been cooked, dried and ground or ensiled with a wide range of foreign material. Faecal material should be heat sterilised before being used in animal feed, although fermentation is an effective process. The immediate drying of poultry waste at between 80-90^{0}C for at least 4-5 days is necessary to avert putrefaction and damage. Level upto 100g per kg in feed did not affect egg production, quality of meat and milk.

Anaerobic Digested Ruminant Manure: Anaerobic Digested Ruminant Manure that result from biogas unit can be used as feed. It is chemically treated with phosphoric acid (2.24g acid/Kg ADM) dehydrated at 90^{0}C can be used as feed ingredient. Ration based on acidified dried ADM and containing barley grains or ground date stone are recommended for growing kids.

Hydrolysed Feather Meal (HFM): HFM is produced from undecomposed feather from slaughtered poultry free of additives under pressure, which will bring about partial hydrolysis to keratin to yield very high protein product. HFM is recommended upto 2.55 in the diet. Feather meal contains approximately 85% crude protein (DM basis) of which 30% is degraded in the rumen. Although HFM has relatively poor balance of amino acid it is a good source of sulphur because of its high cystine content.

Recycled Poultry Bedding: Recycled poultry bedding is a material removed from the floor of poultry houses, particularly broiler houses containing the bedding material, wasted feed, feather and excreta. Recycled poultry bedding may represent alternative, low cost protein source and has been used in monogastric diet, particularly pet food and poultry diet. Before feeding the recycled poultry bedding should be heat processed generally by deep staking to improve its palatability, nutrient availability and to decrease pathogen load. Recycled poultry bedding is relatively low in energy, but is a good source of crude protein, 40-45% of which is NPN and the rest of which is true protein and contains very high concentration of some required minerals.

Constraints in Slaughter House Waste Utilization

Indian meat industry has inherent handicaps which hamper the proper utilization of the animal by-products. At present we do not have major industries based on by-products processing. The major constraints are:

1. **Lack of Modern Abattoir:** Generally in local or panchayat slaughter houses, on an average less than 5 large animals or 15 sheep or goat are slaughtered per day. The clandestine slaughter at various meat shops or family functions is also very common. The quantum of by-products from such small slaughter houses will be small and collection of by-products is difficult. However, the total volume of all these small slaughter houses will be huge but because of lack of facilities it is not collected. It is not economically feasible to have rendering plants or by-products utilization plant, attached to such individual small slaughter houses.
2. **Lack of Collection and Transportation Systems:** The system and facilities (carriage vans) for the collection as well as transportation of animal by-products and fallen animals from small slaughter houses to the processing plants is lacking.
3. **Preference to Hot Meat:** Indians like to purchase hot meat. The sight of poultry birds being slaughtered on the roadside meat shops before the eyes of the customers is verycommon. The heaps of poultry feathers or other poultry by- products on the side of these shops create an obnoxious scene and environment pollution.
4. **Collection of Bones:** In general, the deboning is not done in the slaughter houses. It is being done either at home or restaurants. So it becomes very difficult to collect the bones for further processing.
5. **Unorganized Meat Industry:** Indian meat industry is regulated by unscrupulous uneducated meat traders. They do not know the benefits of processing of animal by-products both in turn of economics as well as pollution and health hazards.
6. **Dead and Fallen Animals/Birds:** It is estimated that around 36 million dead and fallen animals are available in the country every year. Not more than 30% of these being utilized for by-product processing or properly disposed off. It is a major source for spread of diseases.
7. **Lack of Processing Facilities:** There are hardly 183 organised carcass utilization plants (CUPs) in such a vast country processing not even 1% of the raw materials available. The rendering units are attached to upcoming modem abattoirs only.

8. **Lack of Human Resource:** There is also dearth of technically trained and scientific personnel in this area. The Veterinary Education Institutes/ Universities or Veterinary Colleges in State Agricultural Universities lack the programme, facilities as well as the curriculum to train the personnel in by-product processing.
9. **Lack of Research and Development:** There is lack of linkages between laboratory and industry. Even the modern abattoirs and big houses in meat industry do not have proper R&D Section. There is an urgent need for engineering R&D in the development of low inventory, low priced equipments/ rendering units for animal by-product processing.
10. **Diseases:** The problems such as Salmonellosis or recent problems of Bovine Spongiform Encephalopathy (BSE) in Europe especially Great Britain are being linked with feeding of meat meal or meat-cum-bone meal, severely disrupted the market of animal byproducts.
11. **Synthetic Substitutes:** Many synthetic substitutes have come to the market affecting the marketing of inedible by-products. Cellulose, plastic and reconstituted collagens have replaced many of the natural casings which are used for sausages. Vegetable fats have replaced many inedible fats for industrial uses. Inedible fats used in soap industry have been replaced; synthetic insulin produced from animal pancreas is being replaced by biotechnology.
12. **Agitation by Ethical Groups:** Some social ethical groups are agitating to discourage the use of animal by-product for processing into different valuable products. This is also a big hindrance for the development of animal by-product industry.
13. **Identification of Markets:** There is an urgent need to identify markets (domestic as well as international) for both raw and processed animal by-products.

Conclusion

The utilization of animal byproducts are often ignored, however, these items contribute a significant value to the livestock and meat industries. Non-utilization of animal by-products in a proper way may create major aesthetic and catastrophic health problems. Value addition of animal byproducts has two benefits. Firstly, the meat industry gets additional revenue by processing them to livestock feed that otherwise would have been wasted. Secondly, the costs of disposing of these secondary items are avoided. In India, the slaughter house waste management system is very poor and several measures are being taken for the effective management of wastes generated from slaughter houses. Competition is also a strong incentive for meat industries to use by-products more efficiently. This is important, because increased profits and lower costs are required in the future for the meat industry to remain viable. Therefore, the potential and scope of by-product utilization is really great which will result in industrial development, employment generation, environmental management and better returns to the farmers.

References

Irshad A. and Sharma B. D. 2015. Abattoir by-product utilization for sustainable meat industry: A Review. J Anim Pro Adv 2015, 5(6): 681-696

Jayathilakan K., Sultana K., Radhakrishna, K. and Bawa, A. S. 2012. Utilization of byproducts and waste materials from meat, poultry and fish processing industries: a review. J Food Sci Technol 49(3):278–293

Konwar, D and Barman, K. 2005. Potential of utilisation of animal by-product in animal feed. The North East Veterinarian. 5(3): 28-31.

Transforming Rural Areas through Veterinary Science *Pages* **155-160**
Editor: Dipanjali Konwar, Shilpa Sood & Shahid Ahamad
Published by: **ASTRAL INTERNATIONAL PVT. LTD., NEW DELHI**

11 Aquaculture Practices: Significance and Strategies for Increasing Fish Production

Dr. Raj Kumar, Dr. Akhil Gupta & Dr. Sahar Masud

Introduction

Fisheries and Aquaculture are playing an important role in addressing nutritional and livelihood security, especially of the rural poor in developing countries. Fish are rich sources of protein, essential fatty acids, vitamins and minerals. The fats and fatty acids in fish, particularly Omega 3 fatty acids, are highly beneficial and difficult to obtain from other food sources. The growing gap between supply and demand globally will impact on the health and nutrition of low income families, unless efforts are made to increase the production to meet the growing demand. Aquaculture is the culture of Aquatic organisms under controlled conditions. Present concept of aquaculture incorporate culture of all aquatic organisms by following certain management techniques which includes water quality, choice food etc. and to protect them from unwanted predators, diseases, pollutants or any other things which are harmful to them. The aquatic organisms which are normally used for aquaculture for food purpose include fishes, prawns, shrimps, crabs, mussels and some live food organisms like algae and zooplankton.

Aquaculture is essentially an Asian farming practice. India is endowed with vast and varied aquatic resources, of which only about 30% is utilized today for aquaculture. Aquaculture is a new name for what once we called 'fish culture'.

Aquaculture continues to increase in volume and value of output in many countries of the world, filling the gap between the supply and demand for fish and fishery products, improving nutrition and contributing to the household economy, particularly in rural areas. There is immense scope for the betterment of mankind through aquaculture. Currently, China leads in Aquaculture production in the world followed by India, but the difference in production is almost 8-9 times. In India the Aquaculture average growth rate is about 8%.

Importance of Aquaculture

- ✰ Aquaculture has been found to be a productive enterprise compared to traditional agriculture practices.
- ✰ In aquaculture practice, fish can be crowded more closely (200/m^2) and grown as in super intensive fish culture practices like water recirculation system due to their three dimensional utilization of the water column. Through such a practice, a fish yield of 25 tons/ha/yr has been recorded.
- ✰ As the FCR is known to be 1.5 times more in fish compared to chicken and two times more than in cattle and sheep, thus fish production by supplementary feed is higher than that of the livestock.
- ✰ Integration of fish farming with agriculture and/or animal husbandry is known to be more profitable than agriculture alone.
- ✰ Fish culture gives efficient means for recycling agricultural and domestic wastes, in order to help/protect our environment
- ✰ Many high valued and commercially important aquatic items such as prawns, lobsters, frog legs, ornamental fish and many other helps in earning good foreign exchange.
- ✰ Artificial recruitment in the water bodies by fish seed produced in fish hatcheries through aquaculture (ranching), could certainly add new fishery resources or increase existing fish stocks.
- ✰ Aquaculture could help in generating employment for many unemployed and under-employed people. Such a step would help to stop the migration from villages to urban areas.
- ✰ From the point of view of human nutrition, the fish food is not only easily digestive but is also rich in essential amino acids like lysine and methionine. The unique poly unsaturated fatty acids (PUFA) namely, eicosa pentaenoic acid of fish is known to reduce the cholesterol level of blood and save human beings from coronary disease. Further, vitaminsand minerals are also present in good quantities in fish.

Types of Culture Systems

Aquaculture is conducted in all the three types of aquatic environments:

1. **Freshwater aquaculture**: It involves the culture in the water bodies having salinity level of less than 0.5 parts per thousand (ppt).
2. **Brackish water aquaculture**: It involves the culture in the water bodies

having salinity level ranges from 0.5 to 30 ppt, and;

3. **Mari culture or sea farming**: It involves the culture in the water bodies having salinity level of more than 30ppt.

The species of flora and fauna inhabiting the three types of water bodies are accordingly called freshwater species, brackishwater species and marine species. Freshwater which is most extensively used sector of aquaculture, is further divided into two segments.

a. **Cold Waters** of higher altitudes having temperature range of >18°C and

b. **Warm waters** of plains having temperature range of >18°C

Aquaculture practices in these waters are, therefore, called coldwater aquaculture and warm water aquaculture, respectively. Aquaculture is practiced through various methods. Freshwater aquaculture is carried out in fish ponds, fish pens, fish cages, raceways and on a limited scale in paddy fields. Culture of fishes in ponds is the oldest form of aquaculture.

Different Levels of Aquaculture

Depending on the intensity of operation and degree of management, aquaculture practices are classified into following four operations/levels:

1. Extensive aquaculture
2. Semi- intensive aquaculture
3. Intensive aquaculture
4. Super intensive aquaculture

Extensive Aquaculture: In extensive level of aquaculture, low stocking densities of 2000-5000 carp fingerlings are used and no supplemental feed is given. Fertilization may be due to stimulate the growth and production of natural food in the water. In such types of culture system, carp culture does not require water exchange during culture period. The ponds used for extensive aquaculture are usually large (more than 100 ha.). The production is generally low, less than 0.5 ton/ha/yr in the case of carps.

Semi-Intensive Level: Semi-intensive aquaculture uses medium size ponds 0.5 ha each with comparatively higher stocking densities than extensive aquaculture (5000-10000 carp fingerlings/ha). Supplementary feeding is done in moderate amounts. In carp culture, water replenishment is done once or twice a month @10%. The production averages around 3-7 tons/ha/yr of carps.

Intensive Level: In intensive level of aquaculture, the pond size is generally small (about 0.2 ha approximately) with very high density of culture organisms i.e. 20000 to 25000 carp fingerlings/ha are stocked. The system is totally dependent on the use of formulated feeds. Feeding of the stock is done at regular intervals. Water replacement under intensive culture is effected on a daily basis. Production under intensive level of aquaculture is much higher, for example, about 12 to 15 tons/ha/year in carp culture.

Super-Intensive Level: Super intensive aquaculture needs running water supply and complete daily water exchange is performed. This system is mostly practiced in cement tanks, fiberglass tanks and raceways etc. which are fitted with high efficiency biological filters for continues recirculation of water. The size of the tank ranges between 50-100m^3. The cultured organisms are fed with high quality formulated feed. The feed is given through demand feeders. The water quality is regularly monitored with electronic gadgets. Stocking density ranges between 40,000 to 50,000 carp fingerlings/ha. The production ranges between 15-20 tons/ ha/yr in case of carps.

Untapped Potential

- Only one third of freshwater aquaculture and 13% of brackish water resources have been utilized for aquaculture
- Average yield – 2.2 tons/ ha/ yr based on FFDA ponds
- Reservoirs fisheries is highly under-utilized (Av. annual yield – only 20 Kg/ ha)
- Semi-intensive primary production based aquaculture of low – valued food fish has the potential to be adopted by millions of small holders
- At micro-level fish and livestock farming are key source of income and buffer against food insecurity

Objectives for Aquaculture Development

- Commercialization of aquaculture for maximization of production
- Food and nutritional security
- Export earnings
- Employment Generation
- Poverty reduction through livelihood development

Important Cultural Practices of Aquaculture

- Composite fish culture
- Integrated farming system
- Raceway culture
- Cage culture
- Pen culture

Composite Fish Culture

A fish pond is a complex ecosystem as the surface is occupied by the floating organisms such as phyto and zoo plankton; the column region has live and dead organic matter sunk from the surface and the bottom is enriched with detritus or dead organic matter. The marginal areas harbor a variety of aquatic vegetation. The different trophic levels of a pond could be utilized for increasing the profitability of fish culture. Keeping this in mind, the concept of Composite fish culture has been developed. The main objective of this culture system is to select and grow compatible species of fish of different feeding habits to exploit all the types of food available in the different nook and corners of the fish pond for maximizing fish production (New 1995, Gupta et al 2011, Gupta et al 2016).The common species of carps having compatibility and different feeding habits and which comes under composite fish culture are Indian major carps such as catla, rohu and mrigal and exotic carps such as common carp, silver carp and grass carp.

Integrated Farming System

Here, otherwise waste output of one enterprise can be utilized as inputs for other enterprise.

- Wastes/by products produced through agriculture are consumed by cattle and fishes and converted to proteins that build up animal flesh.
- Water from fish ponds can be used as inputs for agriculture/horticulture crops as well as for veterinary enterprises. Mud from fish ponds can be utilized as organic fertilizer for agriculture/horticulture crops.
- All the wastes from veterinary enterprises are utilized as inputs for aquaculture and agriculture.

Cage Culture

Cage aquaculture is a method used for raising aquatic organisms (fish, prawns, molluscs, crabs etc.) within an enclosure, which is installed in suspended state in ponds, reservoirs, lakes, rivers or any other large size water body. In India, it is initiated with the raising of fry (20-25 mm) to advance fingerlings (100-150mm) in water bodies/reservoirs to increase their production. Cages can be of various shapes and sizes. Rectangular cages are however, preferred for easy operation and management.

Pen Culture

Aquaculture in pens implies rising of required aquatic organisms (fish, prawn, molluscs etc.) in an enclosure which is formed by cordoning off areas of an open water body such as inter-tidal areas of the sea or fore shore waters of lakes, reservoirs, river, wet lands etc by net barriers.

Pens are generally constructed on the shore side, in semi-circular, rectangular or square shapes as per the suitability of the site. They are constructed by barricading the other three sides by a wall of nylon netting hung from poles driven to the bottom. The framework is generally made out of bamboo and other locally available wood.

Raceway Culture

Raceways are designed to provide a flow through system to enable the culture/rearing of much denser population of aquatic animals. An abundant flow of good quality, well oxygenated water is essential to provide respiratory needs and to flush out metabolic wastes, particularly ammonia. Raceways are obviously smaller in size than ponds and occupy much less space. Site selection for a raceway farm has to be done with special care. Naturally the most important consideration is the water supply. The main source of water is springs, streams, deep wells and/or lakes.

Future Needs/ Strategies

- ☆ Stocking of yearlings / overwintered fingerlings
- ☆ Making best use of warmer period
- ☆ Periodical harvesting
- ☆ Stocking of species in demand and price
- ☆ Develop Complementarities among the various farming practices
- ☆ Production of low valued carps as well as high valued fish to fulfill the gap between demand and supply
- ☆ Strengthening of domestic markets
- ☆ Develop Aquaculture as the main source of rural livelihoods and income generation
- ☆ Production enhancement through Aquaculture
- ☆ Provision of training and education in Aquaculture
- ☆ Optimum utilization of resources for sustainable increasing production
- ☆ Identification of water bodies/stretches for conservation and replenishment of depleted stocks through ranching
- ☆ Restoration and regular stocking of fingerlings in floodplain wetlands and other natural water bodies
- ☆ Increase the rearing area by establishing more seed rearing units, pen and cage culture systems
- ☆ Strengthening of welfare schemes for the upliftment of community
- ☆ Human resource development in the sector.

Transforming Rural Areas through Veterinary Science *Pages* ***161-168***
Editor: Dipanjali Konwar, Shilpa Sood & Shahid Ahamad
Published by: **ASTRAL INTERNATIONAL PVT. LTD., NEW DELHI**

12 Mitigation of Climatic Stress and Technologies to Reduce Greenhouse Gas Emissions from Livestock

Dr. Jafrin Ara Ahmed & Dr. Nawab Nashiruddullah

Climate duress or the threat of climate change and global warming is now recognised worldwide. Global climate change is primarily caused by greenhouse gas (GHG) emissions that result in warming of the atmosphere (IPCC, 2013). The livestock sector contributes 14.5% of global GHG emissions (Gerber *et al.*, 2013). Climate change will affect livestock production through competition for natural resources, quantity and quality of feeds, livestock diseases, heat stress and biodiversity loss while the demand for livestock products is expected to increase by 100% by mid of the 21st century (Garnett, 2009). Therefore, the challenge is to maintain a balance between productivity, household food security, and environmental preservation (Wright *et al.*, 2004). There is growing interest in understanding the interaction of climate change and agricultural production and it is motivating a significant amount of research (Aydinalp and Cresser, 2008).

Adaptation and Mitigation Practices

Adaptation measures involve production and management system modifications, breeding strategies, institutional and policy changes, science and technology advances, and changing farmers' perception and adaptive capacity.

1. Livestock Production and Management Systems

An adaptation such as the modification of production and management systems involves diversification of animals and crops, integration of livestock systems with forestry and crop production. Improving feeding practices include modification of diets composition, changing feeding time or frequency as an adaptation measure could indirectly improve the efficiency of livestock production.

Mixed farming depends on the management of different feed resources and animal species. A region can consist of individual specialized farms and service systems that together act as a mixed system. The integration of livestock, fish and crops has proved to be a sustainable system through centuries of experience in Asian countries. For example, the integration of fishpond production with ducks, geese, chickens, sheep, cattle or pigs increased fish production by 2 to 3.9 times (Chen, 1996), while there were added ecological and economic benefits of fish utilizing animal wastes. Environmentally sound integration is ensured where livestock droppings and feed waste can be poured directly into the pond to constitute feed for fish and zooplankton. Livestock manure can be used to fertilize grass or other plant growth that can also constitute feed for fish. Vegetables can be irrigated from the fishponds, and their residues and by-products can be used for feeding livestock.

Grazing of livestock under plantation trees such a form of crop-livestock integration that is often found in Southeast Asia. The integration of livestock to utilize the vegetative ground cover under the tree canopy increased overall production and saved the cost of weed control and herbicides. The best integrated mixed farming is probably the mixed crop-livestock systems. Cropping in this case provides animals with fodder from grass and nitrogen-binding legumes, leys (improved fallow with sown legumes, grasses or trees), weeds and crop residues. Animals graze under trees or on stubble, they provide draught and manure for crops, while they also serve as a savings account.

2. Breeding Strategies

Changes in breeding strategies can help animals increase their tolerance to heat stress and diseases and improve their reproduction and growth development. The challenge is in increasing livestock production while maintaining the valuable adaptations offered by breeding strategies. Policy measures that improve adaptive capacity by facilitating implementation of adaptation strategies will be crucial.

3. Farmers' Perception and Adaptive Capacity

Common farmers are not capable to recognize climate change problem and mitigation measures. It is important to collect information about farmers' perceptions to mitigation and adaptation measures. One approach for collecting information about farmers' perceptions that has been used for mitigation and adaptation research is qualitative; using open-ended survey questions or group discussion at workshops to understand individual and group opinions. By understanding farmers' perceptions and including them in rural policy development, there is a greater chance of accomplishing food security and environmental conservation.

4. Mitigation Measures

a. Carbon Sequestration

Carbon sequestration is the process involved in carbon capture and the long-term storage of atmospheric carbon dioxide or other forms of carbon to mitigate or defer global warming. Carbon sequestration can be achieved-

- ☆ Through decreasing deforestation rates, reversing of deforestation by replanting, targeting for higher-yielding crops with better climate change adapted varieties, and improvement of land and water management.
- ☆ Restoring soil organic carbon in cultivated soils through conservation tillage, erosion reduction, soil acidity management, double-cropping, crop rotations, higher crop residues, mulching and more.
- ☆ Improving pasture management by incorporating trees, improving plant species, legume interseeding, introducing earthworms and fertilization
- ☆ By increasing grazing pasture in grasslands that have a lower amount of grazing animals than the livestock carrying capacity

b. Enteric Fermentation

Enteric fermentation is a source of methane emissions that can be reduced through practices such as improvement of animal nutrition and genetics eg. practices for mitigating enteric fermentation are: increasing dietary fat content, providing higher quality forage, increasing protein content, providing supplements (*e.g.* bovine somatotropin, feed antibiotics) and the use of antimethanogens vaccines to suppress methane emissions. Reduction in total and emissions intensity plus increased animal performance can be achieved by feeding supplements that contain levels of lipid to increase dietary concentration of lipids to 6–8% (Grainger *et al.* 2008). Lipids and potentially other supplements that may reduce emissions (e.g. tannins, saponins) can be applied year-round in feedlots and dairy farms where scope exists to modify animal diets on a daily basis. Manipulating microbial populations in the rumen, through chemical means by introducing competitive or predatory microbes, or through vaccination approaches, can reduce methane production. Bacteria introduced to detoxify mimosine in cattle grazing leaucaena have been shown to maintain activity in the herd over 25 years (Jones et al. 2009), and if such persistence and efficacy can be achieved by exogenous reductive acetogens or methane-oxidising organisms on introduction to the rumen, their use as microbial additives may provide a cost-effective mitigation strategy. Ecological change by eliminating organisms from the rumen rather than introducing new organisms can also have long-term impact, with some studies showing that sheep rendered free of protozoa may remain free for 3 years (Bird and Leng 1985). However, defaunation does not always persist or lead to reduced enteric emissions (Bird et al. 2008). The changes in animal productivity associated with these techniques or interventions such as vaccination against methanogens (Wedlock et al. 2010) require further research before consideration as practical mitigation options. Upon vaccination, anti-methanogen antibodies were found in the serum of vaccinated sheep (Wedlock et al. 2010). The first two anti-methanogen vaccines were prepared from whole cells of three and seven selected methanogens in Australia, and these vaccines resulted in no or minimal (only 8% compared to control) decrease in CH4emission (*Wright* et al. 2004). The inefficacy was attributed to the small numbers of methanogen species that the vaccines could target. However, methanogen abundance or CH4 production was not decreased by vaccination using a vaccine that was based on a mixture of five methanogen species representing >52% of the rumen methanogen populations, though the composition of methanogens was altered (*Williams et al.* 2009). It was suggested that anti-methanogen vaccines should be developed based on cell surface proteins that are conserved among rumen methanogens to achieve effective results (*Wedlock et al.* 2013). It should be noted that most antibodies circulate in the blood of a host, and only a tiny amount can enter the rumen through saliva. The amount of antibodies entering the rumen is probably too small to have any effect. Also, antibodies entering the rumen can be rapidly degraded by proteolytic bacteria therein. It stands to reason that vaccination may not be a feasible approach to mitigate CH4 emission from livestock. Routine interventions and feed supplements are difficult or impossible to administer in extensive grazing systems. This severely restricts the use of anti-methanogenic feedstuffs (*e.g.* fats and oils) and feed additives (*e.g.* monensin). Possibilities exist for administering anti-methanogenic compounds in the water supply, in protein/energy/mineral feed blocks and licks, and via drought-fed supplements, but all these options are at the experimental or demonstration stages of development. Reducing emissions intensity per animal through improved efficiency resulting from management change does present a dilemma. Raising cattle more efficiently can enable a property manager to increase stocking rate in response to economic imperatives (Rolfe 2010). Thus, although emissions intensity will decline, emissions per hectare will increase. On a global scale this may be positive as the proportion of low emissions beef in the global supply increases. Alternatively, if carbon sequestration (*e.g.* from woody re-growth occurring in grazed woodlands previously cleared to increase grass production) could also act as an alternative revenue stream, overall profitability could be sustained and carbon balance improved through optimising cattle and carbon production across the landscape (Bray and Willcocks 2009; Donaghy et al. 2010). However, it should be noted that increased carbon sequestration in woody biomass is finite and ceases once the woody vegetation reaches a new biomass plateau, usually within 20–30 years (Donaghy et al. 2010).

Methane is generated in the rumen by methanogenic archaea that utilise hydrogen to reduce CO_2, and is a significant electron sink in the rumen ecosystem. However, reductive aceto genesis has been suggested as an alternative. Not only does this reduce or nullify methane emissions, it can also supply a considerable proportion of the energy needs of the animals. If methane was wholly replaced by acetate in cattle and sheep this would represent an energetic gain of 4 - 15% to the animal. In Australia, marsupials had evolved to fill the niche occupied predominantly by sheep and cattle elsewhere, and like the ruminants, kangaroos developed an enlarged complex forestomach for fermentation of plant material. However, unlike sheep and cattle, kangaroos emit very little methane and appear to possess an alternative mechanism to methanogenesis although their digestive process is analogous to sheep and cattle.

c. Manure Management

Manure is the second largest source of greenhouse gas (GHG) emissions from dairy farms. Livestock urine and manure are significant sources of methane and nitrous oxide when broken down under anaerobic conditions. Most methane emissions from manure management are related to storage and anaerobic treatment. Therefore, most mitigation practices involve shortening storage duration, improving timing and application of manure, used of anaerobic digesters, covering the storage, using a solids separator, and changing the animal diets. Liquid manure found in lagoons or holding tanks releases more methane than dry manure. Pig manure comprises almost half of global manure-related methane emissions. N_2O emissions from manure storage are dependent on environmental conditions, handling systems, and duration of waste management. Manure must be handled aerobically and then anaerobically to release N_2O emissions, which is more likely to occur in dry waste-handling systems. Nitrous oxide is produced during the nitrification–denitrification of the nitrogen contained in livestock waste. Anaerobic conditions often occur where manure is stored in large piles or settlement ponds to deal with waste from large numbers of animals managed in a confined area (for example, dairy farms, beef feedlots, piggeries and poultry farms). Ruminants excrete 75–95% of the nitrogen they ingest. Ruminants on lush spring pasture commonly ingest protein (containing nitrogen) in excess of their requirements but are usually energy limited, resulting in higher ruminal ammonia concentrations being excreted in the urine as urea. Nitrous oxide emissions from ruminants can be minimised by balancing the protein-to-energy ratios in their diets.

Measures to Reduce Livestock Urinary Nitrogen

- ☆ For improved nitrogen efficiency –breeding of animals
- ☆ Using forages that have a higher energy-to-protein ratio
- ☆ Balancing high protein forages with high-energy supplements.

Measures to Reduce Greenhouse Gas Emissions from Livestock Manure

- ☆ Manure stockpile aeration and composting reduces methane emissions
- ☆ Adding urease inhibitors to manure stockpiles can reduce nitrous oxide emissions

Measures to Capture and Use Methane

Livestock industries have shown increased interest in biogas (methane) capture-and-use systems, such as covered ponds and the flaring or combustion of the captured biogas to provide heat or power. The goal is to turn the manure into products such as electricity, fuel, fiber and fertilizers which reduces methane emissions, conserves natural resources and also our dependence on fossil fuels. This benefits not only farmers, but also corporations, communities, and the environment

d. Fertilizer Management

Fertilizer application on animal feed crops increases nitrous oxide emissions Therefore, mitigation measures such as increasing nitrogen use efficiency, plant breeding and genetic modifications, using organic fertilizers, using technologically advanced fertilizers, and combining legumes with grasses in pasture areas may decrease GHG emissions in feed production. Nitrogen use efficiency can be improved by applying the required amount that the crop will absorb and when it needs the nutrients, and placing it where the plant can easily reach it. Regular soil testing can be a part of a nutrient management plan depending on the region and crop, and improve efficiency of nitrogen use (Dickie *et al.*, 2014). Plant breeding and genetic modifications can reduce the use of fertilizers by increasing a crop's nitrogen uptake (Dickie *et al.*, 2014). Increasing the use of organic fertilizers would also decrease emissions because organic fertilizers do not produce as much nitrogen oxide as synthetic fertilizers (Denef *et al.*, 2011). Furthermore, fertilizer technology has improved through regulating the release of nutrients from the fertilizer and inhibiting nitrification to slow the degradation of the fertilizer and maintain the nutrients available for the plant.

References

Aydinalp C. and Cresser M.S. (2008), The effects of climate change on agriculture, Agric. Environ. Sci., 5: 672-676

Bird S.H. and Leng R.A. (1985) Productivity responses to eliminating protozoa from the rumen of sheep. In 'Reviews in rural science: biotechnology and recombinant DNA technology in the animal production industries'. pp. 109–117. (Eds RA Leng, JSF Barker, DB Adams, KJ Hutchinson) (University of New England: Armidale, NSW)

Bird S.H., Hegarty R.S., Woodgate R. (2008). Persistence of defaunation effects on digestion and methane production in ewes. Australian Journal of Experimental Agriculture, 48: 152–155. doi:10.1071/EA07298

Bray S. and Willcocks J. (2009) Net carbon position of the Queensland beef industry. Queensland Department of Primary Industries and Fisheries, Brisbane, Qld.

Burke D. (2001) Dairy Waste Anaerobic Digestion Handbook, Environmental Energy Company, Washington

Chen H., Hayakawa H., Sasaki M. and K. Kimura.(1996) Integrated systems of animal production in the Asian region. Proceedings of a symposium held in conjunction with the 8th AAAP Animal Science Congress, Chiba, Japan, 13-18 October. AAAP and FAO, Rome.

Denef, K., Archibeque, S. and Paustian, K. (2011). Greenhouse gas emissions from U.S. agriculture and forestry: A review of emission sources, controlling factors, and mitigation potential: Interim report to USDA under Contract #GS-23F-8182H.

Dickie A., Streck, C., Roe S., Zurek, M., Haupt F. and Dolginow A.(2014) Strategies for mitigating climate change in agriculture: Abridged report. Climate focus and california environmental associates, prifadred with the support of the climate and land use Alliance.

Donaghy P., Bray S., Gowen R., Rolfe J., Stephens M., Hoffman M. and Stunzner A. (2010) The bioeconomic potential for agroforestry in Australia's northern grazing systems. Small-scale Forestry 9: 463–484. doi:10.1007/s11842- 010-9126-y

Garnett T. (2009), Livestock-related greenhouse gas emissions: impacts and options for policymakers, Environ. Sci. Policy, 12: 491-50

Gerber P.J., Steinfeld H., Henderson B., Mottet A., Opio C., Dijkman J., Falcucci A. and Tempio Tackling G. (2013) Climate Change Through Livestock: A Global Assessment of Emissions and Mitigation Opportunities FAO, Rome

Grainger C., Clarke T., Beauchemin K.A., McGinn S.M. and Eckard R.J. (2008) Supplementation with whole cottonseed reduces methane emissions and can profitably increase milk production of dairy cows offered a forage and cereal grain diet. Australian Journal of Experimental Agriculture 48: 73–76. doi:10.1071/EA07224

IPCC (Intergovermental Panel on Climate Change) (2013).Climate change: The physical science basis. T. F. Stocker, D. Qin, G. K. Plattner, M. Tignor, S.K. Allen, J. Boschung, A. Nauels, Y. Xia, V. Bex, P.M. Midgley (Eds.), Contribution of Working Group I to the Fifth Assessment Report of the Intergovernmental Panel on Climate Change, Cambridge University Press, Cambridge, United Kingdom and New York, NY, USA , p. 1535

Jones R.J.B., Coates D.B. and Palmer B. (2009) Survival of the rumen bacterium Synergistes jonesii in a herd of Droughtmaster cattle in north Queensland. Animal Production Science 49: 643–645. doi:10.1071/EA08274

Rolfe J. (2010) Economics of reducing methane emissions from beef cattle in extensive grazing systems in Queensland. The Rangeland Journal 32: 197–204. doi:10.1071/RJ09026

Wedlock D., Janssen P., Leahy S., Shu D. and Buddle B. (2013). Progress in the development of vaccines against rumen methanogens. Animal. 7: 244–52.

Wedlock D., Pedersen G., Denis M., Dey D., Janssen P. and Buddle B. (2010). Development of a vaccine to mitigate greenhouse gas emissions in agriculture: Vaccination of sheep with methanogen fractions induces antibodies that block methane production in vitro. N Z Vet J. 58: 29–36

Williams Y.J., Popovski S., Rea S.M., Skillman L.C., Toovey A.F. and Northwood K.S. (2009). A vaccine against rumen methanogens can alter the composition of archaeal populations. Appl Environ Microbiol.75:1860–6

Wright A., Kennedy P., O'Neill C., Toovey A., Popovski S. and Rea S. (2004). Reducing methane emissions in sheep by immunization against rumen methanogens. Vaccine.22:3976–85.

Wright I.A., Tarawali S., Blummel M., Gerard B., Teufel N. and Herrero M. (2012), Integrating crops and livestock in subtropical agricultural systems. J. Sci. Food Agric., 92: 1010-1015

Transforming Rural Areas through Veterinary Science *Pages* **169-184**
Editor: Dipanjali Konwar, Shilpa Sood & Shahid Ahamad
Published by: **ASTRAL INTERNATIONAL PVT. LTD., NEW DELHI**

13 Livestock Sector: Contribution and Challenges in Indian Agricultural System

Dr. Anish Yadav, Dr. Pallavi Khajuria, Dr. Shafiya Imtiaz Rafiqui, Dr. Rajesh Godara & Dr. Rajesh Katoch

Animal husbandry is an integral component of Indian agriculture supporting livelihood of more than two-thirds of the rural population. Veterinary science is a multi-disciplinary subject which includes research on diagnosis, control, prevention and treatment of animal diseases as well as on the basic zoology, welfare, and care of animals. All activities of animal science essentially affect human health either directly through biomedical research and public health or indirectly by addressing domestic animal, wildlife, or environmental health. Veterinary research at a fundamental level is a human health activity. Veterinary scientists protect the human health and well-being by ensuring food security and safety, preventing and controlling emerging infectious zoonoses, protecting environment and ecosystem, assisting in bioterrorism and agro-terrorism preparedness, advancing treatment and control of nonzoonotic diseases, contributing to public health, and engaging in medical research. The introduction of the concept of 'One Health' which takes a holistic approach to address human, animal, and ecosystem health, again emphasizes the role of a veterinarian as a leader in present society by addressing the risk and emergence of zoonotic diseases and promoting basic health care needs of the world. Thus, veterinary professionals are key players on bio defense, and thus for national security, food chain safety, and animal and human welfare.

Livestock Sector and its Contribution in Indian Economy

Out of the total livestock in the country, around 38.2 percent are cattle, 20.2 percent are buffaloes, 12.7 percent are sheep, 25.6 percent are goats and only 2.8 percent are pigs. All other animals are less than 0.50 percent of the total livestock population. The composition of livestock population in broad groups like bovine (cattle and buffaloes), ovine (sheep and goats), pigs and poultry, however, has changed over the last two decades. Cattle population that had been increasing until 1992 has started declining and between 1992 and 2003, it declined by 9 percent. The decline in the cattle population is confined to indigenous stock that comprised 87 percent of the total cattle population in 2003. The number of indigenous cattle declined by 15 percent, while that of the crossbred increased by 62 percent. Within the indigenous stock, decline was drastic for males (22%). The main reasons for decline in indigenous cattle population are increasing substitution of draught animals with mechanical power and low milk yield (Birthal and Taneja 2006). The buffalo population has increased from 70 million in 1982 to 98 million in 2003. There has been a small decrease in total bovines in the country by 1.9% between 1997 and 2003. Livestock population as per 19th Livestock Census, 2012 is shown in table below:

<table>
<tr><th>S.No.</th><th>Species</th><th>Population</th><th>Percent Share in World's Livestock</th></tr>
<tr><td>1</td><td>Cattle</td><td>190.9 million</td><td>12.5(Second)</td></tr>
<tr><td>2</td><td>Buffalo</td><td>108.7 million</td><td>56.7(First)</td></tr>
<tr><td>3</td><td>Sheep</td><td>65 million</td><td rowspan="2">2.1</td></tr>
<tr><td>4</td><td>Goat</td><td>135.1 million</td></tr>
<tr><td>5</td><td>Pig</td><td>10.29 million</td><td>1.5</td></tr>
<tr><td>6</td><td>Poultry</td><td>729.2 million</td><td>3.1(fifth)</td></tr>
</table>

*(19th **Livestock Census**, 2012, Source : Department of Animal Husbandry, Dairying & Fisheries, Min. of Agri. GoI.)*

Livestock sector plays a multi-faceted role in socio-economic development of rural households. Livestock rearing has significant positive impact on equity in terms of income and employment and poverty reduction in rural areas as distribution of livestock is more egalitarian as compared to land. In India, over 70 percent of the rural households own livestock and a majority of livestock owning households are small, marginal and landless households. Small animals like sheep, goats, pigs and poultry are largely kept by the land scarce poor households for commercial purposes due to their low initial investment and operational costs. In the recent decade, demand for various livestock based products has increased significantly due to increase in per capita income, urbanization, taste and preference and increased awareness about food nutrition. Livestock sector is likely to emerge as an engine for agricultural growth in the coming decades. It is also considered as a potential sector for export earnings. The importance of livestock goes beyond its food production function (Birthal *et.al* 2002). Livestock sector supplements income from crop production and other sources and absorbs income shocks due to crop failure. It generates a continuous stream of income and employment and reduces seasonality in livelihood patterns particularly of the rural poor (Birthal and Ali 2005). Livestock plays an important role in Indian economy. About 20.5 million people depend upon livestock for their livelihood. Livestock contributed 16% to the income of small farm households as against an average of 14% for all rural households. Livestock provides livelihood to two-third of rural community. It also provides employment to about 8.8 % of the population in India. India has vast livestock resources. Livestock contributes about 40 percent of agricultural GDP. Rapid growth and technological innovation have led to profound improvement in the management of livestock sector, including: a progressive leap from small-holder farming systems towards large-scale specialised industrial production systems; a shift in the geographic locus of demand and supply in the developing world; and an increasing emphasis on global marketing. These changes have put forth the implications for the ability of the livestock sector to expand the production in sustainable ways that promote food security, and public health as well as reduce poverty. The speed of change has often significantly outpaced the capacity of governments and societies to provide the necessary policy and regulations, to ensure an appropriate balance between the provision of private and public goods. The result has been systemic failures apparent in social exclusion, widespread environmental damage and threats to human health. The exponential increase in the fauna population has led to serious implications for the availability, use and management of land and water, forests, and wildlife resources. The change in climate and ecosystems, and the greater human contact with wild animals have resulted in an increased exposure to new disease-carrying vectors and pathogens. The higher density of domestic animals and humans has created a conducive environment for existing and emerging pathogens, and the projected increase in movement of people and animals have increased opportunities for the exchange of pathogens worldwide (FAO, 2010).

In the vast semi-arid or arid areas where crop production is extremely risky, livestock can use vegetation that would otherwise be wasted and convert it to valuable, high-quality products. However, these are environmentally fragile areas. Over the centuries, pastoralists established complex management systems that were sustainable until the relatively recent dramatic increase in population and subsequent livestock density. Overgrazing is the main threat to these areas, and a holistic approach to resource management is necessary to avoid their permanent and irreversible degradation. Crop residues, such as straw, are more efficiently utilized through ruminant feeding, including the production and use of manure and possibly biogas, rather than by burning them, creating pollution and contributing to global warming, or ploughing them back into the soil to improve its structure and water retention. Several hundred million head of cattle and buffaloes are fed throughout the year on rice and cereal straws. Livestock, particularly sheep, are efficient in controlling weeds. They are used in many countries in the Mediterranean basin to reduce forest undergrowth so that the risk of fire during summer is diminished.

Nutrient recycling is an essential component of any sustainable farming system. The integration of livestock and crops allows for efficient nutrient recycling. Animals use the crop residues, such as cereal straws, as well as maize and sorghum stovers and groundnut haulms as feed. The manure produced can be recycled directly as fertilizer. One tonne of cow dung contains about 8 kg N. 4 kg P_2O_5 and 16 kg K_2O

(Ange, 1994). The chemical composition of manure varies, however, according to the animal species (poultry manure appears to be a more efficient fertilizer than cow manure) and also to the nature of their diet. Biogas production from manure is an excellent substitute for fossil fuel or fuelwood for farmers in tropical countries. The best manure for these purposes comes from (in descending order) pigs, cattle, horses, camels and poultry (Kumar and Biswas, 1982). On-farm biogas production reduces the workload of women by eliminating wood collection or fuel purchasing. It is person-friendly because of its convenience and increased hygiene, and it also provides a number of services, such as lighting, warm water and heating. Biogas can also be used to drive machinery such as water pumps. Effluent from biodigesters can be recycled as fertilizer - with even better results than the original manure (Talukder, Ali and Latif, 1988) - or as a fish feed, or it may be used to grow azolla and duckweed.

Bovines, equines, camelids and elephants are all used as sources of draught power for a variety of purposes, such as pulling agricultural implements, pumping irrigation water and skidding in forests. The current number of animals used for draught purposes is estimated at 400 million. Fifty-two percent of the cultivated area in developing countries (excluding China) is farmed using only draught animals and 26 percent using only hand tools (Gifford 1992). During the past ten years, there has been a 23-percent increase in the number of cattle and buffaloes used for draught purposes as well as for meat and milk production. During the same period, the number of equines (horses, mules and asses) used primarily for draught and transport has not changed significantly. Compared with the use of tractors, animal power is a renewable energy source in many developing countries and is produced on the farm, with almost all the implements required made locally. On the other hand, 90 percent of the world's tractors and their implements are produced in industrialized countries and most of those used in developing countries (approximately 19 percent) have to be imported. Animal traction, therefore, avoids the drain of foreign exchange involved in the importation of tractors, spare parts and fuel. Draught animals remain the most cost-effective power source for small and medium-scale farmers. Draught animal power can be even more economic when one bullock is used instead of a pair or when a (cross-bred) cow is used instead of a male, since it reduces the cost of maintaining the larger herd necessary to satisfy both replacement and milk production requirements.

At farm level, dairying is a labour-intensive activity, involving women in both production and marketing. Labour typically accounts for over 40 percent of total costs in smallholder systems. It has been estimated that for each 6 to 10 kg of additional milk processed per day in India, one working day is added for feeding and care. Goat, sheep, poultry and rabbit husbandry, especially in backyard production systems, provides an important source of part-time job opportunities, particularly for landless women and children. The livestock-product processing sector has also been identified as a contributor to employment generation and the reduction of rural depopulation. Small-scale milk processing/marketing is labour-intensive (50 to 100 kg per working day) and generates employment and income from the local manufacture of at least part of the equipment required. The meat sector also provides significant employment opportunities. But the sector has remained under-invested; and neglected by the financial and extension institutions. Livestock markets are under-developed, which is a significant barrier to the commercialization of livestock production. Besides, the sector will also come under significant pressure of increasing globalization of agri-food markets. Milk production is continuously increasing since the initiation of operation flood in the early seventies on account of improved technological changes and creation of market linkages between rural producers and urban consumers through the network of dairy cooperatives (Birthal and Taneja 2006). Yet the productivity is low as compared to many other countries and the world average. Buffalo and cow are important milch species with a share of 55 and 43 percent respectively in total milk output, and goats account for the rest. The milk production grew at a rate of 4.4 percent per annum during the period of 1980-2003. Growth in total milk production, however, declined marginally from 5.3 percent during 1980s to 4.5 percent during 1991-2003.

The growth in meat production has been faster as compared to milk production. Total meat production in the country has increased from 0.9 million tonnes in 1980-81 to 5.9 million tonnes in 2003-04 at an annual rate of 9.3 percent. In early 1980s small ruminants were the major suppliers (44%) of meat, followed by large ruminants (35%), and poultry (19%). The meat production structure however changed drastically during 1990s; monogastrics (poultry and pigs), especially poultry, emerged as the most important meat supplier with significant share of 27 percent in 2003-04. It may be noted that growth in meat production has largely been driven by the increase in number of animals slaughtered as the yield growth was negligible in case of almost all the species. Recent trends, however, indicate improvements in meat yield of cattle, buffalo and sheep, and a decline in meat yield of goat and pig (Birthal and Taneja 2006).

Egg production in the country has increased from 10.06 billion numbers in 1980-81 to 40.4 billion numbers in 2003-04. During 1980-2003, egg production has increased at the rate of 5.8 percent a year. Genetic improvement efforts have contributed substantially to this. About two third of the total egg production in the country, come from improved layers. Average egg yield of an improved layer is 232 eggs/ annum, which is more than double the yield of an indigenous layer. Clearly, there is considerable scope for increasing egg production through substitution of indigenous layers with the improved layers. The average yield of eggs in India is higher than the world average and average yield in developing countries but it is slightly lower than the average yield in developed countries.

Wool production in India has increased from 32.0 million kg in 1980-81 to 48.5 million kg in 2003-04. Annual growth in wool production was 1.7 percent per annum during 1980-2003, which was much lower as compared to annual growth in other livestock products. Domestically produced wool is poorly suited to garment production and fine wool is generally imported from Australia (World Bank, 1999). The wool and hair produced in India mostly with a diameter greater than 30 microns is used for furnishings, carpets and industrial fabrics. The production level of wool in the country is much lower than the existing demand in the wool processing industry.

Challenges and Opportunities in Livestock Sector

i) Germplasm Improvement: India had a very large population of indigenous cows and breedable buffaloes. However majority of them are nondescript low producing animals. Crossbred cows have a good potential for milk production but there is problem of inadequate feeding and management. A new breeding programme - " National Cattle and Buffaloe breeding programme" has been taken by the Government of India with massive financial assistance to the state Livestock Development Boards).Since last several years, massive programmes have been taken up for cross-breeding of local non-descript cattle mainly utilizing semen of two exotic breeds namely Holstein Friesian (for irrigated areas and for farmers with adequate fodder resources) and Jersey (for dry/hilly areas and farmers having low fodder resources). In case of buffaloes the programme is for upgrading of local buffaloes using semen of better dairy breeds like Murrah, Mehasana etc. It is observed that the overall field results of crossbreeding with artificial insemination (A.I.) are still not very satisfactory. For example data of 17 million inseminations done through a large network of about 43782 A.I. centers showed that the number of calves born were only 15% of A.I. done in the field. Only about 10% of the breedable buffaloes were covered by A.I., the rest being covered by natural insemination service from locally available bulls for whom correct pedigree history was not available. Buffalo is the major contributor to India's milk production. Therefore more emphasis is required on buffalo development. Also there is need to improve overall efficiency of bull breeding farms, semen stations, A.I. service including delivery of semen and liquid nitrogen. There is need to select better quality breeding bulls for distribution in the field and introduction of a bull calf rearing scheme by providing incentives to a farmer to purchase and rear a bull calf produced by a high milk yielding dam owned by from an identified breeder farmer. Testing of breeding bulls for possibility of their being carriers of communicable reproductive diseases is necessary. NGOs, progressive farmers as future trainers can be chosen and trained for modern management practices for rearing of dairy animals. Paravets or educated unemployed local village youth for A.I. service and veterinary first aid can also play an important role. Farmers should be taught and encouraged to keep proper breeding records of animals in farm.

ii) **Feed and Fodder Development:** The agrarian economy of the region is fully dependent on agriculture and related activities as clearly revealed by the utilization of land resource in the region. Fodder crop plays vital role in rearing of livestock. Fodder crops are mainly cultivated in kharif (87%) followed by rabi (90%) and jayad (45%). India is the largest producer of milk the world. India covers about one fifth of livestock population of the world, but the milk productivity per milch animal is very low. Almost 70% of arable land is dry or rainfed land having an erratic rainfall, and poor productivity of cereal grains resulting into low output of dry fodder. As a result of rising human population, there is a tremendous pressure on land for its utilization for construction of human housing, roads and industries. The land holdings per farmer -household are getting fragmented and reduced. As and when irrigation facilities are available, the farmers tend to take cash crops and value-added crops. The land for fodder cultivation and availability is a last priority.The cattle population and therefore the demand for fodder is increasing every year. All the above issues have adversely affected the fodder balance for milk production. There is tremendous overall shortage of fodder availability against the nutritional demand for dairy cattle. Crop residues and other cellulosic materials are staple feeds for dairy animals in India. The most abundant residues are cereal straws, sugarcane tops, sugarcane bagasse, pulse straws, millet straws, etc. These feeds are unable to meet the maintenance requirement of animals because of the low digestibility, influenced by high fibre, lignin and silica content.

Supplementation of crop residues with fresh grasses and legumes or concentrate feeds significantly improves feed intake and the performance of animals. Feeding wheat straw with berseem or lucerne is common practice in the Northern region of the country. In dryland farming systems where forages are scarce, crop residues are supplemented with concentrate feeds. Supplementation of the basal diet with good quality forage or concentrates helps to overcome the problem of low palatability. The role of agro-forestry systems in augmenting the supply of green forage needs to be emphasized to farmers. Treating crop residues with 4 percent urea and 45-50 percent moisture improves the nutritive value by increasing digestibility, palatability and crude protein content. The process is simple and can easily be practised by the farmers. Feeding treated wheat straw supplemented with berseem (90:10 mixture on a dry matter basis) ad lib. has shown to support a milk production level of 6 kg/ head/day without concentrates (Agarwal *et al.*, 1988). However urea treatment is not yet used on a wide scale by farmers because of inadequate extension efforts to popularise the technology and the limited availability of liquid cash for farmers to purchase urea.

iii) **Production and Marketing of Milk:** Most of the milk in India is produced in villages. Quantity of milk produced per household is very small. About 56% of milk is available as marketable surplus for urban areas. Fairly large quantity of milk is converted to local milk products (khoa, paneer, butter, ghee etc). The share of organized sector is small (private-11-12%, Government/cooperative sector - 11-12%).There is still a very large portion of milk market in the hands of unorganized sector which has adverse effect on the farm-gate price of the milk. In Government/ cooperative sector, almost 80% milk is marketed as liquid milk and only 20% as milk products. While it is reverse in the private sector - only 30% is marketed as liquid milk and 70% as milk products with value addition.

In absence of properly developed infrastructure for preservation of raw milk in local areas many plants in Govt. sector collect fresh raw milk from the far-flung rural areas (each producer having very small quantities) twice a day , send it over a long distance to towns for processing, incurring high cost on transportation. This erodes the profitability. As a result, many plants have become uneconomical, non-functional or they are working much below their potential capacities. Alternative strategies need to be developed to store raw milk in bulk coolers in the rural area and transport it in bigger volumes at a longer intervals. There is also a need to use alternative and cheaper energy sources to store cool milk, and develop rural markets so that much of the milk produced in the rural areas finds consumption avenue in the nearby local markets. There is a need to set up schemes for diversification and preparation of value added milk products at the production centers instead of sending raw milk over long distances. Depending upon the market demand for a particular product, quantum of raw milk available , and financial position of the milk plant, suitable milk processing and product manufacturing units can be set up.

iv) Drug Resistance: It occurs when an antibiotic has lost its ability to effectively control or kill bacterial growth; in other words, the bacteria are "resistant" and continue to multiply in the presence of therapeutic levels of an antibiotic. With the discovery of antimicrobials in the 1940s, scientists prophesied the defeat of infectious diseases that had plagued humankind throughout history. However, the remarkable healing power of antibiotics invites widespread and often inappropriate use. This misuse and overuse of antibiotics leads to antibiotic resistance among bacteria and consequent treatment complications and increased healthcare costs. Antimicrobial resistance has cast a shadow over the medical miracles we take for granted, undermining every clinical and public health program designed to contain infectious diseases worldwide.

One major class of veterinary antibiotics is the tetracycline group which makes up 40% of the total market. These were one of the first antibiotics to be developed and in many countries have limited use in human patients only. But despite their use in animals, veterinarians have found little evidence of resistant strains causing hard to treat infections in their animal patients. Antibiotic resistance is accelerated by the misuse and overuse of antibiotics, as well as poor infection prevention and control. Steps can be taken at all levels of society to reduce the impact and limit the spread of resistance. To prevent and control the spread of antibiotic resistance, policy makers can ensure a robust national action plan to tackle antibiotic resistance is in place. Also strengthen policies, programmes, and implementation of infection prevention and control measures can play a important role in this regard. Antibiotics to animals should be given under veterinary supervision and antibiotics should not be used for growth promotion or to prevent diseases in healthy animals. Vaccination of animals is necessary to reduce the need for antibiotics and use alternatives to antibiotics when available.

Gastrointestinal nematodes in grazing animals cause major production losses and represent an animal welfare problem worldwide. For decades use of anthelmintics has been central in the control programs of these parasites. This intensive use of anthelmintic drugs has resulted in problems with resistance to the anthelmintic drugs available today. Resistance to all classes of broad spectrum anthelmintics available benzimidazoles (BZ), imidothiazoles-tetrahydropyrines and macrocyclic lactones has been reported (Kaplan, 2004).

Improvement of the grazing management is important in reducing the use of anthelmintics. Reduction of the stocking rate, reducing the grazing season on the pastures and mixed grazing between animal species are all key factors. Furthermore, the animals have to be treated at times when the effect of treatment is best and underdosing is to be avoided. Biological control of nematodes is an interesting way of reducing the use of anthelmintic drugs. The principle of biological control is the use of the natural enemies of the nematodes to reduce the infection level on pastures (Larsen, 2006). These methods have no intention of eliminating the free living larval stages but aim to reduce them to a level where no clinical or subclinical effects are present while stimulating an acquired immune response. Nematode destroying fungi have been a potential candidate in biological control and the fungus Duddingtonia flagrans has shown to be effective. Development of effective vaccines against intestinal parasites will allow the opportunity to reduce the use of antiparasitic drugs. In spite of great efforts making vaccines protecting grazing animals against helminth infections, only a vaccine against the bovine lungworm Dictyocaulus viviparus is commercially available (Smith and Zarlenga, 2004).

v) **Backyard Poultry Farming**: Rural population living in India constitutes 72.2 per cent of the total population, which is predominantly occupied by poor, marginal farmers and landless labourers. Backyard poultry production is an old age profession of rural families of India. It is the most potent source for subsidiary incomes for landless and poor farmers. It is an enterprise with low initial investment but higher economic returns and can easily be managed by women, children and old aged persons of the households. Now-a-days, poultry meat and eggs have been the best and cheapest sources for meeting out theper capita requirement of protein and energy for rural areas of India.

Though India has shown a tremendous growth in poultry production over decades but rural poultry farming is still lagging behind and always found neglected. As it is the best alternative for the small scale farmers to subsidise the income with negligible input, this farming system needs an upliftment with recent advancement of research in the field of rearing of chicks, balanced feeding, disease control and efficient marketing system for the egg and meat. Now-a-days, the backyard poultry can easily start with good egg laying birds of RIR (Rhode Island Red), Chabro, Punjab Red and Partapdhan breeds.

Backyard poultry production system is a low input business and is characterized by indigenous night shelter system, scavenging system, natural hatching of chicks, poor productivity of birds, with little supplementary feeding, local marketing and no health care practice. Poultry development plays a crucial role in increasing egg and chicken meat production. The production of agricultural crops has been rising at a rate of 1.5–2 per cent per annum, where as eggs and broilers has been shown to rise at a rate of 8-10 per cent per annum but the growth has been mainly restricted to commercial poultry. In India, growth in the livestock sector can definitely contribute to poverty reduction, because of the peoples lived in rural areas depends on livestock for their daily livelihoods. It has also been observed that the demand for the animal protein source is increasing rapidly in developing countries. Raising of local poultry breeds in backyard is an important source of livelihood for the rural people. Main interest of the poultry farmers having backyard poultry is not production of eggs, as returns are very low from sale of eggs. They hatch all their eggs and sale them as birds because of broodiness habit of these breeds.

Backyard poultry farming gives employment to the rural small scale and marginal farmers and provides additional income to the rural communities. It also aids in enhancing the soil fertility in backyards (15 chickens produce 1-1.2 kg of manure/day). Products from rural poultry farming fetches high price compared to those from intensive poultry farming. It provides egg and meat with almost no or very less investment through backyard poultry farming in free range system. Birds reared under free range conditions give eggs and meat of low cholesterol concentration compared to those produced under intensive poultry farming. It also lessens protein malnutrition in susceptible groups like pregnant women, feeding mothers and children.

vi) Climate Change and Livestock Production: Climate change may have substantial effects on the global livestock sector. Livestock production systems will be affected in various ways and changes in productivity are inevitable. Increasing climate variability will undoubtedly increase livestock production risks as well as reduce the ability of farmers to manage these risks. At the same time, livestock food chains are major contributors to greenhouse gas emissions, accounting for perhaps 18 per cent of total anthropogenic emissions (Steinfeld et al. 2006). Offering relatively fewer cost-effective options than other sectors such as energy, transport and buildings, agriculture has not yet been a major player in the reduction of greenhouse gas emissions. This will change in the future (UNFCCC 2008), although guidance will be needed from rigorous analysis; for example, livestock consumption patterns in one country are often associated with land-use changes in other countries, and these have to be included in national greenhouse gas accounting exercises (Audsley et al. 2009). Climate change may have impacts not only on the distribution of disease vectors. Some diseases are associated with water, which may be exacerbated by flooding and complicated by inadequate water access. Droughts may force people and their livestock to move, potentially exposing them to environments with health risks to which they have not previously been exposed. While the direct impacts of climate change on livestock disease over the next two to three decades may be relatively muted, there are considerable gaps in knowledge concerning many existing diseases of livestock and their relation to environmental factors, including climate. Similarly, there is a burgeoning literature on mitigation in agriculture. There are several options related to livestock, including grazing management and manure management. The mitigation potential of various strategies for the landbased livestock systems in the tropics amounts to about 4 per cent of the global agricultural mitigation potential to 2030. In the more intensive systems, progress could be made in mitigating GHG emissions from the livestock sector via increases in the efficiency of production using available technology, for the most part, and this may involve some shifting towards monogastric species.

vii) Animal Diseases: Diseases generate a wide range of biophysical and socio-economic impacts that may be both direct and indirect, and may vary from localized to global (Perry & Sones 2009). The last few decades have seen a general reduction in the burden of livestock diseases, as a result of more effective drugs and vaccines and improvements in diagnostic technologies and services (Perry & Sones 2009). At the same time, new diseases have emerged, such as avian influenza H5N1, which have caused considerable global concern about the potential for a change in host species from poultry to man and an emerging global pandemic of human influenza. Globally, the direct impacts of livestock diseases are decreasing, but the total impacts may actually be increasing, because in a globalized and highly interconnected world, the effects of disease extend far beyond animal sickness and mortality (Perry & Sones 2009). For the future, the infectious disease threat will remain diverse and dynamic, and combating the emergence of completely unexpected diseases will require detection systems that are flexible and adaptable in the face of change. Travel, migration and trade will all continue to promote the spread of infections into new populations. Trade in exotic species and in bush meat are likely to be increasing causes of concern, along with large-scale industrial production systems, in which conditions may be highly suitable for enabling disease transmission between animals and over large distances . This has obvious implications for policy-makers and the sheep and cattle industries, and raises the need for improved diagnosis and early detection of livestock parasitic disease, along with greatly increased awareness and preparedness to deal with disease patterns that are manifestly changing. Future disease trends are likely to be heavily modified by disease surveillance and control technologies. Potentially effective control measures already exist for many infectious diseases, and whether these are implemented appropriately could have considerable impacts on future disease trends. Recent years have seen considerable advances in the technology that can be brought to bear against disease, including DNA fingerprinting for surveillance, polymerase chain reaction tests for diagnostics and understanding resistance, genome sequencing and antiviral drugs (Perry & Sones 2009). There are also options associated with the manipulation of animal genetic resources, such as cross-breeding to introduce genes into breeds that are otherwise well-adapted to the required purposes, and the selection via molecular genetic markers of individuals with high levels of disease resistance or tolerance. The future infectious disease situation is going to be different from today's (Woolhouse 2006), and will reflect many changes, including changes in mean climate and climate variability, demographic change and different technologies for combating infectious diseases.

Veterinarian and 'One Health' Concept

More than half of all human diseases are animal originated, caused by multi-host pathogens. Effective prevention and control of infectious diseases at the animal-human-ecosystems interface is the key to prevent the spread of diseases in animals and humans, enhancing food security and fostering poverty reduction. Increased transparency in the animal health situation contributes to better public health. All activities of animal science affect human health either directly through biomedical research and public health or indirectly by addressing domestic animal, wildlife, or environmental health. The Veterinary research transcends species boundaries and includes the study of spontaneously occurring and experimentally induced models of both human and animal disease and research at human-animal interfaces, such as food safety, wildlife and ecosystem health, zoonotic diseases and public policy (Mazet *et al.*, 2009). By its nature, veterinary science is comparative and gives rise to the basic science disciplines of comparative anatomy, comparative physiology, comparative pathology, and so forth; but its ability to reach its peak potential relies on adequate infrastructural, financial, and human resources. These veterinarians partner with zoologists and conservationists, and are often at the fore of emergency relief to treat animals affected by forest fires, oil spills, and other natural disasters, which not only affect wildlife, but also farm and companion animals. Trained veterinary professionals, such as those in Public Service and Food Inspection, work to promote food security and ensure that food from animals is safe to ship and eat (Institute of Medicine, 2012). Through stringent inspections and controls prior and after slaughtering, meat safety is continuously checked. At all phases of the production and distribution of food from animal origin they are involved in preserving its hygiene and safety. The veterinarian is committed professionally and morally with the community, whether rural or urban. Since a born volunteer, he forwards his knowledge to the community as a whole to improve his environmental education and health, to improve the quality of our life.

Since zoonoses can infect both animals and humans, the medical and veterinary communities should work closely together in clinical, public health, and research settings. In the clinical setting, input from both professions would improve assessments of the risk benefit ratios of pet ownership, particularly for pet owners who are immunocompromised. In public health, human and animal disease surveillance systems are important in tracking and controlling zoonoses. The bond between humans and animals has been recognized for many years, and pet ownership has been associated with both emotional and health benefits. However, pet ownership may also pose health risks through the zoonotic transmission of infectious diseases, especially, compromised individuals (Beck and Meyer, 1996).

Since human medicine often does not delve deeply into the role of animals in the transmission of zoonotic disease agents and veterinary medicine does not cover the clinical aspects of human disease, zoonotic disease control requires involvement of both physicians and veterinarians (Glaser *et al*, 1994). It is especially important that both veterinarians and physicians are involved in the control of zoonotic disease because the latter do not usually consider the role of animals in the transmission of disease and the former do not receive extensive training on clinical aspects of human disease (Grant and Olsen, 1999).

In animal clinics, veterinarians work with companion, farm and exotic animals to diagnose and treat acute and chronic diseases, provide targeted vaccines, treat parasitic infection and infestation and perform minor surgeries like dressing wounds, mending broken bones, performing dental work to major ones like caesarean sections and also humanely euthanize whenever necessary. Veterinarians are also key contributors to ethical review processes in vetero-legal cases, speaking with authority and pragmatism as the animals' advocate. That is what these animals deserve, not only the five freedoms- freedom from hunger, freedom from discomfort i.e. having shelter, freedom from pain and suffering from disease, freedom to express its normal behavior, freedom from fear and distress; but proper internationally achievable and respected standards for their whole life.

Animal health is also a critical contributor to both international competitiveness and on-farm profitability. Among the potential adverse impacts from animal diseases and sub-optimal health, include:

- ✰ Adverse effects on food safety and human health, with consequent economic costs including increased health service demands.

- ☆ Major national socio-economic consequences, through very serious international trade losses, national market disruption and very serious production losses in the livestock industries.
- ☆ Less significant national/regional socio-economic consequences, and consequences that mainly affect the industry alone, such as production loss diseases.

Conclusions and Future Strategies

In livestock production, the overriding considerations are the availability and efficient use of local natural resources. A successful livestock development strategy requires the formulation of resource management plans that complement the wider economic, ecological and sociological objectives. Particular attention needs to be given to land-use systems and to the natural resources required for improved livestock production. The strategy should consider the social, cultural, political and institutional elements that affect the management of natural resources. On the policy side, issues relating to land use, common property, legislation, price policies, subsidies, levies, national priorities for livestock development and research capacity have to be addressed. Finally, the implementation of action programmes requires both technical and institutional support and, equally important, government commitment. Developments in breeding, nutrition and animal health will continue to contribute to increasing potential production and further efficiency and genetic gains. Livestock production is likely to be increasingly affected by carbon constraints and environmental and animal welfare legislation. Demand for livestock products in the future could be heavily moderated by socio-economic factors such as human health concerns and changing socio-cultural values. The industrialization of livestock production in many parts of the world, both developed and developing, is either complete or continuing apace. The increasing demand for livestock products continues to be a key opportunity for poverty reduction and economic growth, although the evidence of the last 10 years suggests that only a few countries have taken advantage of this opportunity effectively. There are many cases where the poor have been disadvantaged by the industrialization of livestock production in developing countries, as well as highlighting the problems and inadequacies of commercial, industrial breeding lines, once all the functions of local breeds are genuinely taken into account.

Livestock sector is expected to emerge as an engine of agricultural growth in the 12th plan and beyond in view of rapid growth in demand for animal food products. Considering the existing orientation of livestock production systems and specialized requirements of livestock owners, it's the time to reminisce the role of veterinarians in addressing the constraints and provide extension services towards spreading the awareness about animal health and welfare. This would call for building up an exclusive cadre of livestock extension workers, establishment of Krishi Vigyan Kendra (KVK) exclusively for livestock activities and strengthening Agriculture Technology Management Agency (ATMA) with Animal Husbandry experts. India has about 55000 veterinary institutions including poly clinics, hospitals, dispensaries and livestockman centers. All veterinarians and veterinary para-professionals are licensed to practice by an autonomous Veterinary Council of India and are subjected to legal disciplinary provisions for any professional misconduct. Veterinarians performing official government functions use their best efforts to ensure that any colleagues in clinical practice, either government or private, are kept informed on matters affecting their clients and their animals like an outbreak of notifiable disease. Veterinarian expertised in curing the sick or injured animal will always be in demand as their knowledge in the welfare of animals is unique and they are never reticent in coming forward. Society expects veterinarians to be involved wherever animals are at risk or are about to be placed at risk. They are always pro-active, ask never complacent and willing to be involved. With an increasing global population, they will continue to play an ever more important role in ensuring a healthy world, for animals and humans.

References

Agarwal I. S., Verma M. L., Singh A. K. and Pandey Y. C. 1988.Studies on the effect of urea treated straw on milk production and feeding cost. *Indian Journal of Animal Nutrition*. In press.

Ange, A. L. 1994. Integrated plant nutrition management in cropping and farming systems: a challenge for small farmers in developing countries. Rome, FAO. 7 pp.

Audsley, E., Brander, M., Chatterton, J., Murphy-Bokern, D., Webster, C. and Williams, A. 2009. How low can we go? An assessment of greenhouse gas emissions from the UK food system and the scope to reduce them by 2050.

Beck A. M., Meyers N. M. 1996. Health enhancement and companion animal ownership. *Annual Review of Public Health,* 17: 247-257.

Birthal P. S., Joshi P. K. and Kumar A 2002 Assessment of Research Priorities for Livestock Sector in India, Policy Paper 15, National Centre for Agricultural Economics and Policy Research, New Delhi.

Birthal P. S. 2002. Technological Change in India's Livestock Sub-sector: Evidence and Issues, In: Technology Options for Sustainable Livestock Production in India (P S Birthal and P Parthasarathy Rao, editors). National Centre for Agricultural Economics and Policy Research, New Delhi, International Crops Research Institute for the Semi-Arid Tropics, Patancheru, Andhra Pradesh, and International Livestock Research Institute, Addis Ababa.

Birthal P. S. and Ali J. 2005. Potential of livestock sector in rural transformation, In: Rural Transformation in India: The Role of Non-farm Sector (Rohini Nayyar and A N Sharma editors) Institute for Human Development and Manohar Publishers and Distributors, New Delhi.

Birthal P. S. and Taneja V. K. 2006. Livestock sector in India: Opportunities and Challenges, presented at the ICAR-ILRI workshop on 'Smallholder livestock production in India' held during January 24-25, 2006 at NCAP, New Delhi 110 012.

FAO in One Health, ECTAD Emergency Centre for Transboundary Animal Diseases, 2010. Food and Agriculture Organization of the United Nations, Rome, Italy.

Gifford, R.C. 1992.Agricultural engineering in development.Mechanization strategy formulation.Vol. I: Concepts and principles.FAO agricultural Services Bulletin 99/1. 232.pp.

Glaser C. A, Angulo F. J, Rooney J. A. 1994. Animal-associated opportunistic infections among persons infected with the human immunodeficiency virus. *Clinical Infectious Diseases.* 18: 14-24.

Grant S, Olsen C. W.1999. Preventing zoonotic diseases in immunocompromised persons: the role of physicians and veterinarians. *Emerging Infectious Diseases.* 5: 159-163.

Institute of Medicine (US), 2012. In: Workshop Summary on Improving Food Safety through a One Health Approach, National Academies Press (US), Washington (DC), Workshop Overview.

Kaplan R. M. 2004. Drug resistance in nematodes of veterinary importance. A status report. *Trends in Parasitology*. 20:477-481.

Kumar, S. & Biswas, T. D. 1982. Biogas production from different animal excrete. *Indian Journal of Agricultural Sci*ences, 52(8): 513-520.

Larsen M. 2006. Biological control of nematodes in sheep. *Journal of Animal Sciences*. 84: E133.

Mazet J. A. K., Clifford D. L., Coppolillo P. B., Deolalikar A. B, Erickson J. D. 2009. A "One Health" Approach to address Emerging Zoonoses. In: The HALI Project in Tanzani. PLoS Med., 6(12), e1000190. doi:10.1371/journal.pmed.1000190.

Perry, B. & Sones, K. 2009. Global livestock disease dynamics over the last quarter century: drivers, impacts and implications. Rome, Italy: FAO.

Smith W. D. and Zarlenga D. S. 2006. Developments and hurdles in generating vaccines for controlling helminth parasites of grazing ruminants. *Veterinary Parasitology*. 139:347-459.

Steinfeld, H., Gerber, P., Wassenaar, T., Castel, V., Rosales, M. & de Haan, C. 2006. Livestock's long shadow: environmental issues and options. Rome, Italy: FAO.

Talukder, N. M., Ali, M. S. & Latif, A. 1988. Effect of biogas effluent on the yield and quality of rice. *International Rice Commission. News*. 37: 11-16.

UNFCCC (United Nations Framework Convention on Climate Change). 2008. Challenges and opportunities for mitigation in the agricultural sector: technical paper. United Nation Framework Convention on Climate Change.

Woolhouse, M. 2006. Mathematical modelling of future infectious diseases risks: an overview. Foresight, infectious diseases: preparing for the future, office of science and innovation.

World Bank. 1999. India livestock sector review: Enhancing growth and development, The World Bank, Washington DC, and Allied Publishers, New Delhi.

Transforming Rural Areas through Veterinary Science *Pages* **185-190**
Editor: Dipanjali Konwar, Shilpa Sood & Shahid Ahamad
Published by: **ASTRAL INTERNATIONAL PVT. LTD., NEW DELHI**

14 Conservation of Animal Genetic Resources

Dr. Vikas Mahajan, Dr. Dhirendra Kumar & Dr. Rajan Sharma

Introduction

Sustainable management of animal genetic resources is of vital importance to food, nutrition and environment security. Conservation and judicious use is critical for the survival as well as improved livelihood resource for poor farmers. India is rich in its animal diversity being a mega biodiversity centre. However, currently many unique breeds are facing a threat of extinction for want of an appropriate conservation strategy and its effective implementation at the national/state level.

Animal Genetic Resource

All animal species, breeds & strains which are economic, scientific & cultural interest to the mankind for food & agricultural production, both now & in the future.

Conservation

It means management of the biosphere, so that it may yield the greatest sustainable benefits to present generation while maintaining its potential to meet the needs and aspirations of the future generations (FAO), or it may be also defined as sum of all actions involved in the management of Animal Genetic Resource (AnGR), such that these resources are best utilised & developed to meet immediate and short term requirements for food and agriculture, while maintaining the diversity to meet possible long term needs for future generations.

Factors that Diminish Genetic Diversity are

a. Genetic bottlenecks

b. Random genetic drift

c. Inbreeding

d. Human activities

e. Economic viability

f. Modern agricultural practices

The Food and Agriculture Organization of the United Nations (FAO) has, since the early 1960s, provided assistance to countries to characterize their animal genetic resources (AnGR) and develop conservation strategies.

In 1980, FAO & UNDP considered jointly technical aspect of conservation & laid down definite procedures for conservation. In 1990, FAO's Council recommended the development of a comprehensive programme for the sustainable management of AnGR at the global level. A meeting of experts in 1992, and subsequent sessions of FAO's governing bodies, provided impetus to the development of the Global Strategy for the Management of Farm Animal Genetic Resources, which was initiated in 1993. In 1984, India established National Bureau of Animal Genetic Resources (NBAGR) under ICAR.

Preservation means maintenance of genetic diversity while Conservation is preservation plus upgradation and includes preservation, judicious management, sustainable utilization and restoration and enhancement of natural resources.

Reasons for Conservation

There are many reasons which necessitate the conservation. About 30 to 40% of all AnGR is at risk of extinction. Adequate breed records do not exist, thus the existing data on the number of endangered breeds may be an underestimate. Moreover, animals have multiutility and few are enlisted as under:

1. Economic Potential

a. Opportunities to meet future market demands

b. Insurance against future changes in production circumstances

2. Scientific Use

a. Sustainable crossbreeding schemes requires different viable populations

b. Opportunities for research

3. Cultural Interest

a. Cultural and historical reasons

b. Ecological value

c. Present socio-economic value

Strategies for Conservation: It Includes Following Steps:

a. Identification and listing of all the available animal genetic resources

b. Prioritizing the breed for characterization and conservation based on their population

c. structure, economic utility and genetic diversity
d. Development of technology for collection and freezing of genetic material
e. Documentation and creation of mass awareness

Criteria for Selecting Breeds for Conservation

a. Species a breed belongs to
b. Degree of endangerment
c. Adaptation to a specific environment
d. Traits of economic importance
e. Unique traits
f. Cultural or historical value
g. Genetic uniqueness

It is suggested that breeds with high degrees of endangerment should be given priority (Ruane, 2000).

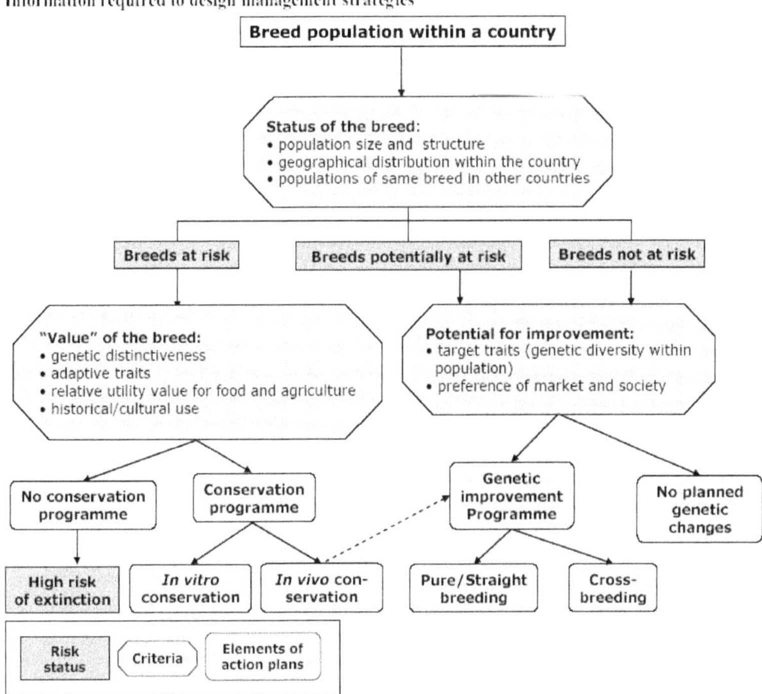

Conservation Methods

In-situ conservation: It refers to conservation of livestock through continued use by livestock keepers in the production system in which the livestock evolved or are now normally found and bred or in simple words, maintenance of breeds within their normal environment.

Key operations for *in-situ* conservation include performance recording, breeding programmes and ecosystem management for sustainable production of food and agriculture.

Minimum number of animals to be maintained should be 150–1500 breeding females in developed countries, & not below 5000 in developing countries.

Advantages of In-Situ Conservation as Under

a. Animals are still being utilized.

b. Performance characteristics can be properly recorded & evaluated.

c. Breeds have opportunity to adapt gradually to changing environment.

Disadvantages of *In-Situ* Conservation as Under

a. Genetic drift may result in unfavourable genetic changes if population is small.

b. Risk of increasing inbreeding & hence homozygosity

c. reduced fitness

d. Animals may be less productive and so more costly to maintain.

2. Ex Situ Conservation

***i. Ex-Situ in Vivo* Conservation:** It refers to conservation through maintenance of live animal populations not kept under normal management conditions (*e.g.* zoological parks and in some cases governmental farms) and/or outside of the area in which they evolved or are now normally found. There is often no clear boundary between *in situ* and *ex situ in vivo* conservation and care must be taken to describe the conservation objectives and the nature of the conservation in each case or in simple way, it means preservation of a sample of a breed in a situation away from its normal production environment or habitat.

***ii. Ex Situ in Vitro* Conservation:** It refers to conservation external to the living animal in an artificial environment, under cryogenic conditions including, the cryoconservation of embryos, semen, oocytes, somatic cells or tissues having the potential to reconstitute live animals (including animals for gene introgression and synthetic breeds) at a later date. It is an important method when there is a critical threat to a breed to become extinct & to ensure adequate gene pool to be retained for future use.

Gene Bank: A physical repository where samples of a genetic resource which are being preserved (*e.g.* embryos, oocytes, semen, tissues, DNA) are kept.

Data Bank: It is the collection of information on characteristics, status, uses *etc.* of genetic resources, stored in a systematic manner (usually electronic) and with provisions for editing and retrieval for viewing and analyses.

Advantages of *Ex Situ* Conservation

a. Parks can be utilised in tourist industry.

b. Free from unintended genetic change.

c. During storage, frozen genetic material is at less risk from diseases and natural disasters.

d. Other options for using cryo preserved materials like DNA-level studies, Supporting *in vivo* populations, Re-establishing extinct populations, Research e.g. identification of major genes.

Disadvantages of *Ex Situ* Conservation

a. Economically not viable & inbreeding if small population is maintained.

b. Reproductive technologies are not uniformly successfull or presently available for all species.

c. Expertise is not always available in the places where it is needed most.

d. Conservation through cryopreservation of semen and embryos is not able to adapt to changes in the production environment.

e. Semen or embyos frozen now may be unable to meet future production requirements.

Choice of Method: Decision will depend on Risk status, Sustainability issues, Costs – long and short-term, Technical difficulty and Risk of failure.

Determining Levels of Threat Used in AnGR as Per FAO, 2007

1. **Extinct**: A breed is categorized as extinct if is no longer possible to recreate the breed population. This situation becomes absolute when there are no breeding males or breeding females remaining.

2. **Critical**: The overall population size is less than or equal to 120 and decreasing and the percentage of females being bred to males of the same breed is below 80%. or simply condition revealing threat to become extinct.

3. **Endangered**: The overall population size is greater than 1000 and less than or equal to 1200 and decreasing and the percentage of females being bred to males of the same breed is below 80%. or simply condition showing threat to become critical.

Some of the scientific and regulatory issues are to be addressed:

a. Biodiversity levels in animal genetic resources.

b. Impact of introduction of exotic germplasm on domestic animal biodiversity

c. Biosafety concerns of introduction of exotic germplasm

d. Conservation methods and strategies

e. Data base management and documentation of animal genetic resources

f. Regulatory mechanisms for handling of animal biodiversity as per the provisions of Biological Diversity Act, 2002

g. IPR issues related to Animal genetic resource biodiversity

h. Patenting

i. Use of biotechnology and genetic engineering for conservation of domestic animal biodiversity and genetic enhancement

Conclusion

Conservation of animal genetic diversity is a global issue, as all countries benefit from the use and development of domestic animals and their many products. Conservation of animal genetic diversity over the long-term, will enable countries and their farmers to better respond to changing environmental conditions and consumer preferences, to pursue new economic opportunities and to reduce their vulnerability to food shortages.

Conservation and sustainable use of animal genetic resources are essential to support and inform the biotechnology industry and other industries that are dependent on genetic resources. Technological developments are increasingly improving our capacity to use and develop genetic resources, and thus, it is imperative that the current rapid erosion of animal genetic resources is addressed. Conservation of AnGR is essential due to rapid loss of varieties and breeds through dilution and breed replacement. Identification and characterization of diversity using available techniques is the first step taken for the conservation. Proper identification of threats and elimination of it through policy and legislations are important. All the available genetic resources cannot be conserved due to high cost involved, conservation should be aimed at the those breeds which are immediately useful to the farmer. *In situ* conservation is the method of choice for conservation. However, *ex situ* methods of conservation (frozen semen etc.) can be complementary to it. Finally, Conservation of AnGR is a multidirectional activity which encompasses not only preservation & maintenance of existing breeds but also their improvement & proper management. The overall aim is sustainable utilization, restoration & enhancement of resources so as to meet needs of mankind at present & in future.

Referrences

Acharya, R.M. and Bhat, P.N. 1984. Livestock and poultry genetic resources in India. Indian Veterinary Research Institute, Izatnagar, India

Ruane, J. 2000. A framework for prioritizing domestic animal breeds for conservation purposes at the national level: a Norwegian case study. Conservation Biology, 14(5): 1385–1393.

Kannaiyan, S and A. Gopalam, 2007. Biodiversity in India- issues and concerns (S.) Associated Publishing Company, New Delhi. p. 421.

Transforming Rural Areas through Veterinary Science *Pages* **191-202**
Editor: Dipanjali Konwar, Shilpa Sood & Shahid Ahamad
Published by: **ASTRAL INTERNATIONAL PVT. LTD., NEW DELHI**

15 Sperm Quality Biomarkers: Advanced Diagnostic Tools

Dr. Sanjay Agarwal & Dr. Dhirendra Kumar

Introduction

Since the first attempts to freeze human semen (Spallanzani, 1776) there have been many improvements in the methodological approaches and freezing of spermatozoa, among which one major achievement was the use of glycerol as a cryoprotectant (Polge *et al.*, 1949).

For a successful conception the fertilizing sperm should have functional competent membranes, organelles and an intact haploid genome. In assisted reproductive techniques (ART), such as artificial insemination (AI) and in vitro fertilization (IVF), sperm is not directly introduced in the female genital tract after ejaculation but first collected by the use of an artificial vagina, by manual stimulation or by electroejaculation (Franco and Baruffi, 2002; Senger, 2002). The collected sperm is diluted, cooled or frozen and stored for extended time prior to introduce in the female genital tract (AI). All sperm processing steps may introduce damage to sperm DNA, membranes and organelles. In order to be able to obtain better fertilization results it is necessary to assess the quality of sperm just before their use in ART.

Recently the fluorescent probe methods for sperm analysis has totally replaced the conventional methods used in past decades. Through fluorescent markers the plasma membrane, acrosomal status, mitochondrial activity, lipid peroxidation and chromatin or DNA integrity *etc.* is assessed with great accuracy these markers are also known as molecular makers in sperm analysis.

Cryopreservation techniques induce detrimental problems like:

- **Capacitation-Like Changes**: after freezing/thawing, sperm behaves as if capacitated, which decreases its ability to survive within the female genital tract and to fuse with the oocytes.

• **Motility Impairment**: a decrease in the motility is observed in post-thawed spermatozoa, which tend to exhibit a variable degree of motility weakening, with subsequent hampering of sperm progression till the oviducts and a decrease on the fertility potential.

• **Oxidative Damages**: which may trigger apoptosis and DNA damage when reaching a given threshold. Apoptosis compromises the mitochondrial function, motility and predispose to DNA fragmentation.

• **Membrane and Acrosome Integrity**: loss of membrane integrity lead to altered ionic transport to the cell, in particular the calcium and water balance, with subsequent loss of the sperm ability for volume regulation and osmoadaptation. Also, it will compromise protein location and/or exposition on the cell's surface, which negatively affects sperm survival, sperm binding to oviductal epithelium and interaction between male and female gametes. In addition, restrain of the acrosome integrity may compromise sperm competence to penetrate the oocyte layers at fertilization;

• **DNA and Chromatin Changes**: which may not be directly related to fertilization but are often reported to impair sustainable post-syngamy embryonic development and pregnancy.

Membrane and Organelle Integrity

1. Plasma Membrane

The plasma membrane surrounds the entire sperm cell holding together its organelles and intracellular components and by its semi-permeable features maintains the chemical gradient of ions and other soluble components. Specific plasma membrane proteins facilitate transport of glucose and fructose from the extracellular environment into the sperm (Angulo *et al.*, 1988; Burant and Davidson, 1994; Schurmann *et al.*, 2002). These transporters are indispensable energy source substrates: in the mature sperm approximately 90% of ATP is produced by glycolysis (anaerobic) indicating the importance of monosaccharides as substrates for ATP production (Marin *et al.*, 2003; Mukai and Okuno, 2004). If the sperm plasma membrane is not functionally intact the sperm is considered deteriorated (dead) and in vivo is not capable to fertilize.

A. Plasma Membrane Integrity is Usually Assessed after Staining Cells with:

(a) Membrane-Impermeable Dyes: cells that are capable to exclude these dyes can be considered to be alive. An array of membrane-impermeable fluorescent probes with affinity for DNA is currently used for this purpose. Different probes that work on this principle with distinct excitation (ex) and emission (em) properties are:

- ☆ **Hoechst 33258** (ex/em of 358/488 nm wavelength (Hong *et al.*, 1988; McLaughlin *et al.*, 1992);
- ☆ **YoPro-1** (ex/em of 488/515 nm wavelength [Harrison *et al.*, 1996]);
- ☆ **Propidiumiodide** (Garner *et al.*, 1986; Pintado *et al.*, 2000) **or**

Ethidiumhomodimer-1 (Cheng *et al.*, 1996) (both have an ex/em of 488 and 568/ >620 nm wavelength);

- ☆ **ToPro-3 and TOTO** (ex/em of 647/670 nm wavelength [Haugland, 2004]).

(b) Acylated Membrane Dyes (AM Loading): these membrane probes are amphipathic and thus can pass the intact membrane and enter the living sperm. Entered probes are immediately deacylated by intracellular esterases leaving the probe membrane impermeable. Thus, living sperm cells will get loaded with probes that become entrapped in the cell, whereas, the entered probes easily leak out of deteriorated cells with damaged membranes.

- ☆ **Fluorescein diacetate (CFDA)**
- ☆ **Carboxy(methyl) derivatives:**
    - SYBR-14 (ex/em 488/515 nm wavelength).

B. Lipid Organization

The capacitation status of sperm usually is assessed with:

- ☆ **CTC (Chlortetracyclin) Test**: It is routine test to assess the occurrence of the capacitation and acrosome reaction. Principle is that the fluorescence is activated when there is bounding of free calcium ions. The following patterns are obtained:
- ☆ ***F pattern***- uncapacitated and acrosome intact i.e. an overall staining of the sperm head.
- ☆ ***B pattern***- capacitated and acrosome intact i.e. a more prominent staining of the apical area of the sperm head and decreased staining at the posterior area of the sperm head (Ward and Storey, 1984).
- ☆ ***AR pattern***- capacitated and acrosome reacted (Saling and Storey, 1979).
- ☆ **Merocyanine 540:** is a useful fluorescent hydrophobic probe for lipid packing because it binds preferentially to membranes with highly disordered lipids. It is also sensitive to heat-induced changes in the organization of membrane lipids, thus allowing the monitoring of alterations in the lipid architecture of the cells (Rathi *et al*, 2001).

C. Lipid Peroxidation

The lipid peroxidation of sperm is assessed with:

- ☆ **BODIPY581/591-C11** (4,4-difluoro-5-(4-phenyl-1,3-butadienyl)-4-bora-3a,4a-diaza-s-indacene-3-undecanoic acid): It is a fatty acids sensitive fluorescent probe which is a fluorescent analog for unsaturated fatty acids, the main targets for reactive oxygen species (ROS). Essentially, C11BODIPY581/591 changes its fluorescent properties after peroxidation. The intact probe is red fluorescent but turns into green fluorescence when peroxidized by ROS and into orange when peroxidized by peroxynitrite (Drummen *et al.*, 2004). This green and orange emission shift indicates the presence of reactive oxygen and nitrogen species in the hydrophobic part of lipid bilayers of sperm membranes. The ratio of green + orange fluorescence versus total fluorescence (an indication of the degree of probe peroxidation) correlates well with the degree of endogenous phospholipid peroxidation (Brouwers and Gadella, 2003).

2. Acrosome

The acrosome is a large Golgi/ER derived acidic secretory organelle. It is filled with hydrolytic enzymes that are organized in a kind of enzyme matrix and most enzymes are heavily glycosylated (Ramalho-Santos *et al.*, 2002). Initial sperm-zona binding trigger the acrosome reaction resulting in the release and activation of acrosomal enzymes. This together with the acquired hyper-activated motility helps the sperm to penetrate the zona pellucida (Honda *et al.*, 2002). The acrosome must remain intact before and during the transit of the sperm to the isthmus until zona binding has been accomplished. Early acrosome reactions render sperm infertile, and therefore, it makes sense to assess acrosome integrity before ART.

Acrosome Integrity is Commonly Measured with

(a) Fluorescent Conjugated Lectins: The lectin conjugates bind to specific carbohydrate moieties of glycoproteins that are exclusively localized in the acrosome. Absence of fluorescence in the living sperm indicates an intact acrosome, whilst fluorescent is indicative of acrosome disruption or reacted sperm. Depending on the mammalian species the most commonly used lectin conjugates used are-

- ✰ **Pisum Sativum** (green pea; PSA)
- ✰ **Arachis Hypogaea** (peanut; PNA)
- ✰ **Concanavalin A Lectins** (conA) (Holden *et al.*, 1990)

Acrosome-specific lectins can be conjugated with an array of fluorescent groups:

- ✰ **PNA-FITC** (ex/em 488/515 nm wavelength (Szasz *et al.*, 2000)
- ✰ **PNA-TRITC** (ex/em 568/590 nm wavelength (Malmi *et al.*, 1987)
- ✰ **PNA-RPE** (ex/em 488/620 wavelength (Gadella and Harrison, 2000; 2002)

(b) Lysosomal Stains: acrosome is similar to the lysosome, which is an acidified organelle with an internal pH of 5. Therefore, specific probes normally used to stain lysosomes, such as

- ✰ **Lysotracker Green TM** (ex/em 488/515 nm wavelength): can be used to specifically stain the sperm acrosome (Thomas *et al.*, 1997; 1998). A variety of other are
  - Orange TM 488/550,
  - Red TM 568/590,
  - Deep Red TM 628/650

3. Mitochondria

Sperm mitochondria are localized in the mid-piece area enrolled over the principal part of the flagellum. Mitochondria produce ATP by oxidative phosphorylation, its activities are correlated with sperm motility, and thus with fertilization potential.

The Functional Integrity of Mitochondria can be Stained with Specific Dyes:

- ☆ **Rhodamine 123:** it is used to selectively stain functional mitochondria. The principle of this probe is that it only fluoresces red when the proton gradient over the IMM is built up. When the proton gradient collapses, the aerobic production of ATP fails, and mitochondria remain unstained, whereas, positive stained cells are aerobically functional (Garner *et al.*, 1997). Remarkably, an individual sperm either has a fully fluorescent mid-piece or is not fluorescent indicating that depolarization of the IMM is an orchestrated event occurring at once over the entire mid-piece (Mukai and Okuno, 2004).
- ☆ **Mitotracker Dye:** it selectively binds to the respirating mitochondria and become fluorescent after oxidation. Since this process is only relevant in functional mitochondria these probes are suitable to discriminate sperm with deteriorated mitochondria from aerobically capable sperm (Gadella and Harrison, 2002; de Veris *et al.*, 2003).
  - Mitotracker Deep Red TM (628/650)
  - Mitotracker Red TM (568/595)
  - Mitotracker Orange TM (488/550)
  - Mitotracker Green TM (488/515)
- ☆ **JC-1** (5,5′, 6,6′-tetrachloro-1,1′,3,3′-tetraethylbenzimidazolyl carbocyanine iodide): change their fluorescent properties due to changes in the potential of the IMM (JC-1 switches from orange fluorescence in the aerobic functional mid-piece towards green fluorescent after IMM depolarization) (Garner and Thomas, 1999; Gravance *et al.*, 2000). JC-1 can be used to report depolarization of the IMM and thus to report on mitochondrial functionality.

4. Multiple Sperm Parameter Staining

It is possible to stain sperm cells simultaneously with four dyes to discriminate:

i. Viable sperm from plasma membrane deteriorated sperm (using PI and SYBR-14),

ii. Acrosome integrity (using PNA-PE),

iii. Functional status of mitochondria (using Mitotracker Deep Red TM) and

iv. Non-sperm events (Nagy *et al.*, 2003). The wide range of spectral variations of each class of membrane and organelle probes makes it possible to design assays to detect multiparametric features of sperm deterioration.

5. DNA Damage Assessments

An association between infertility and the integrity of DNA content in sperm has been suggested.

The integrity of male DNA is of utmost importance for embryo development and offspring production (Glimore *et al.*, 1995). DNA damage (abnormal chromatin structure) may arise from different processes: deficient recombination or packaging during spermatogenesis, apoptosis and oxidative stress. DNA loss of integrity does not always impair fertilization, but compromises sustainable embryo development, predisposing to embryo losses and abortion (Holt and North, 1984; Drobuis *et al.*, 1993).

DNA damage can be assessed mainly by three different approaches:

A. DNA Condensation

Firstly, the DNA of matured sperm cells (probably the fertilization competent subpopulation) is extremely highly condensed on protamines in a toroid structure. The DNA loops around 500 times around the DNA/ protamine toroid structure and extends to approximately 50,000 base pairs per toroid (Sotolongo *et al.*, 2003). The sperm's head contains about 50,000 of such structures (for arrangement of DNA-protamine toroids in the sperm head (Ward, 1993; Brewer *et al.*, 1999; Balhorn *et al.*, 2000; Fuentes-Mascorro *et al.*, 2000; Sotolongo *et al.*, 2003). Condensation takes place during spermatid development where histones are removed from nucleosomes by transition nuclear proteins (Zhao *et al.*, 2001; Brewer *et al.*, 2002; Meistrich *et al.*, 2003). The stripped DNA is coated with protamines and repacked in late-step spermatids in two transition phases (Bellve *et al.*, 1975; Goldberg *et al.*, 1977; Balhorn *et al.*, 1984; Fuentes-Mascorro *et al.*, 2000). Proper condensation probably stabilizes the DNA and makes it less vulnerable for oxidative damage. However, repair of DNA damage is not possible in the mature sperm (Dadoune, 2003).

The condensation status of individual sperm cells can be assessed using:

(a) COMET assay: This is used to identify both condensation of DNA and breaks and nicks. It detects single stranded (SS) and double stranded (DS) DNA in a single sperm. Using a single cell DNA gel electrophoresis assay (COMET) discrimination can be made between fluorescently labeled DNA of normally condensed sperm nuclei (minimal migration) and more loosely packed DNA (tailing of DNA) after allowing DNA migration on an agarose gel under an electric field. Protamines are the key proteins involved in final condensation of sperm DNA (Ward, 1993; Brewer *et al.*, 1999; Balhorn *et al.*, 2000; Brewer *et al.*, 2002; Corzett *et al.*, 2002; Brewer *et al.*, 2003; Meistrich *et al.*, 2003).

(b) Chromomycin A3 (ex/em of 440 and 470 nm wavelength): can be used to follow the last compaction steps of DNA to protamines. This fluorescent dye binds to deprotaminated DNA (at GC specific regions) but fails to do this after protamination of DNA (Bianchi *et al.*, 1993). The probe is used to detect protamination defects in sperm (Sakkas *et al.*, 1995).

B. DNA Breaks and Nicks

The second level is to detect whether sperm DNA is double stranded (intact) or whether single stranded DNA (damaged, for example, in nicks) are formed.

(a) Acridine Orange can be used to stain single stranded DNA (red fluorescent) and double stranded DNA (green fluorescent).

(b) TUNEL: fluorescent sperm cells contain single stranded DNA that were labeled by dUTP nick-end labeling (TUNEL) at the 3-OH termini (Gadella *et al.*, 1999; Benchaib *et al.*, 2003; Sakkas *et al.*, 2003; Seli *et al.*, 2004). The proportion of TUNEL+ cells appears to correlate well with decreased pregnancy rates using ART (Benchaib *et al.*, 2003). The proportion of TUNEL+ cells may increase after cryo-preservation (Anzar *et al.*, 2002).

C. Nuclear Fragmentation

The third level to detect DNA damage is to look at nuclear/ DNA fragmentation (the latter is defined as a result from double strand breaks in DNA. The resulting nuclear fragments can be imaged by TEM or a fluorescent microscope after staining the sperm with a DNA probe.

Conclusions

Conventional methods used in sperm quality assessment are unsatisfactory to correctly predict sperm fertility potential and do not provide sufficient information for diagnosing and overcome some clinical infertility situations. The major advantages of biomarker approach over conventional semen analysis are the proficiency to accurately measure biomarker levels and to expose hidden sperm defects, which go undetected during current sperm morphology assessment. Newer, diagnostic tests of sperm function have the increased potential to deliver relevant information and to have an effective predictive role in male reproductive medicine. Sperm deterioration can be measured at the membrane and organelle level and an increase of sperm with compromised membranes/ organelles will lead to reduced fertility rates. Sperm deterioration at the DNA level may not affect fertilization rates as long as sperm membranes and organelles remain functionally intact. However, the DNA damage leads to a reduced embryo development after the onset of the embryonic genome. Thus, on one hand, intact functional sperm membranes are essential to achieve fertilization in vivo, but do not essentially contribute to later processes after conception. On the other hand, sperm DNA has no function in achieving fertilization but becomes importantly involved in embryonic development from the onset of embryonic DNA expression (i.e. after the first cleavages). Thus, both deterioration of sperm membranes and DNA are probably important factors involved in male subfertility or infertility. Finally, objective high-throughput multi-parameter sperm assessments (preferably with the aid of flow cytometric detection of fluorescent staining) provide statistically stronger data which will be required for future studies to be able to get correlations between sperm quality parameters and fertility results. This may lead selection of top male animals with respect to high quality.

References

Anzar, M., He, L., Buhr, M. M., Kroetsch, T. G. and Pauls, K. P. (2002). Sperm apoptosis in fresh and cryopreserved bull semen detected by flow cytometry and its relationship with fertility. *Biol. Reprod.*, **66:** 354–360.

Angulo, C., Rauch, M. C., Droppelmann, A., Reyes, A. M., Slebe, J. C. and Delgado-Lopez, F. (1988). Hexose transporter expression and function in mammalian spermatozoa: cellular localization and transport of hexoses and Vitamin C. *J. Cell Biochem.*, **71:** 189–203.

Balhorn, R., Brewer, L. and Corzett, M. (2000). DNA condensation by protamine and arginine-rich peptides: analysis of toroid stability using single DNA molecules. *Mol. Reprod. Dev.*, **56:** 230–234.

Balhorn, R., Weston, S., Thomas, C. and Wyrobek, A. J. (1984). DNA packaging in mouse spermatids. Synthesis of protamine variants and four transition proteins. *Exp. Cell Res.*, **150:** 298–308.

Bellve, A. R., Anderson, E. and Hanley Bowdoin, L. (1975). Synthesis and amino acid composition of basic proteins in mammalian sperm nuclei. *Dev. Biol.*, **47:** 349–365.

Benchaib, M., Braun, V., Lornage, J., Hadj, S., Salle, B. and Lejeune, H. (2003). Sperm DNA fragmentation decreases the pregnancy rate in an assisted reproductive technique. *Hum. Reprod.*, **18:** 1023–1028.

Bianchi, P. G., Manicardi, G. C., Bizzaro, D., Bianchi, U. and Sakkas, D. (1993). Effect of deoxyribonucleic acid protamination on fluorochrome staining and in situ nick-translation of murine and human mature spermatozoa. *Biol. Reprod.*, **49:** 1083–1088.

Brewer, L. R., Corzett, M. and Balhorn, R. (1999). Protamine-induced condensation and decondensation of the same DNA molecule. *Science*, **286:** 120–123.

Brewer, L., Corzett, M. and Balhorn, R. (2002). Condensation of DNA by spermatid basic nuclear proteins. *J. Biol. Chem.*, **277:** 38895–38900.

Brewer, L., Corzett, M., Lau, E. Y. and Balhorn, R. (2003). Dynamics of protamine 1 binding to single DNA molecules. *J. Biol. Chem.*, **278:** 42403–42408.

Brouwers, J. F. and Gadella, B. M. (2003). In situ detection and localization of lipid peroxidation in individual bovine sperm cells. *Free Radic. Biol. Med.*, **35:** 1382–1391.

Burant, C. F. and Davidson, N. O. (1994). GLUT3 glucose transporter isoform in rat testis: localization, effect of diabetes mellitus, and comparison to human testis. *Am. J. Physiol.*, **267:** R1488–1495.

Cheng, F. P., Fazeli, A., Voorhout, W. F., Marks, A., Bevers, M. M. and Colenbrander, B. (1986). Use of peanut agglutinin to assess the acrosomal status and the zona pellucida-induced acrosome reaction in stallion spermatozoa. *J. Androl.*, **17:** 674–682.

Corzett, M., Mazrimas, J. and Balhorn, R. (2002). Protamine 1:protamine 2 stoichiometry in the sperm of eutherian mammals. *Mol. Reprod. Dev.*, **61:** 519–527.

Dadoune, J. P. (2003). Expression of mammalian spermatozoal nucleoproteins. *Microsc. Res. Tech.*, **61:** 56–75.

de Vries, K. J., Wiedmer, T., Sims, P. J. and Gadella, B. M. (2003). Caspase-independent exposure of aminophospholipids and tyrosine phosphorylation in bicarbonate responsive human sperm cells. *Biol. Reprod.*, **68:** 2122–2134.

Drobnis, E. Z., Crowe, L. M., Berger, T., Anchordoguy, T. J., Overstreet, J. W. and Crowe, J. H. (1993). Cold shock damage is due to lipid phase transitions in cell membranes: a demonstration using sperm as a model. *J. Exp. Zool.*, **265:** 432-437.

Drummen, G. P., Gadella, B. M., Post, J. A. and Brouwers, J. F. (2004). Mass spectrometric characterization of the oxidation of the fluorescent lipid peroxidation reporter molecule C11-BODIPY(581/591). *Free Radic. Biol. Med.*, **36:** 1635–1644.

Flesch, F.M. and Gadella, B. M. (2000). Dynamics of the mammalian sperm plasma membrane in the process of fertilization. *Biochim. Biophys. Acta.*, **1469:**197–235.

Franco, Jr. J. G. and Baruffi, R. L. (2002). Introduction to methods for collecting human gametes in assisted reproduction. *Reprod. Biomed. Online*, **5:** 187–197.

Fuentes-Mascorro, G., Serrano, H. and Rosado, A. (2000). Sperm chromatin. *Arch. Androl.*, **45:** 215–225.

Gadella, B. M. and Harrison, R. A. (2000). The capacitating agent bicarbonate induces protein kinase A-dependent changes in phospholipid transbilayer behavior in the sperm plasma membrane. *Development*, **127:** 2407–2420.

Gadella, B. M. and Harrison, R. A. (2002). Capacitation induces cyclic adenosine 30, 50-monophosphate-dependent, but apoptosis-unrelated, exposure of aminophospholipids at the apical head plasma membrane of boar sperm cells. *Biol. Reprod.*, **67:** 340–350.

Gadella, B. M., Miller, N. G. A., Colenbrander, B., van Golde, L. M. G. and Harrison, R. A. P. (1999). Flow cytometric detection of transbilayer movement of fluorescent phospholipid analogues across the boar sperm plasma membrane: elimination of labelling artefacts. *Mol. Reprod. Dev.*, **53:** 108–125.

Garner, D. L. and Thomas, C. A. (1999). Organelle-specific probe JC-1 identifies membrane potential differences in the mitochondrial function of bovine sperm. *Mol. Reprod. Dev.*, **53:** 222–229.

Garner, D. L., Pinkel, D., Johnson, L. A. and Pace, M. M. (1986). Assessment of spermatozoal function using dual fluorescent staining and flow cytometric analyses. *Biol. Reprod.*, **34:** 127–138.

Garner, D. L., Thomas, C. A., Joerg, H. W., DeJarnette, J. M. and Marshall, C. E. (1997). Fluorometric assessments of mitochondrial function and viability in cryopreserved bovine spermatozoa. *Biol. Reprod.*, **57:** 1401–1406.

Gilmore, J. A., McGann, L. E., Liu, J., Gao, D. Y., Peter, A. T., Kleinhans, F. W. and Critser, J. K. (1995). Effect of cryoprotectant solutes on water permeability of human spermatozoa. *Biol. Reprod.*, **53:** 985-995.

Goldberg, R. B., Geremia, R. and Bruce, W. R. (1977). Histone synthesis and replacement during spermatogenesis in the mouse. *Differentiation*, **7:** 167–180.

Gravance, C. G., Garner, D. L., Baumber, J. and Ball, B. A. (2000). Assessment of equine sperm mitochondrial function using JC-1. *Theriogenol.*, **53:** 1691–1703.

Harrison, R. A., Ashworth, P. J. and Miller, N. G. (1996). Bicarbonate/CO2, an effector of capacitation, induces a rapid and reversible change in the lipid architecture of boar sperm plasma membranes. *Mol. Reprod. Dev.*, **45:** 378–391.

Haugland, R. P. (2004). Assays for cell viability, proliferation and function. In: Handbook of fluorescent probes and research products 9th ed., Eugene: Molecular Probes Inc., 2004 (chapter 15).

Holden, C. A., Hyne, R. V., Sathananthan, A. H. and Trounson, A. O. (1990). Assessment of the human sperm acrosome reaction using concanavalin A lectin. *Mol. Reprod. Dev.*, **25:** 247–257.

Holt, W. V. and North, R. D. (1984). Partially irreversible cold-induced lipid phase transitions in mammalian sperm plasma membrane domains: freeze-fracture study. *J. Exp. Zool.*, **230:** 473-483.

Honda, A., Siruntawineti, J. and Baba, T. (2002). Role of acrosomal matrix proteases in sperm-zona pellucida interactions. *Hum. Reprod. Update*, **8:** 405–412.

Hong, C. Y., Huang, J. J., Wu, P., Lo, S. J. and Wei, Y. H. (1988). Fluorescence supravital stain of human sperm: correlation with sperm motility measured by a transmembrane migration method. *Andrologia*, **20:** 516–520.

Kawase, Y., Araya, H., Kamada, N., Jishage, K. and Suzuki, H. (2005). Possibility of long-term preservation of freeze-dried mouse spermatozoa. *Biol. Reprod.*, **72:** 568–573.

Keskintepe, L., Pacholczyk, G., Machnicka, A., Norris, K., Curuk, M. A. and Khan, I. (2002). Bovine blastocyst development from oocytes injected with freeze-dried spermatozoa. *Biol. Reprod.*, **67:** 409–415.

Kusakabe, H. and Kamiguchi, Y. (2004). Chromosomal integrity of freeze-dried mouse spermatozoa after 137Cs gamma-ray irradiation. *Mutat. Res.*, **556:** 163–168.

Liu, J. L., Kusakabe, H., Chang, C. C., Suzuki, H., Schmidt, D. W. and Julian, M. (2004). Freeze-dried sperm fertilization leads to full-term development in rabbits. *Biol. Reprod.* **70:** 1776–1781.

Malmi, R., Kallajoki, M. and Suominen, J. (1987). Distribution of glycoconjugates in human testis. A histochemical study using fluorescein- and rhodamine-conjugated lectins. *Andrologia*, **19:** 322–332.

Marin, S., Chiang, K., Bassilian, S., Lee, W. N., Boros, L. G. and Fernandez-Novell, J. M. (2003). Metabolic strategy of boar spermatozoa revealed by a metabolomic characterization. *F.E.B.S. Lett.*, **554:** 342–346.

McLaughlin, E. A., Ford, W. C. and Hull, M. G. (1992). Motility characteristics and membrane integrity of cryopreserved human spermatozoa. *J. Reprod. Fertil.*, **95:** 527–534.

Meistrich, M. L., Mohapatra, B., Shirley, C. R. and Zhao, M. (2003). Roles of transition nuclear proteins in spermiogenesis. *Chromosoma*, **111:** 483–488.

Mukai, C. and Okuno, M. (2004). Glycolysis plays a major role for adenosine triphosphate supplementation in mouse sperm flagellar movement. *Biol. Reprod.*, **71:** 540–547.

Nagata, S., Nagase, H., Kawane, K., Mukae, N. and Fukuyama, H. (2003). Degradation of chromosomal DNA during apoptosis. *Cell Death Differ.*, **10:** 108–116.

Nagy, S., Jansen, J., Topper, E. K. and Gadella, B. M. (2003). A triple-stain flow cytometric method to assess plasma- and acrosome-membrane integrity of cryopreserved bovine sperm immediately after thawing in presence of egg-yolk particles. *Biol. Reprod.*, **68:** 1828–1835.

Pintado, B., de la Fuente, J. and Roldan, E. R. (2000). Permeability of boar and bull spermatozoa to the nucleic acid stains propidium iodide or Hoechst 33258, or to eosin: accuracy in the assessment of cell viability. *J. Reprod. Fertil.*, **118:** 145–152.

Polge, C., Smith, A.U. and Parkes, A.S. (1949) Revival of spermatozoa after vitrification and dehydration at low temperature. *Nature*, **164:** 666–676.

Ramalho-Santos, J., Schatten, G. and Moreno, R. D. (2002). Control of membrane fusion during spermiogenesis and the acrosome reaction. *Biol. Reprod.*, **67:** 1043–1051.

Rathi, R., Colenbrander, B., Bevers, M. M. and Gadella, B. M. (2001). *Biology of Reproduction*, **65**: 462.

Sakkas, D., Manicardi, G. C. and Bizzaro, D. (2003). Sperm nuclear DNA damage in the human. Adv. Exp. Med. Biol., 518: 73–84.

Sakkas, D., Manicardi, G., Bianchi, P. G., Bizzaro, D. and Bianchi, U. (1995). Relationship between the presence of endogenous nicks and sperm chromatin packaging in maturing and fertilizing mouse spermatozoa. Biol. Reprod., 52: 1149–1155.

Saling, P. M. and Storey, B. T. (1979). Mouse gamete interactions during fertilization in vitro. Chlortetracycline as a fluorescent probe for the mouse sperm acrosome reaction. J. Cell Biol., 83: 544–555.

Schurmann, A., Axer, H., Scheepers, A., Doege, H. and Joost, H. G. (2002). The glucose transport facilitator GLUT8 is predominantly associated with the acrosomal region of mature spermatozoa. Cell Tissue Res., 307: 237–242.

Scovassi, A. I. and Torriglia, A. (2003). Activation of DNA-degrading enzymes during apoptosis. Eur. J. Histochem., 47: 185–194.

Seli, E., Gardner, D. K., Schoolcraft, W. B., Moffatt, O. and Sakkas, D. (2004). Extent of nuclear DNA damage in ejaculated spermatozoa impacts on blastocyst development after in vitro fertilization. Fertil. Steril., 82: 378–383.

Senger, P. L. (2002). Reproductive behavior. In: Pathways to pregnancy and parturition2nd ed., Ephrata: Cadmus Professional Communications Science Press Division, 2003 (chapter 11).

Sotolongo, B., Lino, E. and Ward, W. S. (2003). Ability of hamster spermatozoa to digest their own DNA. Biol. Reprod., 69: 2029–2035.

Spallanzani, L. (1776) Osservazioni e spezienze interno ai vermicelli spermatici dell'uomo e degli animali. In Opusculi di Fisica Animale eVegetabile, Opusculo II. Modena, Italy.

Szasz, F., Sirivaidyapong, S., Cheng, F. P., Voorhou, W. F., Marks, A. and Colenbrander, B. (2000). Detection of calcium ionophore induced membrane changes in dog sperm as a simple method to predict the cryopreservability of dog semen. Mol. Reprod. Dev., 55: 289–298.

Thomas, C. A., Garner, D. L., DeJarnette, J. M. and Marshall, C. E. (1998). Effect of cryopreservation of bovine sperm organelle function and viability as determined by flow cytometry. Biol. Reprod., 58: 786–793.

Thomas, C. A., Garner, D. L., DeJarnette, J. M. and Marshall, C. E. (1997). Fluorometric assessments of acrosomal integrity and viability in cryopreserved bovine spermatozoa. Biol. Reprod., 56: 991–998.

Ward, C. R. and Storey, B. T. (1984). Determination of the time course of capacitation in mouse spermatozoa using a chlortetracycline fluorescence assay. Dev. Biol., 104: 287–296.

Ward, M. A., Kaneko, T., Kusakabe, H., Biggers, J. D., Whittingham, D. G. and Yanagimachi, R. (2003). Long-term preservation of mouse spermatozoa after freeze-drying and freezing without cryoprotection. Biol. Reprod., 69: 2100–2108.

Ward, W. S. (1993). Deoxyribonucleic acid loop domain tertiary structure in mammalian spermatozoa. Biol. Reprod., 48: 1193–1201.

Zhao, M., Shirley, C. R., Yu, Y. E., Mohapatra, B., Zhang, Y. and Unni, E. (2001). Targeted disruption of the transition protein 2 gene affects sperm chromatin structure and reduces fertility in mice. Mol. Cell Biol., 21: 7243–7255.

Transforming Rural Areas through Veterinary Science *Pages* **203-216**
Editor: Dipanjali Konwar, Shilpa Sood & Shahid Ahamad
Published by: **ASTRAL INTERNATIONAL PVT. LTD., NEW DELHI**

16 Major Constraints and Strategies for Milk Production in Hilly and Kandi Areas of Jammu

Dr. Surinder K. Gupta & Dr. Suraj Amrutkar

Introduction

As per 2012 census, total milk production in our country is more than 140 million tons. Rank of India in milk production is 1st with 18.5% share of world production. Per capita availability of milk in India is 337 gram per day. Uttar Pradesh has 1st in milk production. India has 2nd in cattle population with 190.9 million and 1st rank in buffalo population with 108.7 million.

Milk may be defined as the whole, fresh, clean, lacteal secretion obtained by the complete milking of one or more healthy milch animals, excluding that obtained within 15 days before or 5 days after calving or such periods as may be necessary to render the milk practically colostrum free and containing the minimum prescribed percentage of milk-fat and milk-solids-not-fat. The major constituents of milk are water, fat, protein, lactose, sterols, vitamins, enzymes, pigments, *etc.* All milks contain the same kind of constituents, but varying amounts. Milk from individual cows shows greater in small herds than in large ones. In general, milk fat shows the greatest daily variation, and then comes protein, followed by ash and sugar.

Major Constraints for Milk Production in Kandi Areas

Insufficient fodder and lack of water supply are the primary factors limiting livestock development in Kandy areas. Others have identified the lack of high yielding animals in the traditional herds and the low prices for fresh milk which create a disincentive to producers as additional limiting factors. Other important factors which constraint domestic milk production are the competition from imported dairy products, insufficient technical and extension service, inadequate labour supply as well as ecological factor.

- ☆ **Green Fodder:** In kandi areas, upto 99% of cattle feed under traditional management is derived from bush grazing.The cattle are fed through free range systems in communal grazing lands or from residues which may or may not belong to the owner of the herd. The natural fodder last the rainy season. As the dry season approaches, scarcity of fodder arises. The consequences of inadequate feed are low milk yield, low resistance to disease, and high mortality, particularly during the dry season.
- ☆ **Water Supply:** As a management practice, herdsman does not fetch water for their cattle. Rather, they move with their herds to where they will find water in streams, dams, rivers. During the dry season, and particularly in summer, most of such sources of water dry up in kandy areas. Some of the cattle may not survive the movement due to excessive heat and thirst.
- ☆ **Low Milk Yield in Stock:** Majority of cattle in kandy areas are traditional desi cattle herd. This means that there are no exotic breeds or cross-breeds in traditional herds. The yield from the traditional herds is low only because of the type of stock kept.
- ☆ **Low Milk Price:** Cost of production of milk at farm is approximately 35 rupees per liter, but at milk collection center, cost of milk is only 25-30 rupees per liter due to less fat content which is below cost of production of milk.
- ☆ **Competition from imported dairy products:** Imported dairy products are adversely competing with local dairy products. Hence the cost of raw milk is decreasing day by day.
- ☆ **Insufficient Technical and Extension Services:** In kandy areas of the state has a eve team of technical and extension staff consisting of one Veterinary surgeon with sub ordinary staffs. But they are not operational due to lack of mobility, lack of sense of duty and the generally unfavorable attitude of staff to work in rural areas. With this type of shortage of extension and technical services, cow die from preventable diseases while milk production from the cows in milk fall much below what would be expected from the application of improved animal health and husbandry practices.
- ☆ **Inadequate Labour Supply:** Government provides lot of subsidy to the farmers and people below economical poor level including ration with 2 rupees per kg. Hence, they don't have any need to earn money. Whole day they are playing with card and other things in villages, but not ready to go for work. Young generation is also not ready to work of labour. The herds of the most absentee stock owners are milked only to meet the needs of the herding households because of shortage of labour.

- ☆ **Ecological Factor:** There are the technical factors which make it difficult for cattle production to expand to all the kandyareas of the state. Climatic factors as well as the prevalence of flies in the would require the introduction of cattle breeds adopted the conditions of the ecological zone of kandy area.
- ☆ **Other Constraints:** There are number of other constraints includes such as high requirement of commercial supplementary feed for modem dairy production, poor pasture management and grazing control *etc.*

Factor Affecting Milk Yield (Quantity)

Species

The milk yield varies from species to species. Buffalo yield more than average Indian breed milch animals.

Breeds

Among major factors, breed is one of the most important constituents. Animal belonging to the milch breeds produce more milk (*Viz.* Sindhi 1135 litres/lactation) as compared to dual purpose breed *Viz.* Haryana (1100 litre/lactation).

Individuality of Animals

The strain and the cows within a breed also are different in producing total yield. Larger cows normally secrete more milk. Cows normally will not secrete more milk daily than the equivalent of 8-10 % of their body weight, whereas goats may secrete enough milk daily to equal 20 or more percent of their body weight.

Stage and Persistency of Lactation

There is considerable variation in the persistency of milk secretion following peak production within 2 months after lactation. Some cows are very persistent and their rate of milk secretion declines slowly (6-8 % of their previous month). The production of other cows may decline very rapidly (8-12 %), so that they show poor persistency.

Frequency of Milking

As milk accumulates in the lumen of the alveoli and fills the storage areas of the udder, pressure develops inside those areas. This tends gradually to inhibit further milk secretion. The more frequent removal of milk permits maximum intensity of milk manufacturing process. Therefore, frequent evacuation of udder is essential for maximum milk production. It has been shown that milking cow three-times-a-day increases milk production (10-25 percent) over two-times daily milking. Milking four-times-a-day instead of three-times results in another 5-15 percent increase in production. Of course, this will involve some more expenditure.

Pregnancy

During the first 5 months of pregnancy, the decline in milk yield in pregnant cows is similar to the equivalent lactation period in non-pregnant cows. However, following the fifth month of pregnancy, cows begin to decline more rapidly in milk yield.

The average gestation period of dairy cows is 283 days. The aim is to have each cow mated about 85 days after calving. If mated earlier than 85 days, the total yield for the lactation is reduced as in case after about 20th week of pregnancy milk yield will start falling more rapidly.

Age

It is believed that there is a slight additional growth of secreting cells of dairy cattle during each pregnancy until cows reach about 7 years of age. This is manifested by the increase in yearly milk.

Estrus

The activity of a cow when in heat generally reduced milk secretion, however, this is temporary. To minimize milk loss during estrus, cows should be controlled.

Dry period

Cows are normally bred 70 to 90 days (average of 85 days) after parturition. It is expected that they will lactate about 305 days and then be given a 60 day dry period before the next calving. The dry period is important for replenishing body supplies including regeneration of secretion tissue. Allowing dairy cows a dry period has been shown a result in significantly higher production during the succeeding lactation.

Gestation

A significant reduction of milk yield occurs towards the end of pregnancy. Although the exact reason is not yet known but according to one hypothesis it has been suggested that level of nutrient required for foetal development are highest; however, this appears to be only 1 to 2 percent of the daily requirement of the cow. Another convincing explanation is that a change in hormone production, in which large amounts of estrogen and progesterone are released into blood stream, which are detrimental to high milk yield. During fourth to fifth months of gestation, there is an increase of SNF.

Temperature and Humidity

Severe weather conditions drastically affect milk production. Temperature between 40-75°F has no effect on the milk production. In this range (Comfort Zone), no body processes are directly involved in maintaining body temperature. At a very high temperature feed consumption is greatly reduced, there is an increase in water intake, an increase in body temperature and respiration decrease in milk yield with lowered milk fat, SNF and total solids.

High relative humidity accentuates the problem of high temperature.

Changes Occurring During a Normal Lactation

Some changes can also occur during the normal lactation.

Feed

The speed of synthesis and diffusion of various milk constituents is dependent on the concentration of milk precursors in blood, which reflects the quality and quantity of the food supply. Nature provides for maintenance, growth and reproductive needs before energy is made available for lactation. Inadequate feed nutrients probably limit the secretion of milk more than any other single factor in a dairy cow. Although good nutrition alone can't guarantee high milk production, poor nutrition can prevent attainment of a cow's full potential just as poor management, low genetic potential on an unfavorable environment. The maintenance of lactation is closely related to an adequate feed intake by the lactating animals.

Stress

Recently more attention has been focused on the role of stress in the secretion of milk. As animals are selected to secrete higher levels of milk, any sort of stress will play an increasingly important role in lactation.

Effect of Milker

The amount of milk drawn from a cow is definitely influenced by the change of milker. Due to change of milker, the slight variation in milking process, upsets cow and thereby affects milk yield.

Diseases

Any one of the many diseases may significantly reduce the amount of milk secreted. Disease may affect heart rate, and therefore, the rate of blood circulation through the mammary gland; which influences milk secretion.

Factors Affecting Composition of Milk

The variation in composition and daily yield of milk is a regular phenomenon in any milking animal. Broadly, the factors which are responsible for such variation can be divided into

1. **Physiological:** which will be governed by the genetic makeup
2. **Environmental:** such as age, number of previous lactations, pregnancy, nutrition status *etc.*

The dairy man has hardly got any control over the physiological factors but he has some control over the environmental factors. A thorough understanding of the factors those change the environment of the dairy cattle can be used to take advantage of some of the changes in milk composition and yield that occurs during a normal lactation.

Variation in the composition of milk may result from one or more of a number of causes described below:

Species

Each species yields milk of characteristic compositions.

Breed

In general, if breeds producing the largest amounts of milk yield, then produce milk of a lower fat percentage. The composition of milk varies with a number of non-nutritional factors, one of the most marked being the effect of breed. The within breed variation in milk composition is very common. The fat and crude protein content of the milk is inversely to the lactation yield. Lactose values tend to be slightly higher in the milk from breeds with high fat content and thus the SNF content (Protein+Lactose+Ash) are also higher. Because of this fairly close relationship between fat and SNF contents, the selection of the cows producing a higher fat content should also ensure a high SNF content.

Individuality

Each cow tends to yield milk of a composition that is characteristic of an individual.

Interval of Milking

In general, a longer interval is associated with more milk with a lower fat content. The ideal interval between milking should be at 12 hours which is hardly followed by any dairymen. Uneven milking intervals affect the fat more than the protein or SNF percentage. With a long interval, the milk will be lower in fat and lactose, it will be slightly higher protein and as a result of counterbalancing, the SNF content will remain stable.

Completeness of Milking

If the cow is completely milked, the fat content is normal; if not, it is usually lower.

Frequency of Milking

Whether a cow is milked two, three or four times a day, it has no great effect on the fat content.

Day-to-Day Milking

May show variation from theindividual cow. Percentage composition of milk as well as yield varies considerable from day-to-day. In general daily variation of milk yield is caused by excitement, estrus, incomplete milking, and other irregularities previous to milking, disease under feeding and related factors.Depression in milk yield that last for several days are usually accompanied by higher fat tests as because there is inverse relationship between milk yield and fat test. An incomplete milking fails to obtain the last drawn milk, which extremely high in milk fat. First drawn milk, or foremilk may be as low as 1 percent milk fat. The milk yield at the next milking is higher in milk fat content since it contains the leftover milk from the last milking with a high fat content from the present milking.

Fat test may again vary upto 1 percent between the night and morning milking when the cows are milked at 14 and 10 hours intervals. The explanation for this variation will involve probably two factors: 1) due to relationship of pressure to milk and fat secretion, in which milk produced during a long interval and against a higher udder pressure which has a lower fat test, 2) due to exercise, which has a tendency to increase the level of milk fat. Consequently the evening milk of cows at equal intervals produces milk that has a slightly higher fat test than does that obtained from morning milking.

Disease and Abnormal Conditions

This tends to alter the composition of milk, especially when they result in a fall in yield. Very little is known about the influence of certain diseases on protein and SNF. An increase in body temperature frequently will be accompanied by an increase in fat % and a decrease in milk yield and SNF content. Udder infections, such as mastitis cause a decrease in milk fat, SNF, protein, lactose and a notable increase in the mineral and chlorides.

Ketosis reduces milk yield and also markedly increases the fat content of the milk. The effect of other diseases on milk composition is not so clear.

Portion of Milking

Fore-milk is low in fat content (less than 1 percent), while strippings are highest (close to 10%). The other milk constituents are only slightly affected on a fat free basis.

Changes Occurring During a Normal Lactation

Lactation period of an animal is the period from the time animal gives birth to a young one till she goes dry. Throughout this period which generally considered for about 305 days, there is a variation of both in composition and total yield.

Stage of Lactation

The first secretion after calving (colostrum) is very different from milk in its composition and general properties. The change from colostrum to milk takes place within a few days. Immediately after the young one is born, the cow produces secretion which is quite different from the normal milk and is known as colostrum, lasts for 3 to 5 days after parturition. It has a high content of fat and protein, and a low content of lactose, the contents of all protein fractions are high but there is an exceptionally high proportion of globulins, mainly in immunoglobulins, which persists for 1 or 2 days only. As lactation progresses and milk yield increases, there is rapid reduction in fat and protein contents and an increase in lactose content, changes which continue up to or beyond the peak (4 to 8 weeks) in yield.

During the post-peak period, milk yield initially declines at a more or less constant rate of about 2-2.5% per week and there is definitely a slight reversal of the previous changes in milk composition. This becomes more marked as the milk yield decline is accelerated towards the end of lactation.

The size of fat globules is bigger during the first few months and it remains fairly constant during the fifth, sixth and seventh months of lactation and again become smaller during the last month of lactation period.

The fatty acid composition of milk fat also changes throughout lactation. The fat of colostrum removed at first milking has a lower proportion of short-chain fatty acids, especially butyric acid and a higher proportion of palmitic acid than the fat of milk removed at subsequent milking throughout the 1st week of lactation. The relative proportion of short chain fatty acids, except butyric acid, increase throughout the first 8-10 weeks of lactation, that of palmitic acid is fairly constant and the proportion of stearic and octadecanoic acids tends to decrease. Subsequent changes associated with stage of lactation are small.

Pregnancy

There is an increase of SNF and protein in late lactation which must be associated with pregnancy, since open (non-pregnant) cows do not show increases in these components with advancing lactation. Pregnancy has no apparent effect on the fat content of milk.

Yield

For a single cow, there is a tendency for increased yields to be accompanied by a lower fat %, and vice versa.

Feeding

Has temporary effect only.

- **Changes in Milk fat Content:** One of the most marked changes in milk composition due to diet is the effect on fat content. Milk fat is highest when the fermentation in the rumen favors the production of acetic acid, and thus diets which depress this acid will depress the content of milk fat. These are the follows:
    - High concentrate ration
    - Low roughage rations
    - Grass from lush (tender and full of juice) pasture
    - Finely ground hay
    - Heat treated feeds
    - Feeds in pelleted form
    - Fish oils will depress the fat content of milk from 1 to 0.5% for as they are fed.

It has been noted that the above rations decrease milk fat by decreasing the acetic acid production on the other hand by increasing propionic acid content.

Research findings suggest that the fat depression in milk can partially be rectified by feeding the following materials:

- Sodium or potassium bicarbonate
- Calcium hydroxide
- Magnesium carbonate
- Magnesium oxide

- Sodium bentonite
- Partially delactosed whey

Some of the above compounds increase the rumen pH and other decrease propionate production and increase rumen acetic acid production. The drawback is using these substances is that most of them are unpalatable and decrease appetite.

- Feeding of ration having at least 17% fibre
- Use of screen that is more than 1/8 inch in diameter if ground forage is used
- Feeding of unground forage at a minimum rate of 1.5 kg hay per 100 kg body weight per day.
- Vegetable oils have been shown to cause a temporary increase in milk fat

Changes in Milk Flavor

Several weeds such a wild onion, and garlic when fed to the milch animals results into objectionable flavor in milk.

Changes in Protein and SNF Content

Changes in protein and SNF contents of milk is less pronounced by environmental factors, while the mineral and lactose contents content are not at all variable under normal farm conditions. Underfeeding of dairy cows results in a 0.2 percent reduction in protein and SNF percentage and a depression of milk yield. Increasing the plane of nutrition to 25 percent above normal standards results in an increase in SNF and protein percentage to the same event. High level of nutrition results in an elevated propionic acid production in the rumen.

Changes in Mineral and Vitamin Contents

Among minerals, the major elements (calcium, phosphorus, potassium, chlorine and sodium) can't be changed by altering the levels of these elements in the ration of a cow. Trace minerals with the exception of iron and copper can be increased by increasing the levels of those minerals in the ration upto a certain extent. For iodine, which is transferred in maximum amount, it is only 3-5 percent of the amount present in the ration appeared in milk.

Among vitamins, some of the fat soluble vitamins, A,D and E can be increased in milk through dietary process. Marked seasonal variation occurs in the vitamin A content is increased when the cow is exposed the enough of green forages specially during rainy season. The carotene content in all green forages are converted into vitamin A. Vitamin D content of milk can similarly be increased by providing sun-cured roughages or by exposing the cows to direct sunlight.

Changes in Specific Gravity of Milk

When the dairy cows goes off feed there is a decrease in the volume of milk produced, accompanied by increase in the fat, mineral, protein and total solids with a simultaneous reduction in lactose and specific gravity of milk.

Season

The percentage of both fat and solid-not-fat show slight but well defined variations during the course of the year. Temperature above 70°F (21°C) and below 30°F cause an increase in the fat content of milk, whereas protein and SNF quantities decline at higher temperature and increase at lower temperature. Milk production is usually less during the summer because of the higher environmental temperature and the prevalence of green forage scarcity. Thus the season of calving has got a marked effect on the total production. Cows freshening shortly before winter months produce total yield than those calving at other times of the year. The increase is probably due to more favorable temperature and more digestible feed available during the winter.

Age

The fat percentage in milk declines slightly as the cow grows older. Protein, fat and SNF decline with age. Analysis of results has indicates that in case of fat and SNF (mainly lactose) progressively reduce averaging approximately 0.2 to 0.4 % respectively over the first five lactation. If the cow produces milk with 5.2 % fat in the second and third lactation, the fat content may be about 4.5 % when the animal is about 11 or 12 years of age.

Condition of Cow at Calving

If the cow is in good physical condition when calving, it will yield milk of a higher fat percentage than it would if its physical condition was poor.

Excitement

Both yield and compositions of milk are liable to transient fluctuations during periods of excitement, for whatever reason. This may result in incomplete milk removal and thus a lower fat test. The SNF content remains unchanged.

Administration of Drugs and Hormones

Certain drugs may effect temporary change in the fat percentage; injection or feeding of hormones results in increase of both milk yield and fat percentage.

Exercise

Slight exercise apparently increases the fat content from 0.2 to 0.3 %without reducing the quantity of milk secreted. Moderate to heavy exercise in high producing cows, however, will result in reduced milk secretion and a corresponding increase in fat content. Exercisecauses no apparent change in the SNF content of milk.

Dry Period and Body Condition

The length of the dry period and the body condition at calving are related. Cows must be in good body condition at calving and must have a dry period to attain maximum production. The dry period is important for replenishing body supplies if the cow is in poor body condition at calving and also to generate milk secretory tissue.

Calving Interval

The interval between calving is another important management problem. The farmer must deal with. The decision should be made on the basis of individual factors such as feed.

Residual Milk

The residual milk is the amount of milk left in the udder after a normal milking. It can be obtained only after the injection of oxytocin and re-milking the animal. The amount of residual milk is proportional to the amount of milk present in the udder at the beginning of the milking. On an average, it has been observed that it is about 13.9 and 17.8 percent for a cow milking only once a day and for a cow when milking intervals were 10 and 14 hours respectively. Older cows have higher percentage of residual milk have a lower persistency of lactation. The percentage residual milk is also higher in low producers that high producers.

Udder Pressure and Secretion Rate

The pressure required to stop the secretion process has not been definitely determined and it probably varies from cow to cow. In general after the pressure reaches a certain point, the rate of milk secretion decreases. Secretion totally stops at about 35 hours after the last milking.

The effect of unequal milking intervals indicates that cows milked at either 9 and 15 hours or 8 and 16 hours daily intervals produce 1 to 3 percent less milk per lactation that cows milked at equal intervals. Increasing the frequency of milking to three or four times daily increases the level of milk production. Three times a day milking increases the milk production by 15-25 percent, but only about 5-10 percent of this is due to better feeding and management. Most of the increase in four-times-a-day milking over three-times-a-day milking is due to better feeding and management of the cows.

Thus milking at regular intervals should always be the aim of all dairy farmers. Three-times-a-day milking over twice-a-day milking (at equal intervals) although yields high, but the farmers before adopting the method should first compare the cost for extra management and the feed with that of the extra production due to thrice –a-day milking.

Strategies for Increase Milk Production

There are number of factors which influence the quantity and quality of milk. By studying all the factors responsible for milk production, we can increase the production of milk. Proper management and nutrition play important role in production of milk.

Start Cow with Successful Dry Period

Dry period (60-90 days) nutrition and management affects health and performance after birth. Thus, evaluate your dry cow programme if you are unhappy with milk cow performance.

Prevent Subclinical Milk Fever

Reduce the risk of subclinical milk fever (low blood calcium) during the first week of lactation.

Optimize Feed Intake Immediately after Calving

- ☆ Provide warm water with drinkable drench.
- ☆ Allow access to fresh total mixed ration.
- ☆ Provide grass hay.
- ☆ Keep the feed bunks clean and fresh.

Optimize Cow Comfort

To optimize cow comfort in the fresh cow group:

- ☆ Use a stocking rate at 80 to 85 percent of capacity
- ☆ Keep cows in a fresh cow group for 14 to 21 days
- ☆ Provide 30 to 36 inches of bunk space per cow
- ☆ Reduce social stress (especially for first calf heifers)
- ☆ Prevent cows from separating from the normal herd mates
- ☆ Invest in cows cooling for dry and lactating cows

Maintain Rumen Health and Prevent Ruminal Acidosis

- ☆ Provide a flake of grass hay for the first five days after calving. Early lactation diet should contain plenty of good quality digestible fiber (31 to 35 percent neutral detergent fibre)
- ☆ Minimize the risk of slug feeding or diet sorting that may result in rumen acidosis

Identify Cows with a History of Metabolic or Health Problems

Cows with a history of milk fever, ketosis or mastitis are likely to face these problems again. Keeping an eye on cows prone to health problems allows you to help prevent these problems.

Position of Feed Additives

Fresh cow groups are most likely to offer a return on investments for feed additives.

- ☆ Ionophores increase glucose availability
- ☆ Rumen protected choline improves liver health and function
- ☆ Protected amino acids meet amino acid requirements without overfeeding protein
- ☆ Supplemental protected fat increases energy intake
- ☆ Yeast culture stabilizes rumen fermentation

Anti-Nutritional Factors

Anti-nutritional factors include feeds containing mold, wild yeasts and poorly fermented feeds.

Feed Correct Amount of Antitoxins

Antioxidants (for example vitamin E and selenium) help reduce the impact of oxidative stress. Oxidative stress could be too much fat mobilization, poor air quality or injury. These all decrease the efficiency of immune system function.

Provide adlib green fodder such as Lucern and Berseem to productive animal.

References

Handbook of Animal Husbandry (2011).3rd revised edition, 1233 pp.

Banerjee, G. C. (1998). A text book of Animal Husbandry, 6th edition, 1079 pp.

Sastry, N.S.R. & Thomas, C.K. (2005). Livestock Production Management, 4th revised edition, 642 pp.

Chakrabarti, A. (2011) Text Book of Clinical Veterinary Medicine, 3rd edition, 701 pp.

Verma, D.N. (1999) A text book of Livestock production Management in tropic, 1st edition, 748 pp.

Transforming Rural Areas through Veterinary Science *Pages* **217-224**
Editor: Dipanjali Konwar, Shilpa Sood & Shahid Ahamad
Published by: **ASTRAL INTERNATIONAL PVT. LTD., NEW DELHI**

17 Managemental Problems under Animal Husbandry Practices in Kandi Areas of Jammu

Dr. Surinder K. Gupta & Dr. Suraj Amrutkar

Introduction

Dairy farming is very profitable business if started with proper training and proper knowledge about local market problems which are faced or the reasons for loss in this business may be just because of poor management, lack of labour, lack of feed, improper care of cattle. Livestock is one of the widely expanding sectors and over the years, this sector has established it's important in development of rural economy. This sector not only supplements income of the farmers but also provides gainful employment on the hand and supplements the vital and varied nutritional requirements of the individual. Dairying has become an important secondary source of income for millions of rural families and has assumed a most important role in providing employment and income generating opportunity.

In Kandi areas of Jammu region, farmers are already poor due to low rainfall. Farmers can't get profit from their field. They are totally dependent upon natural rainfall. All over India, all marginal farmers are poor in condition in kandi areas because they totally depend upon their luck, in lot of ways like for rain, for market rate, for disease of plant. Because of this reason, day by dayfarmers becomes poor and poor. Our honorable Prime minister has goal to doubling the farmer's income within five years. Is it possible? We can increase our production in field but at a certain limit. At the same time, fertilizer and other cost increases multiple times. But farmer's grain can't get that much prize. So for doubling farmer's income, integrated farming with the help of livestock is the last option in front of farmers. In this condition, they are rearing domestic animals for getting additional income. In this way, in same field they can increase their income in multiple times by rearing cattle, poultry, pig, sheep and goat. But due to lack of education and finance, they are facing lot of problem in animal husbandry practices.

Present Status of India in Dairy Farming (2012 Census)

Total livestock (Cattle, Buffalo, Sheep, Goat, Pig, Horse, Mules, Donkey, Camel, Mithun and Yak) population of India is 512.2 million. India has 2nd rank in cattle population with 190.9 million. In Buffalo population, India has 1st rank with 108.70 million. Total milk production in our country is more than 140 million tons. Uttarpradesh has 1st rank in milk production with 23.33 million tons. Rank of India in milk production is 1st with 18.5% share of world population. Per capita availability of milk in India is 337 gram per day.

Some of the Practical Dairy Farming Challenge in Kandi Areas of Jammu Region

Small Dairy Farms

Majority of dairy animals are kept by small farmers and the number can vary from 1 to 5 animals per farm. It might not be suitable to call them as dairy farms.

Feeding of Dairy Animals

The dairy farming in Kandy areas is a supplementary business to agriculture. Means the dairy animals are raised on the residues (left over) of agriculture mainly. Very few farmers have separate fodder cultivation fields. Other constraints in feeding are:

- No awareness about balanced feeding of cattle. *i.e.* knowledge of how much of what should be fed to animals.
- Water only given in limited amount/times.
- A supplement feeding is very minimal or absent.

Health Issues

Good hygiene largely determines the health and production of cows. In animal health, there are following challenges like:

- Availability of qualified veterinarian in rural areas.
- Frequent disease incidence like FMD which has negative impact on dairy production. It also affects many animals in village.
- Absence of preventive health care measures like vaccination and deworming.
- Dystokia is also the major problem in exotic cross breed of dairy.

Management of Animals

In management there are challenges like:

- ✰ Hygienic animal shed
- ✰ Teat washing and dip before milking
- ✰ Dis-infestation of animal shed regularly

Farm Economics

- ✰ Dairy farmers are not aware of proper record keeping and dairy farm economics
- ✰ This has a negative impact on the income of the farmers and his spending on dairy animals.

Scarcity of Green Fodder

- ✰ Green fodder is very essential for maintenance of milk production. In kandi areas, due to low rainfall, farmers can't get fodder crop over a year.
- ✰ Weeds also the major problem in fodder crop production. Weeds compete with fodder crop like *Berseem* and *Lucern*. Hence final production of fodder crop decreases.

Reproductive Problems

- ✰ Repeat breeding is the main problem in Kandi areas.
- ✰ Retention of placenta is also the problem.
- ✰ Mineral and vitamin deficiency is also the major reason behind repeat breeding / anoestrus.
- ✰ Veterinary specialist facility is not available mostly in the hilly and interior areas.
- ✰ Artificial Insemination facility is readily not available
- ✰ Local bulls are the only option in front of farmers for breeding purpose, they get infected due to work load of natural insemination. Most of the time, infected bulls spread the reproductive diseases in local areas.

Clinical Management of Reproductive Problems in Dairy Cows for Kandi Areas

Reproductive herd health programs are effective in maintaining and improving the reproductive efficiency of dairy herds resulting in increased net income. Unobserved estrus, ovarian cysts, conception failure, uterine disease, abnormal pregnancy, and observed abortions are common reproductive abnormalities in dairy cows that may be controlled effectively with improved management practices and appropriate administration of pharmacological and biological agents. Prostaglandin F_2-alfa is effective in the management of unobserved estrus, uterine disease, and abnormal pregnancy whereas gonadotropin releasing hormone is a reliable treatment for ovarian cysts and may be useful to improve conception in repeat breeders. Incidence of uterine disease can be minimized by eliminating or reducing factors that predispose to retained placenta and appropriate treatment of affected cows. Immunizing agents should be selected for each herd based on risks of exposure to infectious diseases that cause infertility or abortion.

Problem Related to Milking in Kandi Areas

For the end consumer, obtaining milk that is clean and free of harmful bacteria is a must. But how can dairy farms ensure that high standard of hygiene is upheld? Using innovative techniques and high quality milking machinery is one thing. The milk must be tested and analyzed regularly. Milking place can be rinsed regularly ensuring that the level of hygiene remains very high. Even though the site where the milking actually takes place is the most critical when it comes to the sanitation and hygiene, studies has shown that there are other factors which can influence the quality of the milk. To achieve the best end results and maintain the highest level of hygiene in the milking process, it is important to be sure to work with the best equipment and smart milking monitoring measures.

Methods of Milking

Hand Milking

The following are the different methods of hand milking in Kandi areas.

- **Stripping:** Firmly holding the teat between the thumb and fore finger and drawing it down the length of the teat and at the same time pressing it to cause the milk to flow down in a stream.
- **Full hand Milking:** Grasping the teat with all the five fingers and pressing it against the palm does full hand milking.
- **Full hand milking followed by stripping**
- **Fisting (Knuckling):** This is the worst method of milking adopted by some kandi area farmers. In this method, they bend their thumb against the teat. Knuckling should always be avoided to prevent injuries of the teat tissues.

The recommended method is full hand milking followed by stripping.

Machine Milking

Due small herd size and low productive cows, negligible (very few) farmers using machine milking. The advantage of milking machine are manifold. It is easy to operate, costs low, saves time as it milk 1.5 litre to 2 litres per minute. It is also very hygienic. All the milk from the udder can be removed. The machine is easily adaptable and gives a suckling feeling to the cow and avoids pain in the udder as well as leakage of milk.

Mastitis in Dairy Cattle

Mastitis is also the main problem due to faulty management in front of farmers in Kandi areas. Mastitis is the inflammation of the mammary gland and udder tissue, and is a major endemic disease of dairy cattle. It usually occurs as an immune response to bacterial invasion of the teat canal by variety of bacterial sources present on the farm, and can also occurs as a result of chemical, mechanical or thermal injury to the cow's udder.

Milk secreting tissues and throughout the udder can be damaged by bacterial toxins, and sometimes permanent damage to the udder occurs. Severe acute cases can be fatal, but even in cows that recover there may be consequences for the rest of the lactation and subsequent lactation.

Practices such as close attention to milking hygiene, the culling of chronically infected cows, good housing management and effective dairy cattle nutrition to promote good cow health are essential in helping to control herd mastitis levels. Mastitis is most often transmitted by contact with the milking machine, and through contaminated hands or other materials, in housing, bedding and other equipments.

Tips to Overcome Problems in Cattle Rearing

Lack of awareness on aspects of farm management in livestock hampers the full productivity of dairy animals. Some of the problems that are usually encountered in dairy livestock and their possible remedial measures are:

- ✰ **High Mortality in Calves and Poor Growth:** Remedial measures to be taken up are colostrum feeding within an hours after birth, deworming, feeding antibiotics, early introduction to concentrates and green (creep feeding).
- ✰ **Low Milk Yield:** Numerous factors responsible for low milk production. It can be improve the production by providing green fodder, concentrate mixture as well as mineral mixture, adlib water, stress free environment, high quality species selection, free from infection and by maintaining hygiene.
- ✰ Main problems among milking animals are reproduction based problem mainly anoestrus, repeat breeding, long calving intervals, low milk performance and mineral deficiencies. In this cases proper heat detection, feeding balanced rations and mineral supplementation, protection against thermal and ecto and endo parasitic infestation can help averts the problem.
- ✰ The productive performance of a dairy farm is viable if cows calve every year and produce milk for atleast 300 days with high production efficiency. If there are 20-30 cows, they should all in the milking. Proper recording of body weight gain, physiological activities and milk production can help in judging the performance of individual animals. From this one can identify the poor producing animals and undertake the remedial measures in time. The animals which do not respond to improved feeding and management should be removed.
- ✰ **Management:** Milking management is very important task in dairy because it is the quality and the production of milk which matters most. Farmers should follow good milking management practices, especially cleanliness and hygiene at the milking place. Practice regular milking hours as far

as possible and equal milking intervals. After washing the udder with antiseptic like $KMnO_4$ and wiping it with a clean cloth, practice dry and full hand milking method followed by stripping. Complete the milking within 5-7 minutes gently without much noise.

☆ **Tick Control Strategies in Dairy Farm:** Ticks are economically the most important pests of cattle and other domestic species in tropical and subtropical countries. They are the vectors of a number of pathogenic microorganisms including haemo-protozoans (***Babesiosis, Tropical theileriosis***), rickettsial (*Anaplasmosis*), virals as well as bacterial (***Pastuerella, Brucella, Listeria, Staphylococcus***) and *Spirochaetes*. The ticks are voracious blood suckers, loss of blood for their rapid development impoverishes the hosts. In heavy tick infestation cattle must have more feed merely to meet the demands of the parasites; the growth of young animals is retarded and they may remain thin, weak and stunted.

An integrated control strategy based on the following measures is recommended for the control of ticks in cattle and buffaloes.

- Housing in tick proof building
- Slow burning of the wastes near the walls of the animal sheds
- Separate housing for cattle and buffaloes
- Quarantine
- Pasture spelling and rotational grazing
- Manual removal of ticks
- Clearance of vegetation
- Use of acaricides:

At present, periodic application of acaricides (agents used to kill ticks and mites) is the most widely used method of tick control in dairy farming. Control of ticks with acaricides may be directed against the free living stages of ticks in the environment or against the parasitic stages on host. Acaricides can be applied by dipping, washes, spraying, pour-on, spot-on or by injections. Dipping is an expensive operation but is desirable when a large number of cattle are to be treated or when a tick eradication programme is in place. Butox is a range of formulations containing the synthetic pyrethroid Deltamethrin as an active ingredient. It is for the control of ecto-parasitic infestations in cattle and sheep caused by ticks, lice, flies, mites, midges and keds.

Following precaution should be observed while dipping animals for tick control and treatment.

☆ Wound should be attended to thoroughly before resorting to dipping, otherwise dipping causes discomfort to animals and toxicity may occur.

☆ Avoid dipping on cloudy, rainy, windy or cold days.

☆ The animals to be dipped should not be thirsty.

☆ Animals that are fatigue due to any reason should not be dipped.

- To the extent possible, avoid contamination of the dipping tank with organic matter (e.g. dung) as it lowers the concentration of insecticides in the dip.
- The animals must actually swim in the tank and have one or two dips of their head in the acaricidal solution. For this purpose, two attendants with forked blunt sticks should direct the operation.
- Let the animals drain properly before they are sent out to the fields, otherwise the insecticides will cause pollution of feed, fodder or other items coming in contact with insecticides. Design the dipping area with a good drain back to the dipping bath.
- The concentration of the dip should be very carefully adjusted and may be same as recommended for the spray but in no case higher than that.
- Weak animals less than three months old should not be subjected to dipping.
- Human safety against insecticides is of paramount importance. While handling any acaricide, avoid repeated or prolonged contact with skin and inhalation of dust and mist. Wear clean clothing and wash hands and face before eating or smoking. Keep the antidote (generally Atropine sulphate injection @ 0.2-2 mg/kg) ready for use in the case of acaricide poisoning.

Retention of Placental Membrane

Retention of placenta is also the problem of kandy areas farmer. It **causes** may be due to abortion, dystokia, premature delivery, lack of exercise, deficiency of hormones like oxytocin and / or estrogen, infections like brucellosis, ***Vibriosis*** and ***Trichomoniasis***. Symptoms of this condition / malady is placenta retained even after 12 hours of parturition, straining, foul smelling discharge, fever, loss of appetite, dullness and depression.

Treatment

- Remove placenta manually.
- Administration of injection Oxytocin I/M at approximately 12 hours after parturition.
- Keep 2-4 furea boluses intrauterine for 1-2 days.
- Give orally Replanta powder @50 gm/day for 3-4 days.
- Parenteral administration of antibiotics for atleast three days.

Prophylaxis

- Breed at proper age.
- Avoid injury or unnecessary tractions at delivery.
- Provide adequate nutrition.
- Control of infectious diseases.

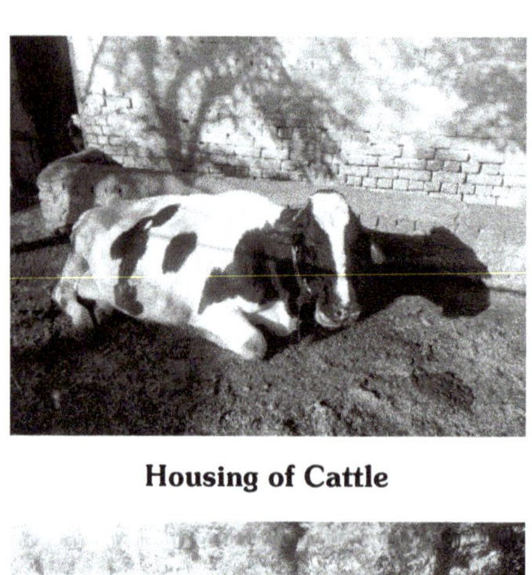

Housing of Cattle

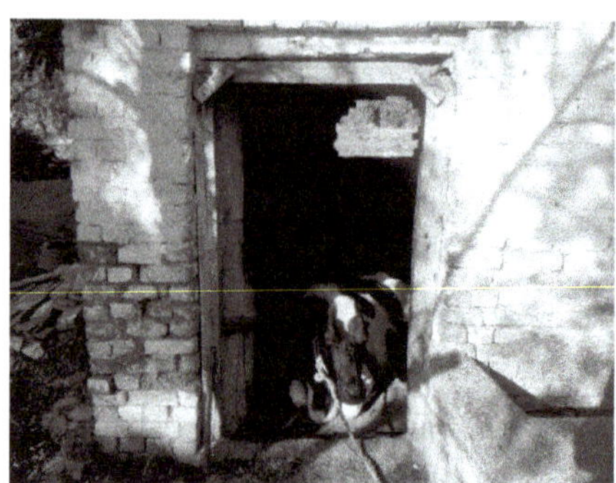

Housing of Cattle

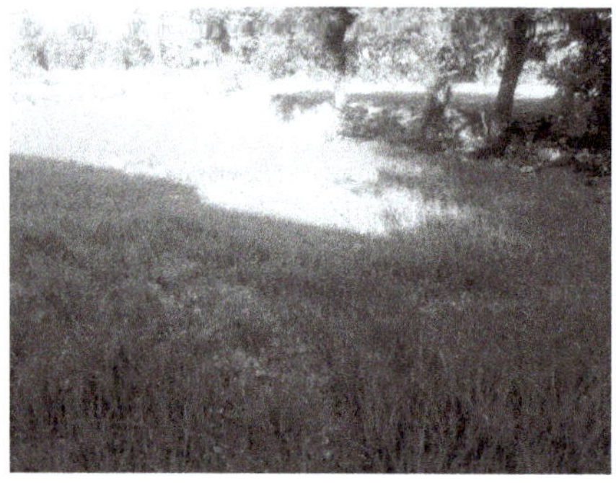

Fodder Crop

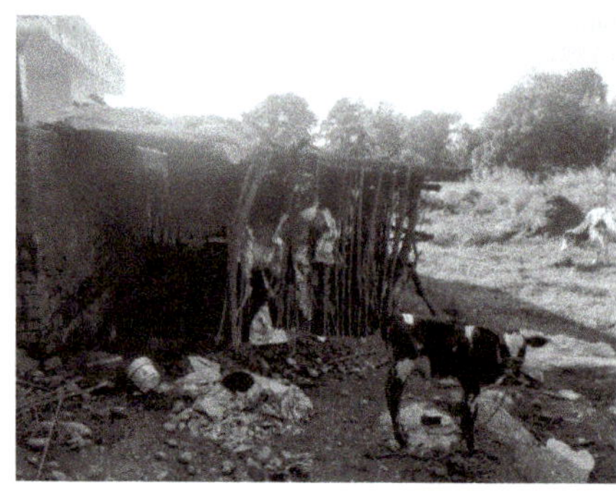

Housing of Cattle

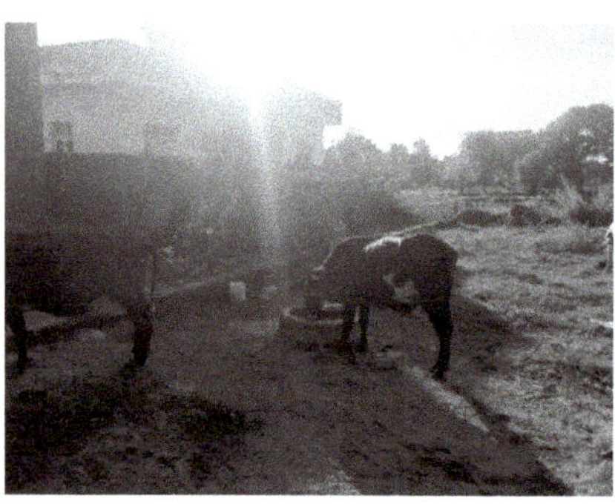

Housing of Fodder

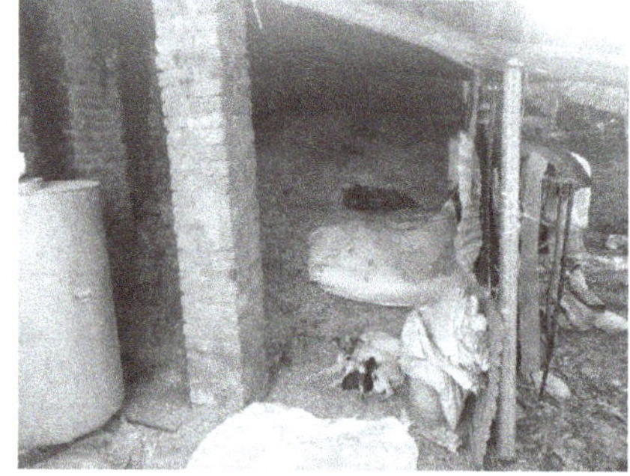

Storage of Wheat Straw

These photographs depicts the ground reality and condition of farming community of Kandi areas of Jammu region rearing Livestock for their earning.

Transforming Rural Areas through Veterinary Science *Pages 225-238*
Editor: Dipanjali Konwar, Shilpa Sood & Shahid Ahamad
Published by: **ASTRAL INTERNATIONAL PVT. LTD., NEW DELHI**

18 Common diseases of Cattle in Kandi areas of Jammu

Dr. Surinder K. Gupta & Dr. Suraj Amrutkar

Introduction

Tropical and subtropical climatic conditions provide most suitable environment for the proliferation and spread of several types of diseases. It can be said that about one fourth losses in production are due to diseases. A large number of diseases of domestic animals and man are caused by minute organisms, invisible to naked eye, named microbes. Although India is a major producer of livestock products, the average productivity of livestock is quite lower compared to world average. Inadequate availability of feed and fodder, insufficient coverage through artificial insemination, low conception rats, non-availability of quality males for breeding, poor management practices, high mortality and morbidity losses due to diseases, inadequate marketing infrastructure and unorganized marketing are the other major concern.

A large number of infectious and metabolic diseases prevalent in our Indian livestock have serious implication for animal productivity, export potential and safety/quality of livestock products, and many of the diseases have zoonotic implications. The current efforts of prevention and control of livestock diseases needs to be strengthened. There is a shortage of veterinary and para-veterinary manpower and facilities including mechanism for diagnosis, treatment, tracking and prevention of the diseases. Adequate infrastructure for ensuring bio-security, proper quarantine systems and services to prevent the ingress of diseases across the states and national borders is not available.

As per 2012 census in J & K states, there is decrease in livestock population over 2007 to 2012 from 10.98 million to 9.20 million (excluding 0.008 million stray cattle) registering a decline of 16.25% in the total number of animals of various species. Cattle population in J & K is 2798 thousand.

Bacterial Diseases of Cattle

1. Haemorrhagic Septicemia: Galghotu – in Hindi.

This disease is also known as Pasteurellosis-in-cattle, shipping fever, Shipping pneumonia, HS. It is usually an acute, less frequently sub-acute, febrile of cattle and buffaloes characterized by sudden onset, high temperature, edematous swellings of sub cutaneous tissue, particularly of the throat and acute gastro enteritis caused by *Pasteurellaboviseptica.*

Prevalence

It may occur sporadically, usually enzootically in India.

Species Affected

Cattle, buffaloes and deer. The disease is more common in buffaloes than cattle.

Mode of Transmission of Disease

- ☆ Contaminated water, soil and utensil, etc.
- ☆ Contact of diseased animal with healthy animal
- ☆ Insect vectors like flies may transmit the disease
- ☆ Climatic factors are of great importance for high incidence of diseases in tropical and subtropical area.

Incubation Period :1-3 days

Symptoms

- ☆ High fever (rectal temperature rises up to 104 to 106°F)
- ☆ Dullness, depression, anorexia, off feed and standing in one place.
- ☆ Head, throat, dewlap and neck become swollen. The swelling is hard, hot, tense and painful
- ☆ Tongue is swollen and protruded outside, salivation and difficulty in swallowing.
- ☆ Breathing becomes difficult on account of oedema of the pharynx.
- ☆ Blood sometimes seen from the nose.
- ☆ At first, there is constipation, soon followed by diarrhea accompanied with straining, grunting and symptoms of colic.
- ☆ Difficult breathing with pneumonia
- ☆ Acute conjunctivitis with lachrymation

Virulence: 50 percent to 100 percent mortality. It is more fatal for buffaloes.

Diagnosis

- ☆ High temperature

- ☆ Swelling of head, throat and dewlap
- ☆ Blood smear reveals the bipolar gram-negative bacteria.
- ☆ Inoculation of blood in the rabbit cause death within 24 hours.
- ☆ Post mortem examination shows that swelling and hemorrhagic spot in the lymph gland and serous membrane and in the organs. Spleen is normal in size. Gastrointestinal tract is severely inflamed and the contents mixed with blood. Lungs are inflamed, the pleura is oedematous and haemorrhagic.

Treatment and Control

General

- ☆ Good feeding and adequate housing for animals during monsoon season are highly desirable.
- ☆ Isolation and disinfection should be carried out.

Prophylaxis

- ☆ **HS Antiserum:** is used for the passive immunity; Dose: Cattle, 10 to 20 cc, S/c
- ☆ **HS Vaccine (dead):** Vaccination should be done two months before the onset of disease
- ☆ **HS Oil Adjuvant Vaccine (Bain's Vaccine):** is a dead vaccine, prepared from a highly antigenic strain of *P. Septica* killed by formalin; Dose: Cattle, 2 to 3 cc. I/m.

Curative Treatment

- ☆ **Bacteriostatic:** Sulpha drugs such as Sulphamerazine, Sulphamethazine, Sulphanilamide, Sulphathiazole, etc. have been widely employed.
- ☆ **Antibiotics:** Broad spectrum antibiotics viz: dehydro-streptomycin, terramycin, Auremycin, Chloromycetin, bacitracin, I/m or I/v may be tried. Penicillin may also be given.
- ☆ **HS Antiserum:** may be given in therapeutic doses, S/c, 50cc.
- ☆ **Antiseptic:** Potassium permanganate half to one drachm in water, carbolic acid one drachm or lugol's iodine I/v also tried.

2. Black Quarter(Black-Leg)

It is an acute infectious and highly fatal, bacterial disease of cattle. Buffaloes, sheep and goats are also affected. Young cattle between 6-24 months of age, in good body condition are mostly affected. It is soil borne infection which generally occurs during rainy season. In India, the disease is sporadic (1-2 animal) in nature.

Causal Organism

It is a bacterial disease caused by clostridium chauvoei.

Symptoms

- High Fever (106-105°F), loss of appetite, depression and dullness.
- Suspended rumination
- Rapid pulse and heart rates
- Difficult breathing (dyspnoea)
- Lameness in affected area
- Crepitation swelling over hip, back and shoulder
- Swelling is hot and painful in early stages whereas cold and painless inter
- Recumbency (prostration) followed by death within 12-48 hrs

Treatment

- Penicillin @10000 unit/kg body weight IM (locally daily for 5-6 days)
- Oxytetracycline in high doses i.e. 5-10 mg/kg body weight IM or IV
- Incise the swelling and drain off
- B.Q. antiserum in large does, if available
- Injection Avil/ Cadistin @5-10 ml IM

3. Brucellosis

It is also called Contagious abortion or Bang's disease. It is a specific contagious disease of cattle, pigs, goats etc. Characterized by abortion in the female and orchitis in the male by *brucellaabortus.*

Prevalence

Throughout the world.

Species Affected

Cattle, buffalo, sheep and goat. It causes disease in man-undulated fever but this disease can be caused also by B. suis and B. melitensis.

Etiology

Is Brucellaabortus, a small gram-negative, non-spore forming rod.

Natural Transmission

- Through ingestion of organism which is present in large number of aborted foetus, foetal membranes and uterine discharge.
- The bovine habit of licking of young, eating of placenta and licking the genitalia causes rapid spread of disease.
- Bull gets infection through infectious cow.
- Brucella may enter through the unbroken skin or through injured area.
- Disease can be transmitted through milk.

Incubation Period

Is variable, about 21 days

Symptoms

- Abortion are more common during the middle or last 6 months of pregnancy
- The act of abortion is preceded by uneasiness, secretion of colostrum and other normal signs of parturition.
- The placenta is usually characteristically altered and it is streaked with a yellowish slime and the cotyledons which normally are firm and red, become flaccid and covered with creamy yellow coating.
- The surface is necrotic. An infected dam may retain the placenta for as long as three to four week, vaginal discharge changes reddish to brown through-out the period.
- In bull, there is a swelling and permanent induration and thickening of the testicles.
- Working bullock may be affected with hygroma of the knee-joint.
- Sometimes chronic infection takes place causing permanent sterility in bull.

Diagnosis

- **Clinical Symptoms:** The disease is suspected when number of cows abort at a time. The placental lesion is sufficient for a diagnosis.
- Identification of organism in microscope.
- Culture can be made from stomach content, intestinal content, placenta, uterine exudate and milk of the infected animals.
- Serological tests: Blood Serum Agglutination Test
- Brucella isolation can be made from the foetal stomach contents, lung or rectum.

Treatment and Control

General Treatment

- Removal of infected animals from the herd
- Placenta and foetus should be burnt
- Disinfection should be done for infected byres, etc.

Prophylaxis

- Br. Abortus strain 19 vaccine is widely used in calves.Dose: Heifers: S/c 5 cc.

Curative Treatment

- Broad spectrum antibiotic, Viz: Streptomycin and Aureomycin may be tried.

- ☆ **Sulphadiazine** or triple **Sulphonamides** may also be used.

4. Tuberculosis

It also known as "Pearl disease, Phthisis, consumption, Piner's disease, T.B." T.B. is a chronic infectious disease, characterized by the slow progressive development of tubercleT.B. is a chronic infectious disease, characterized by the slow progressive development of tubercle or nodules in almost any organ of the body except the skeletal muscles. It is a zoonosis and in the past has been one of the greatest scourges of mankind. It is of great economic importance in cattle, pigs and poultry including man caused by *Mycobacterium tuberculosis.*

Prevalence

It is probably present in almost all countries. But few countries are now free from this disease.

Species Affected

All warm blooded animals.

Etiology

is mycobacterium tuberculosis of which there are three main types, viz: Bovine, Avian and Human, that is M. bovis, M. avian and M. tuberculosis in cattle, poultry and man respectively. M. bovis is a cylinder rod-shaped microorganism which has specific characteristics of being acid fast, gram positive, aerobic and non-motile organism.

- ☆ Mode of transmission
- ☆ Inhalation of infected droplets.
- ☆ By ingestion of infected discharges, from faeces, milk or urine and from open lesions in lymphocytes.
- ☆ Through drinking water
- ☆ Infection via skin abrasion can occur, but less likely
- ☆ Animal may retain the microorganism for many years in encapsulated lesions in the lungs, then under certain conditions the capsule may break down and release micro-organism into the surrounding causing disease.
- ☆ The drinking of milk from infected udders by calves and pigs is the most common method of transmission to these animals.

Symptoms

Because almost any organ in the body may become involved there are no clear cut symptoms which are indicative of the presence of disease, these symptoms exhibited depending on the organ affected.

- ☆ **Pulmonary Tuberculosis:** is usually a chronic disease and is known as "consumption " or "phthisis". In the beginning slight cold with a short dry cough are present. Feeding or exercise may bring on the cough. After a time the cough becomes more frequent, harsh and moist. Temperature is not usually present in early stages, later on fluctuations in temperature occur. It gradually increases in quantity and become purulent.

- ☆ **Intestinal Tuberculosis:**The intestines, the mesenteric lymph gland, liver, peritoneum and pancreas become affected. These may beaffected in conjunction with the lungs.There is a persistent diarrhea. Occasional tympany. Emaciation is so marked that the affected animals are called "piners".
- ☆ **Mammary Tuberculosis:** May be primary from external infection of milk ducks but is usually secondary to generalized tuberculosis. The udder is affected with a hard painless enlargement of gland.
- ☆ The symptoms consist of a hard swelling and disturbance of function. If it affects the vertebral column which can be cut with a knife.
- ☆ **Tuberculosis of the Meninges:** The animal make erratic movement, appears blind, walk in circles and may be comatose before death.
- ☆ **Skin Lesions:** are rarely emaciated. They consist of small encapsulated abscesses along the lymphatic's.
- ☆ **Eye Lesions:** There is an iritis or opacity of the cornea.
- ☆ **Genital Tract:** The testicles are enlarged, hard and painless. The bull is often sterile. The ovaries, the fallopian tube, and uterus may be affected, resulting in Chronic Metritis, Sterility and nymphomania.

Diagnosis

- ☆ **Clinical Diagnosis:** of tuberculosis from the symptoms is possible only after the disease has reached a very advanced stage.
- ☆ **Radiology:** is frequently used for diagnosis in man, seldom in animal.
- ☆ **Demonstration of Tubercle Bacilli:**
  - Microscopical examination of sputum, milk, faeces, urine etc.
  - By cultural examination
  - By animal inoculation
- ☆ **Tuberculin Test:** 0.1cc concentrated tuberculin injected intradermally into the skin on the side of neck in two successive doses. In non-reacting animals there is practically an insignificant increase in skin thickness. These is no heat or tenderness and no oedema around the firm nodule left by the injection.

Treatment and Control

General Treatment

- ☆ All animals with clinical signs of tuberculosis are to be slaughtered, especially those showing signs of pulmonary, intestinal, udder or uterine tuberculosis. The remainder are to be tested with tuberculin and then divided into herds, viz: reacting and non-reacting. In India slaughtering of reacting cases are not possible in cattle, therefore a third group of clinical cases is essential which should be under-strict segregation till they die a natural death.

- ☆ The milk from tuberculous cows may contain tubercles bacilli even when the udder is not visibly tuberculous.

Prophylaxis

- ☆ **BCG vaccine** is a living but almost avirulent strain of bovine tuberculous bacilli.
- ☆ Dose: I/v, cattle 5 to 50 mg moist weight of bacilli in a appropriate volume, repeated every two years and S/c in cattle 50-100 mg weight of bacilli in a appropriate volume, repeated annually.

Curative Treatment

- ☆ **Antibiotics:** Streptomycin is tried in human beings with good results
- ☆ **Tuberculin:** Was at one time tried as a curative but its use is not free from risk.
- ☆ Nourishing diet and cod liver oil may be given to improve the resistance of the animal.

5. **Mastitis:** Thanela Rog in Hindi.

It is an acute or chronic inflammation of the mammary gland chiefly of bovines usually affecting the secondary cells and frequently causing total suppression of milk on account of specific microorganism, *streptococcus agalactiae*, or it may occur sporadically in one or a number of animals in a herd due to any one of a variety of microorganism which has been identified with the disease.

Prevalence

It is reported in bovines from almost every country in the world, but is of course much more important where dairy farming has been or is being developed. Nevertheless sum on, its important in buffaloes, sheep and goat where these species are maintained for milk production should not be under estimated.

Causes

A large number of micro-organism have been implicated in mastitis and although it is not feasible to describe in details the disease caused by each one separately. They are divided into two groups:

Infective Group

- Streptococcus agalactiae
- Staphylococcus aureus

Pathogenic Group

- Streptococcus dysgalactiae

- Streptococcus uberis
- Cornebacteriumpyogenes
- Escherichia coli
- Microbacterium tuberculosis
- Actinomycesbovis

Predisposing Factor

- ☆ Bad sanitation of byre
- ☆ Sudden change of diets
- ☆ Irregularity and bad method of milking
- ☆ Contamination of the hand of milker
- ☆ Incomplete stripping and retention of milk in the udder.
- ☆ Secondary infection such as brucellosis, Cowpox, FMD and other infections of the gastro-intestinal tract and genital tract such as metritis etc.

Mode of Transmission

Infection nearly always occurs by microorganism gaining access to the udder through the teat canal. The predisposing factors may be in the individual cow or the herd as a whole. They include:

- ☆ Age of the animal
- ☆ Stage of lactation
- ☆ Milk yield
- ☆ Hereditary factors
- ☆ Trauma or injury of the udder or teats
- ☆ Hygienic measure
- ☆ Unknown factors

Symptoms

Clinically, the disease is approximately divided into several forms:

Sub Clinical Mastitis

This can only be identified by laboratory examination of milk drawn from the udder. There are no visible signs. This is also *latent mastitis.*

Chronic Mastitis

This is characterized by repeated mild attack of mammary swelling, with the production of clotted milk.

Acute or Severe Clinical Mastitis

It is usually sporadic and is characterized by rapid onset of a diffuse swelling in a quarter that has been normal previously. There is a pain on palpation. The milk is not normal in appearance. High fever and anorexia is noticed.

Gangrenous Mastitis

It is characterized by cold bluish discoloration of teats and udder which may require amputation.

Diagnosis

The symptoms are diagnostic in acute cases. The destruction of carriers of latent cases is of importance in eradicating the disease from a herd.

The following tests are used for detecting the latent cases:

Dish test

Little milk is drawn into a flat dish with a blackened bottom surface. The presence of fine clots suggests infection.

Sediment Test

the amount of sediment obtained by centrifuging normal milk at 5000rpm is 0.1in 100ml of grayish white colour. In infected milk, the amount will be about0.25 or more in 100 ml of yellowish colour.

Chemical Reaction Test

Normal milk has a pH slightly on acidic side of neutrality whereas, blood serum is alkaline. Infected animals have slightly alkaline milk pH.

Bacteriological Examination

Bacterial culture can be made and examine the specific characters of the organisms examined.

Cultural Examination

Infected milk can be examined culturally.

Treatment

General

- Elimination of predisposing factors
- Protect the teats from injury
- Wipe the teat dry with cloth after milking
- Isolation of infected animals
- Udder, teats and milker's hand should be washed with antiseptic.
- A cream containing 0.5% Zinc oxide applied on teats abrasions.

Curative Treatments

- **Procaine Penicillin:** Dose: 2000 unit/pound body weight I/m daily
- **Intra-Udder Infusion**

  Ry Crystalline penicillin G 1000000 units

  Duhydro streptomycin, 1 gram

Distilled water, 40 cc

Sig. Infuse the udder

- **Antibiotic Cream** Viz: Masticillin M, Strypen fort; Neothion; Mastalon may be infused in infected udder through teat cannulae
- Hot formulation may be given
- Mag. Sulph; Fomentation may also be useful.
- Tetracyclines 1-3 g every 24 hours or 10-11mg of streptomycin /1kg body weight every 24 hours will destroy microorganism in the udder.

6. Calf Scours

It also known as Bacterium coli infections, White scours, Diarrhoea in new born calves. It is an acute highly infectious disease of calves characterized by marked prostration and profuse diarrhea caused by *Escherichia coli.*

Species Affected

Calves, lambs and piglets

Causes

is *E. coli* causes calf scours. In addition to calf scour, *E.coli* may causes abortion in sheep and mares, mastitis in cows, pyelitis, cyctitis, cholecystitis and peritonitis.

Predisposing Causes Are

- ☆ Failure to receive colostrum appears to be most important factor. Colostrum is rich in antibodies.
- ☆ Vitamin A deficiency in the dam
- ☆ Over feeding of milk with high fat percentage

Mode of Transmission

- ☆ Calf sucking contaminated udder
- ☆ Intra-uterine infection
- ☆ The disease is a first sporadic, later becomes an enzootic massive infection of the surrounding.

Symptoms

- ☆ **Acute Forms:** There isanorexia, and the animal is unable to move. Severe uncontrolled foetid clay coloured diarrhea, temperature, colic, grinding of teeth, salivation, spasmodic muscular contraction, fits, pain on palpation of abdomen, coma and death within 24 hours.
- ☆ **Mild Form:** Symptoms may not go beyond the appearance of diarrhea with a slight anorexia.
- ☆ **Chronic Form:** The calf become thin, pot bellied, plastered with faeces but surviving for a week.

Period of Incubation

From few hours to several days.

Treatment and Control:

General

- ✰ Feeding of colostrum
- ✰ Proper sanitation should be made

Prophylaxis

Administration of vitamin A in the form of shark liver oil.

Curative Treatment

- ✰ Antibiotic:
    - Streptomycin orally, Dose 0.5 g to 1.0g daily
    - Terramycin orally, 200 mg daily for three days
    - Aureomycin 25 ml/lbs body weight
- ✰ **Bacteriostatic:**Sulphaguanidine and sulphamerazine etc. are of value
- ✰ **White scour antiserum:**Dose I/m. 20 cc to 40 cc.

Viral diseases of Cattle

1)Foot and Mouth Disease: Khura Mu Pacca Rog in Hindi

The foot and mouth disease is a highly communicable disease affecting cloven-footed animals. It is characterized by fever, formation of vesicles and blisters in the mouth, udder, teats and on the skin between the toes and above the hoofs. Animals recovered from the disease present a characteristically rough coat and deformation of the hoof. In India, the disease is wide spread and assumes a position of importance in livestock industry. The disease is spread by direct contact or indirectly through infected water, manure, hay and pastures. It is also conveyed by cattle attendants. It is known to spread through recovered animals, field rats and birds.

Symptoms

- ✰ Fever with 104-105°F
- ✰ Profuse salivation ropes of stringy saliva hangs from mouth
- ✰ Vesicles appears in mouth and in the inter digital space
- ✰ Vesicle appear in mouth and in the inter digital space
- ✰ Lameness observed
- ✰ Cross bred cattle are highly susceptible to it

Treatment

- ✰ The external application of antiseptic contributes to the healing of the ulcers and wards off attacks by flies.

- A common and inexpensive dressing for the lesions in the feet is a mixture of coal-tar and copper sulphate in the proportion of 5:1.

Precautions

- Heavy milch animals and exotic breeds of cattle bred for milk should be protected regularly
- It is advisable to carry out two vaccinations at an interval of six months followed by an annual vaccination programme.
- Isolation and segregation of sick animals. It should be informed immediately to the veterinary doctors.
- Disinfection of animal sheds with bleaching powder or phenol.
- Attendants and equipments for sick animals should be ideally separate
- The equipments should be thoroughly sanitized
- Proper disposal of left over feed by the animal
- Proper disposal of carcasses
- Control of flies

Major Reproductive Problem in Kandi Areas of Jammu

1) Repeat Breeding Syndrome

A repeat breeder is a cow that is cycling normally, with no clinical abnormalities, but has failed to conceive after at least two successive inseminations.

Cause and Symptoms

In practice, some will have been inseminated at the wrong time, others may have pathological changes in the bursa or oviduct that are difficult to palpate, or undiagnosed uterine infections.

An early repeater is an animal's whose luteal function has been shorter than normal or typical for the physiological oestrus cycle in non bred cow. In these cows the most probable event is either failure of fertilization (delayed ovulation, poor semen quality etc.) or early embryonic death (delayed ovulation, poor embryo quality, unfavorable uterine environment, precocious luteolysis).

The cows will come into heat within 17-24 days after AI. A late repeater is a cow that comes into heat later than 25 days after AI. In these animals, the luteal function was maintained for longer than the physiological luteal phase in non bred cows. Fertilization and initial recognition of pregnancy probably took place but for some reason (i.e. inadequate luteal function, inadequate embryo signaling, infectious diseases, induced luteolysis) luteolysis was induced and pregnancy lost.

Good heat detection and records are key to identifying these cows.

Treatment

- Repeat breeders should be carefully evaluated in order to define the most probable reason for the failure to conceive (early repeat) or failure in pregnancy maintenance (early and late repeats).

- Initially heat records should be evaluated to classify the cows as early or late repeat.
- Cows that have had three services and are not pregnant should be checked before serving again by a veterinarian.

Prevention

- Ensure you are serving cows at the correct time. This means that all staff should know the signs of heat. Milk progesterone testing is also useful; cows in a true heat will have very low progesterone.
- Ensure insemination techniques are as good as possible. This is particularly important.
- Do not serve cows previously diagnosed as pregnant without doing a cow-side progesterone test to confirm it has low progesterone means not pregnant.
- If the cow is pregnant, AI may cause foetal loss.
- Identify and treat cows with infection before starting to serve them.
- Don't start serving too soon after calving because it resulted into lower pregnancy rates and so more repeat breeder cows.
- Minimize stress at service. For example, try and avoid serving around turnout or when you change the diet.

Suggested Reading

Sastry, A.S. (1983). Veterinary Pathology, 6th edition, CBS publisher and distributor, pp780.

Handbook of Animal Husbandry (2011).3rd revised edition, pp. 1233.

Banerjee, G. C. (1998). A text book of Animal Husbandry, 6th edition.pp, 1079.

Sastry, N.S.R. & Thomas, C.K. (2005). Livestock Production Management, 4th revised edition, pp. 642.

Chakrabarti, A. (2011) Text Book of Clinical Veterinary Medicine, 3rd edition, pp.701.

Verma, D.N. (1999) A text book of Livestock production Management in tropic, 1st edition, pp748.

Bikane, A.U. & Kawitkar, S.B. (2010).Handbook for Veterinary clinician.Third edition.pp.422.

Transforming Rural Areas through Veterinary Science *Pages* **239-252**
Editor: Dipanjali Konwar, Shilpa Sood & Shahid Ahamad
Published by: **ASTRAL INTERNATIONAL PVT. LTD., NEW DELHI**

19 Recent Trends for Teat and Udder Surgery in Ruminants

Dr Md Moin Ansari

Historical changes in the demand for milk products have been largely driven by human population growth, income growth and urbanization and the production response in different livestock systems has been associated with science and technology as well as increases in animal numbers (Philip, 2010). Unscientific milking and management practices are the main cause for teat and udder affections and cause a great loss to the poor farmers. The farmers are less aware about clean milk production and teat or udder health. Further, they also do not pay enough attention on udder care and sometimes even mishandle the udder which always leads to teat and udder affections (Chakrabarti *et al.*, 2014). Udder and teat health are increasingly important for dairy producers and any disease condition involving udder or teat ultimately affects the productivity and the farmer's economy. The udder and teats are vulnerable to external trauma or injury because of their anatomical location, increase in size of udder and teats during lactation, faulty methods of milking, repeated trauma to the teat mucosa, injury by teeth of calves, accidentally stepped on teat, paralysis resulting from metabolic disturbances at parturition (Tiwary *et al.*, 2005). The disease conditions of teats and udder not only cause discomfort to the animals with painful milking but also make teats and udder prone to mastitis. Milk flow disorders are a central problem in the field of udder health. Teats of milked farm animals are parts of the udder, serving the role of both a valve regulating milk outflow as well as that of a natural barrier for exogenous infections, affecting the quality traits of milk. It give rise to different kinds of mastitis, which consequently leads to a loss in milk production, detrimental changes to the milk components and raw milk quality, increased costs for the treatment of the animal, early culling, and hence, a negative economic impact. In addition, anomalies of the udder and teats may preclude or interfere with milk outflow and may predispose to mastitis (Abdel Hady, 1993, 2015).

The diseases of udder can be congenital anomalies are known at the time of first calving but acquired anomalies can affect any stage of lactation. Congenital and acquired surgical conditions of udder and teats can be grouped into three main categories. (i). Conditions of epithelial surface of udder and teats includes supernumerary teats/extra teats, bovine ulcerative mammitis/ sore teats, udder and teat abcess, teat lacerations and fistulae. (ii). Conditions of glands and tea cistern or canal includes lactoliths/milk stones, teat canal polyp, teat spider, fibrosis of teat canal, tumour of mammary gland. (iii). Conditions of teat sphincter includes teat stenosis/hard milker, teat leaker/free milker, blind teats. Congenital aberrations in the mammary gland of the cows include many structural defects; however, the only one of significance is supernumerary teats. Supernumerary teats may be located on the udder behind the posterior teats, between the front and hind teats, or attached to either the front or hind teats (Aiello, 1998). In India, some reports on the congenital abnormalities of the udder and teats in buffaloes were published (Rambabu *et al.*, 2011). Congenital condition is usually associated with improper development of the teat cistern or teat canal. Whereas acquired obstructions are caused by injury, tumor or infections. The resulting membrane, obstructing the milk flow, is either thin or thick, and is located high at the base of the teat or lower down in the cistern. Palpation reveals fluctuating milk above the obstruction but milking is not possible. In case of congenital cases with improper development of the teat cistern, it may impossible to feel the milk pocket. Treatment of such cases is not recommended, the quarter is usually allowed to atrophy and become non-functional. If the pocket of milk can be palpated, prognosis is usually considered good to favorable. According to Alacam *et al.*,1990, Singh *et al.*,1993, surgical treatment through the teat orifice was successful in 84% of the operated cases. After rectification with Hudson's teat spiral or small teat bistuory. Complete milking from the affected quarter is not recommended for 2-3 days in an order to avoid a stricture. Flow of the milk itself keeps the teat cistern patent (Singh *et al.*,1993, Athar *et al.*,1999).

In teat laceration and fistulae condition is mostly observed in those animals that have long teats and pendulous udder (Tyagi and Singh, 2012 and Kashyap *et al.*,2014) . When animal tries to jump over the barbed wire or pass through the thorny bushes, their teat get teared due to laceration of skin and muscles. If this laceration is deeper, then even teat canal gets opened and milk will start flowing through the teared portion. This condition is called as teat fistula. The cases of teat fistula are considered as emergency because any delay in repair of such teat will cause development of mastitis or necrosis of the teat. For repair of such teat, all aseptic precautions should be taken into considerations. A full coverage of systematic antibiotic is required and for proper drainage Larson's teat plug is used. Different suture techniques are used to repair the teat fistula but double layer simple continuous suturing with Polyglycolic Acid (PGA) 3-0 and in between simple vertical mattress simple interrupted suturing of skin with nylon 1-0 is found suitable for repair of teat fistula. Modransky and Welker (1993) reported that penetrating teat lacerations and fistula in goat were repaired by suturing in 3 layers. A simple continuous pattern of 4-0 or 5-0 synthetic absorbable suture was used in the mucosa and muscularis layer, separately. To close the skin, various patterns like vertical mattress, simple interrupted or simple continuous with 3-0 non absorbable, stainless steel staples or tissue adhesives were used. Non penetrating teat lacerations were repaired by simple continuous sutures using fine (4-0) synthetic absorbable suture material in muscular is and skin was closed by simple interrupted or vertical mattress sutures of 3-0 non absorbable material. Couture and Mulon (2005) reported that injuries to the end of the teat were frequent and frustrating to treat in goat. Treatment of these injuries evolved from being aggressive using teat knives to a more conservative approach employing rest nonreactive teat inserts. The process of milking seems simple, but it involved fine-tuned mechanics. Teat fibrosis, even when small, had a disastrous effect on the production life of an animal. There was no place for error; any surgical intervention should be precise and aim for perfection.

Tyagi and Singh (2012) and Kashyap *et al.* (2014) opined that the fencing was the predisposing factor for teat laceration and wounds and it may be due to pendulous udder and long teats. They also observed that teat obstruction was due to faulty milking and suckling that causes trauma of teat and obstruction of milk flow due to growth inside the teat canal. Laying down on sharp objects or inflicted by long untrimmed claws of the cow itself or by another cow trotting a recumbent one. Non penetrating wounds may be handled as any other lacerations, keeping in mind that large amount of scar tissue or flaps of skin may interfere with milking or have undesirable cosmetic effect. Penetrating wounds of the udder with exposed parenchyma should be closed with catgut and antibiotic should be administered by intramammary infusion. According to Nichols (2008) teat lacerations are classified according to the duration from time of trauma, the localization and conformation of the laceration and the thickness of the lesion (full or partial thickness). Wounds in the area of the teat sphincter may lead to stenosis. If there are flaps of skin that protrude, they should be sutured or removed. Portions of non viable skin should be trimmed back to conform to normal contour of the teat. Sutured wounds of the teat may be protected by an adhesive elastic bandage.

Kashyap *et al.* (2014) also opined that potential risk factors for pathology of mammary glands include previous mastitis history, increased parity, poor body conditions etc. He also observed that cases of udder fibrosis could be attributed to the negligence by the owners with delayed presentation in the clinics or not noticed that lead to chronic mastitis resulting in fibrosis of the udder. O'Connor (2005) also opined that chronic mastitis may arise independently or follow the acute form, infection usually occurs by the secretary ducts, rarely by way of the blood and lymph stream. Tyagi and Singh (2012) also observed that it may sometimes lead to gangrenous mastitis. In this study the incidence of teat laceration may be due to crossing of thorny fencing which are applied by the farmers to protect their crops. The pendulous udder comes in contact with fencing and lead to teat laceration.

Teat obstruction involves the intraluminal lesions that partially or completely hinder the milk outflow. These lesions have been identified and classified in literatures (Ducharme *et al.*,1987, Johnson, 1988, Alacam *et al.*,1990, Singh *et al.*,1993, Athar *et al.*,1999). Teat spider condition is usually due to congenital absence of teat cistern or canal. Teat spider is met with in buffaloes and cows as a congenital as well as acquired anomaly [Johnson, 1988, Alacam *et al.*,1990, Singh *et al.*,1993). It can be acquired in cases of injury, tumour or inflammation of mammary tissue resulting in formation of thin or thick membrane, situated either at the base or middle of the teat. This membranous obstruction removed by teat scissor, Huges teat tumour extractor, teat bistouries or Hudson spiral teat instrument. Fibrosis of teat canal is commonly observed in most of the lactating animals where a hard fibrous cord like structure is observed in the teat. Exact cause of this condition is not clear. However, repeated trauma due to mechanical injuries, thumb milking and calf suckling are the main contributory factors. Sometimes mastitis can also result into fibrosis of quarter followed by teat canal. Tumour of mammary gland is infrequently in lactating animals however, fibro adenoma reported in heifer. The growth can be surgically removed under caudal block or local infiltration analgesia.

Teat stenosis/Contracted sphincter or teat orifice "hard milker" may be congenital in origin or may be acquired as a result of trauma to the end of the teat. There is a small stream of milk, and prolonged milking time. There may be loss of milk due to incomplete milking or trauma to the teat due to attempts for strenuous milking methods (Singh *et al.*,2003). Teat stenosis resulting from mucosal lesions in the region of the streak canal or Furstenberg's rosette may be successfully treated via theloresectoscopy (Bleul *et al.*, 2005). Stenosis of streak canal without acute inflammation can be treated successfully by incising the sphincter in three directions with teat knife, Bard parker blade No.11, Udall's teat knife, McLean teat knife. Teat leaker/Free milker is just reverse of teat stenosis. It can be due to injury or relaxation of teat sphincter. In this case milk will go on leaking and sometimes infection may gain entry leading to mastitis. This condition is treated by injection of 0.25 ml of lugol's iodine around the orifice or scarification and suturing with one or two stitches with monofilament nylon. Blind teats may be congenital or acquired due to any trauma near the teat sphincter. Such cases generally reported just after parturition on palpation milk thrill found in teat cistern on pressing milk passed backward toward milk udder cistern. Imperforated teat treated by 15 gauze needle, after creating opening, it is further dilated using hugs teat tumour extractor, milk canula fixed for 24 hour after that frequent milking advised at 4 to 6 hours intervals to prevent adhesion. Administration of proper antibiotics is done for a minimum period of 3-5 days.

Lactolith/milk stone is a conditions of gland and teat cistern or canal. They are formed into the teat canal when the milk is rich in minerals and salty in taste due to super saturation of salts. The stone moves freely in teat canal and hinder the milk flow, if large in size. They usually get washed out along with ilk but if large in size then it can be crushed with small forceps or cutting the sphincter with Litchy teat knife or teat bistouries and milked out. Teat canal polyp are small pea sized growths attached to the wall of teat canal. The polyps hinder the milking process and sometimes even block the passage of teat canal. Teat polyps can easily take out by Huges teat tumour extractor. If its location is above the teat canal thelotomy is the best method for resection of excessive tissue. Postoperative gentamicine and prednisolone infusion for five consecutive days found suitable to check infection as well as helpful in checking further growth of the polyp.

Supernumerary teats were found to be congenital in nature by O, Conner (2005), Bemji and Popoola (2011), Adebayo and Chineke (2011). Supernumerary or extra teats are often seen on the posterior surface of udder and in-between the teat. They may be functional or nonfunctional, functional activity can be determined only after parturition of the animal. They frequently interfere with free milking process and are objectionable on show animals. Surgical removals of supernumerary teats are best in young animals and in case of older cow in dry condition. Surgery performed under local infiltration analgesia with two elliptical incisions at the junctions of teat and udder and skin wound closed with interrupted suture using non-absorbable suture material.

In bovine ulcerative mammitis (sore teats), teats become painful due to presence of crakes, traumatic injuries, lesions due to disease conditions such as pox, Foot and Mouth Disease etc. If these lesions are not treated well in time, the animal will not allow touching the affected teat for milking. These lesions become ulcers in due course of time and the condition are then known as bovine ulcerative mammitis. Ulcerative thelitis is a disease affecting primarily the high-yielding primiparous graded Murrah milch buffaloes and causing serious economic losses to the farmers in coastal districts of Andhra Pradesh (Lokanadhamu *et al.*,2005). The disease is characterized by acute inflammation of one or more teats with subsequent thickening, narrowing or closure of teat canal leading to incomplete drainage of milk. The quality of milk appears to be normal unlike in clinical mastitis. This is followed by ulceration, focal necrosis, and either partial or complete sloughing off the affected teat. Oozing of blood from injured teat causes contamination of milk while milking thereby making it unfit for human consumption. In such cases, sterilized teat siphon should be used to drain the milk out. For treatment of such painful lesions, the wound should be washed with light potassium permanganate solution and then soothing preparation such as iodized glycerin, bismuth iodoform paraffin paste, zinc oxide ointment or antiseptic dressing with soothing emollient may be continued till the complete healing of the lesion occurs. Healing may be delayed due to the trauma of milking and secondary bacterial infections. Similar signs were reported by many workers in ulcerative mammillitis of cows (Gibbs *et al.*,1970, Turner *et al.*,1976, Chauhan *et al.*,1989, Janett *et al.*,2000) and in buffaloes (Sharma *et al.*,1998, Malleswara *et al.*,2003). As primiparous animals were most commonly affected with this condition, there is lot of impact on milk production due to loss of teats, resulting in great economic loss to the farmers.

Bolbol and Gasnawy (1991) treated twenty-seven udder wounds in lactating goats and ewes and closed with synthetic tissue adhesive. Twenty-four healed by primary intention (89%), two wounds were partially healed by primary intention and partially by second intention and a wound failed to heal and developed milk fistula. In general, non suture closure of skin wounds using tissue adhesive proved to be satisfactory and highly efficient in small ruminants. Al-Sadi *et al.* (1994) reported ectopia of mammary tissue in a female goat. The ectopic tissue was in the form of two subcutaneous masses, one on either side of the vulval opening. Surgical excision of the masses was performed. Grossly, the excised tissues were lobular and contained milky fluid. Microscopically, each lobule consisted of alveoli, intralobular ducts and loose cellular connective tissue. Many of the alveoli were filled with amorphous pink material mixed with neutrophils. Spindle-shaped myoepithelial cells were noted in the walls of both the alveoli and the intralobular ducts. Each lobule was surrounded by a thick connective tissue capsule containing interlobular ducts and blood and lymph vessels. Lactiferous ducts and an external skin opening were not seen. These results indicated an ectopic mammary tissue. This report may well be one of the extremely rare reports of ectopia of the mammary tissue. Concerning the teat lumen granuloma, Blowey and Weaver (1991), described the teat granuloma (pea) as a freefloating, irregular rubbery mass of fibrocollagenous material covered by mucosa which may develop in the teat cistern and pass down to the sphincter, thus obstructing the milk flow. Weaver (1986) adopted manual expression from a surgically dilated teat orifice for the small and mobile masses but in cases which produce clinical signs, vertical incision in teat wall opposite to the mass was indicated with surgical resection followed by suturing of the teat wall.

Ruptured suspensory ligaments are of two types, 1) rupture of the medial ligaments: is the most common type of rupture and results in a lateral displacement of the right and left haves of the udder. When viewed from the rear this is recognized by the teats splaying outwards. The teats are no longer perpendicular to the ground or parallel with each other. Sudden change in the udder conformation may notice, and there is a loss of the dividing curvature between the two halves of the udder. 2) rupture of the lateral ligaments: is the most easily recognized and results in a dramatic lowering of the udder below the hocks (Jackson and Jackson PGG, Cockcroft, 2002). Anderson *et al.* (2002) stated that udders in goat with poor suspensory ligament or long teats can be injured during grazing activities. Barbed wires, dog attacks and horn punctures can tear the skin of teat and udder. Treatment of these affections includes cleansing and debriding to bleeding tissues, the facial layer of udder or inner teat lining was closed with a fine absorbable suture material. Non absorbable sutures were placed on the skin. Teat injuries had drawn more attention more recently. Surgical interventions were better planned, and blind treatment with unsuitable teat knives was avoided. Treatment of superficial of full-thickness teat lacerations did not require a high level of anatomic or surgical knowledge, although basic surgical principles should be applied. Hemostasis, delicate débridgement and tissue handling, and appropriate suture materials and patterns were key to success. Appropriate sedation, anesthesia, and analgesia were essential to achieve this goal and should never be neglected. Therefore, a rapid and accurate diagnosis and prognosis is mandatory in patients with udder diseases, and requires the use of state-of-the-art examination techniques and therapeutic treatments.

In udder and teat abscess formation occurs more often on the udder than the teat, mastitis especially due to resistant microbes suddenly develop abscessation on side of affected udder. Udder abscesses are clinically manifested either in a form of chronic suppurative mastitis caused by the common environmental pathogens (Contreras *et al.*,2007; Schroeder, 2009) or in a circumscribed localized swelling anywhere of the udder and most commonly seated on craniolateral and posterior aspects of the udder quarters (Misk, 2008). Such cases can easily be diagnosed by exploratory puncture of the swollen part which revealed the presence of pus and necrotic tissues. The abscess cavity is opened for complete drainage of pus. After drainage of the pus, the cavity is dressed with tincture iodine followed by application of soothing agents until obliteration of abscess cavity. In case of necrosis of teat or udder, amputation of teat or affected quarter is recommended followed by daily dressing till complete healing of wound occurs. Treatment by a stab incision was performed on the lateral aspect of affected quarters and complete evacuation of the contents was performed in chronic suppurative form (Paape *et al.* 2001), whereas the localized form was treated similar to those elsewhere in the body. Hematomas of the udder are considered as inflected by the cow itself or by external trauma from butting or kicking by other cows but injuries from these sources seldom are confirmed by Lisie *et al.* (2008). Balhara *et al.* (2014) reported that, hemolactia in buffaloes usually occurs immediately after calving as a result of rupture of many small congested blood vessels or seepage of blood into teat canal by diapedesis. Hematomas are diagnosed as subcutaneous, mixed and parenchymatous. Matthew *et al.* (1990) who reported a case of acute gangrenous mastitis due to clostridium perfringens type A and Escherichia coli in a five-year-old Holstein cow.

Hussein and EI-Maghraby (2001) described two different techniques for mastectomy carried out on 14 goats with gangrenous mastitis. The animals were randomly assigned to one of two groups containing seven goats each. The first group was operated via a classical surgical mastectomy technique (either bilateral (n=5) or unilateral (n=2)). The second group was operated via vascular ligation of the external pudendal blood vessels and milk vein and amputation of the affected teat (either bilateral (n=3) or unilateral (n=4)). Comparison between the two groups was carried out. Vascular ligation and teat amputation proved to be an effective, quick, safe, and less expensive technique for mastectomy in goats. Ligation of udder vasculature was less traumatic than surgical amputation and the stress on the patient was minimal.

Milk flow disorders/disturbances are the main indication for ultrasound imaging (ultrasonogrphy) of the mammary gland in ruminants (Franz *et al.*,2009) and particularly the teat is an important application. Ultrasound imaging techniques and minimally invasive surgery help the surgeon to make the best decision. Finally, more investigation was needed to treat varicose veins to understand the origin and develop better treatment. Ultrasonography is also useful for monitoring the healing process after surgical removal of proliferative tissue. Additionally, it aids in the diagnosis of mastitis and thus promotes efficient therapy. It is a non-invasive method, allowing the visualisation of the separate structures of the mammary gland (teat and parenchyma). B-mode ultrasonography is used extensively as a safe and non-invasive diagnostic technique as a method of choice for detecting reproductive disorders in large domestic animal species (Ali *et al.*,1992**)**. Physiology and diseases of the udder are an important facet of reproduction and production of sheep and goat. Mammary gland function is also very important for the health and growth of newborns since udder diseases are known to have a negative impact on both these factors and can impose public health hazards for populations consuming their milk. Echography of the mammary gland parenchyma in ruminants is performed primarily through the direct contact technique (transcutaneous echography) with a low-frequency linear, sector or convex transducer (3.5–5 MHz) and horizontal scanning. Examination of the teat is done primarily through the water bath technique and vertical scanning. A high quality image can be achieved by using a high frequency probe (at least 7.5 MHz). Teat injuries and the milking technique are the main reasons for disturbed milk secretion (Bleul *et al.*,2002; Geishauser *et al.*,2005; Condino *et al.*,2010). Echographic scanning of the teat is used primarily on cows and sheep for the diagnostics of stenoses, obstructions and fibrous changes in the area of the teat canal, the rosette of Furstenberg or the boundary between the teat and gland cisterns (Saratsis, 1991; Trostle & O'Brien, 1998; Dinç *et al.*,2000; Flöck *et al.*,2004; Mavrogianni *et al.*,2004; Couture & Mulon, 2005). Echography is used for examination of the mammary gland parenchyma in cases of inflammatory processes (mastitis), oedema of the udder without mastitis symptoms, pathological formations localised deep within the parenchyma (abscesses, haematomas, tumours, foreign bodies, connective tissue buildups), which cannot be detected through clinical examination (Flöck & Winter, 2006; Franz *et al.*,2009). Banting (1998) used the echostructure of the mammary gland in cows with induced staphylococcal mastitis (Staphy- lococcus aureus), in order to determine the prognosis and the choice of treatment. Flöck & Winter (2006) found out the characteristic echographic image in cows' mammary glands inflammation caused by Arcanobacterium pyogenes and some Gram-negative bacteria of the Enterobac- teriaceae family. They described the changes in the udder parenchyma in cases of abscesses and haematomas. Franz *et al.* (2009) observed a penetrating foreign body in the parenchyma as a hyperechoic linear structure causing a strong acoustic window. O'Brien *et al.* (2002) found gases during the echographic examination of an oedematous mammary gland in cows. Our echographic studies on the mammary gland in goats suffering from acute mastitis, revealed a non-homogenous and hypo- to hyperechoic mammary gland parenchyma structure, with a lack of clear visualisation of the mammary canals and the blood vessels (Fasulkov and Koleva, 2011). The echography of the teat in these animals exhibited a thickened hyperechoic teat wall, as well as numerous hyperechoic structures in the teat cistern, representing milk coagula. Because of the more severe clinical expression and the major change in the echogenicity of the udder of goats with acute mastitis caused by Staphylococcus aureus, we believe that the severity of the inflammation and the type of the etiological agent possibly affected the echographic image for these animals (Fasulkov & Koleva, 2011). The echographic examination of the mammary gland is also for the determination of the dimensions of structures within the area of the teat. It allows for detailed measurements of the length and diameter of the teat canal, cistern, and the thickness of the teat wall (Gleeson *et al.*,2002; Slosarz *et al.*,2010). A number of authors established a connection between mastitis in cows, the stage of lactation, the characteristics of the teat, and the visualisation of the teat canal (McDonald, 1975; Seykora & McDaniel, 1985; Grindal *et al.*,1991; Seyfried, 1992; Scherzer, 1992; Celik *et al.*,2008). Teat endoscopy is an excellent diagnostic procedure for covered teat injuries. Minimal invasive surgical therapy with the help of teat endoscopy. The teat endoscopy provided exact condition of the mucosa, intensity/grade and eventual duration of pathological changes Rathod *et al.*(2009). Theloscopy requires minimum time for giving accurate diagnosis about the internal teat injuries. By using theloscopy milk flow disorder can be diagnosed easily and precisely. Theloscopy allows to treat injuries according to a precised diagnosis and to monitor the treatment Rathod *et al.* (2009).

Suggested Reading

Abd-El-Hady AAA. 1993. Studies on the surgical udder and teat affections in dairy farms. M.V.Sc. Cairo University, Egypt.

Abd-El-Hady AAA. 2015 Clinical observations on some surgical udder and teat affections in cattle and Buffaloes. Scholars Journal of Agriculture and Veterinary Sciences. Sch J Agric Vet Sci 2015; 2(4A):270-281.

Adebayo JO, Chineke CA. 2011.Evaluation of West African Dwarf goat for some qualitative traits inSouthwestern Nigeria. Afr.J.Agric.Res.6: 6204-6207.

Aiello SE. 1998. Udder diseases. In the merk veterinary manual, 8th edition, Whitehouse Station, NJ, USA, P. 1028.

Alacam E, Dinc DA, Guler M. 1990. Diagnosis and treatment of various teat problems in dairy cows with special reference to radiographic techniques. Doga, Turk Veterinerlik ve Hayavncilick Dergisi, 1990; 14: 1-10.

Ali, A.M., el-Sanousi, S.M., al-Eknah, M.A., Gameel, A.A., Dafalla, E.A., Homeida, A.M., Radwan, Y.M. 1992.Studies on the infundibular cysts of the uterine tube in camel (Camelus dromedarius). Rev. Elev. Med. Vet. Pays. Trop. 45:243-53.

Al-Sadi HI, Lssa MJ and Al-Badrany.1994. Ectopic mammary tissue in a black goat. Small Ruminant Research 14(2):181-183.

Anderson DE, Hull BL and Pugh DG.2002. Diseases of mammary gland in sheep and goat. Sheep and Goat Medicine. pp 341-358.

Athar M, Muhammad G, Shakoor A. 1999. Acquired contralateral teat spider in a cow and its successful treatment. Pakistan Vet. J., 19 (1): 49-50.

Balhara AK, Rana N, Phulia SK. 2014. Blood in milk- Causes and Control. (Online). Available form: http://www.buffalopedia.cirb.res.in

Banting, A., 1998. Ultrasonographical exami- nation of the mammary gland in cows with induced S. aureus mastitis: A criteria for prognosis and evaluation of therapy. Cattle Practice, 6, 121–124.

Bemji MN, Popoola SA.2011.A note on the incidence of udder abnormalities in West African Dwarf goat inSouth Western Nigeria.Livestock Research for Rural Development 23.

Bleul UT, Schwantag SC, Bachofner C, Hassig MR, Khan WK. 2005. Milk flow and udder health in cows after treatment of covered teat injuries via theloresectoscopy: 52 cases (2000 – 2002). JAVMA, 226(7):1119 – 23.

Bleul, U. T., S. C. Schwantag, C. Bachofner, M. R. Hässig & W. K. Kähn, 2005. Milk flow and udder health in cows after treat- ment of covered teat injuries via thelore- sectoscopy: 52 cases (2000–2002). Jour- nal of American Veterinary Medical Asso- ciation, 226, 1119–1123.

Blowey RW, Weaver AD. 1991. A color atlas of diseases and disorders of cattle. London provider, Nolfe, Chapter II, Udder and teat disorders. 177 –188.

Bolbol AE and Gasnawy YA.1991. Clinical use of tissue adhesives in the closure of udder wounds in lactating ewes and goats. Rev. Elev. Med. Vet. Pays. Trop. 44(4):409-11.

Celik, H. A., I. Aydin, M. Colak, S. Sendag & D. A. Dinc, 2008. Ultrasonographic eva- luation of age related influence on the teat canal and the effect of this influence on milk yield in Brown Swiss cows. Bulletin of the Veterinary Institute in Pulawy, 52, 245–249.

Chakrabarti A, ChandranPC, KumarP, Dey, A. 2014. Teat and udder disorders in goats (Capra hircus) in Bihar, India. S. Asian J. Life Sci.2 (2):20–22

Chauhan HVS, Gupta MK, Jha GJ, Pandey RS, Singh KK, Sinha RP, Prasad A. 1989. Studies on the bovine herpes mammillitis (BHM) in cattle. Indian Veterinary Journal, 66: 106-109.

Condino, M. P., K. Suzuki, K. Sato, K. Hya- kutake & K. Taguchi, 2010. Evaluation of a milk-flow assessment technique in dairy cows with normal teat canals or stenotic teat canals. American Journal of Veteri- nary Research, 71, 1123–1126.

Contreras A, Luengo C, Sanchez A, Corrales JC. 2003. The role of intramammary pathogens in dairy goats. Livest. Prod. Sci., 79, 273-283.

Couture Y and Mulon PY.2005. Procedures and surgeries of the teat. Vet. Clinical. North. Am. Food Anim. Prac. 21(1):173-204.

Couture, Y. & P. Y. Mulon, 2005. Procedures and surgeries of the teat. Veterinary Clinic of North America, Food Animal Practice, 21, 173–204.

Dinç, D. A., S. Şendağ & I. Aydin, 2000. Di- agnosis of teat stenosis in dairy cattle by real-time ultrasonography. Veterinary Re- cord, 147, 270–272.

Ducharme NG, Arighi M, Horney FD, Livesey MA, Hurtig MH, Pennock P. 1987. Invasive Teat Surgery in Dairy Cattle. I. Surgical Procedures and Classification of Lesions. Can Vet J, 28(12):757-762.

Fasulkov, I. & M. Koleva, 2011. Ultrasound imaging findings in acute mammary gland inflammations in goats. Journal of Moun- tain Agriculture on the Balkans, 14, 210– 221.

Flöck, M. and P. Winter, 2006. Diagnostic ul- trasonography in cattle with disease of the mammary gland. The Veterinary Journal,171, 314–321.

Flöck, M., D. Klein and M. Hofmann-Parisot, 2004. Ultrasonographic findings of patho- logical teat changes in cattle. Wiener Tierärztliche Monatsschrift, 91, 184–195.

Franz, S., M. Floek and M. Hofmann-Parisot, 2009. Ultrasonography of the bovine udder and teat. Veterinary Clinic of North Ame- rica, Food Animal Practice, 25, 669–685.

Geishauser, T., K. Querengässer and J. Quer- engässer, 2005. Teat endoscopy (thelo- scopy) for diagnosis and therapy of milk flow disorders in dairy cows. Veterinary Clinics of North America: Food Animal Practice, 21, 205–225.

Gibbs EPJ, Johnson RH. and Osborne AD. 1970. The differential diagnosis of viral skin infections of bovine teat. Veterinary Record, 87: 602-609.

Gleeson, D. E., E. J. O'Callaghan and Rath, MV. 2002. Effect of milking on bovine teat tissue as measured by ultrasonography. Irish Veterinary Journal, 55, 628–632.

Grindal, R. J., A. W. Walton & J. E. Hillerton, 1991. Influence of milk flow rate and streak canal length on new intramammary infection in dairy cows. Journal of Dairy Research, 58, 383–388.

Hussein M and El-Maghraby. 2001.Comparison of two surgical techniques for mastectomy of goats. Small Ruminant Research 40(3):215-221.

Jackson PGG. and Cockcroft PD. 2002. Clinical examination of the udder. In: Clinical Examination of Farm Animals. 1st edition Blackwell Science; Chapter 12, P.154-166.

Janett F, Stauber N, Schraner E, Stocker H, Thun R; Bovine herpes mammillitis clinical symptoms and serological course. Schweiz Arch Tierheilkd,2000; 142: 375-380.

Johnson L. 1988. Mammary gland. In: Text book in Large Animal Surgery, 2nd Ed. (ed. Oehme, F.W.). Williams and Wilkins. Baltimore, USA, pp. 220 – 227.

Kashyap DK, Giri DK, Dewangan G.2014. Prevalance of udder and teat affections in non-descript goats in Rajasthan. Ind.J.small Ruminants Res.. 20(1): 131-133.

Lisie W; George, Thomas J. Divers, Norm Ducharme, and Frank L.W.2008. Diseases of the Teats and Udder. In: Rebhuns Disease of Dairy Cattle. 2nd edition. Elsevier Health Sciences, Saunders W.B, Thomas J. Divers. 327-394.

Lokanadhamu M, Sreedevi B, Venkata RT. 2005.Studies on etiology, symptomatology, diagnosis and therapy in ulcerative thelitis of buffaloes in Andhra Pradesh (INDIA). Buffalo Bulletin, 24: 56-69.

Malleswara Rao UVN, Sreedevi B, Venkata Reddy T. 2003. Studies on ulcerative mammillitis of buffaloes in Andhra Pradesh (India). Buffalo Bulletin, 2003; 22 (4): 80-90.

Matthew S, Ila M, Lewis, John A, Scholten. 1990. Acute gangrenous mastitis due to Clostridium perfringens type A and Escherichia coli in a cow. Can Vet J, 31: 523-524,

Mavrogianni, V. S., G. C. Fthenakis, A.R. Burriel, P. Gouletsou, N. Papaioannou and I. A. Taitzoglou, 2004. Experimentally induced teat stenosis in dairy ewes: Clinical, pathological and ultrasonographic features. Journal of Comparative Pathology, 130, 70–74.

McDonald, J. S. 1975. Radiographic method for anatomic study of the teat canal:

Cha- racteristics related to resistance to new in- tramammary infection during lactation and the early dry period. The Cornell Veteri- narian, 65, 492–499.

Misk NA. 2008. Atlas of Veterinary Surgery, 2008; Faculty of Veterinary Medicine, Assiut University, Egypt

Modransky P and Welker B.1993. Management of teat lacerations and fistulae. Veterinary Medicine 88(10):995-1000.

Nichols S. 2008. Teat Surgery in cattle. In: Current Veterinary Therapy: Food Animal Practice. Chapter 82.

O Connor J. J. 2005. In: Dollar's Veterinary Surgery. CBS Publishers and Distributors. New Delhi, p. 771.

Paape M.J., Poutrel B, Contreras A, Marco JC, Capuco AV; Milk somatic cells and lactation in small ruminants. J. Dairy Sci., 2001; 84(E. Suppl) E237-E244.

Philip K.T.2010. Livestock production: recent trends, future prospects. Philos Trans R Soc Lond B Biol Sci. 365(1554): 2853–2867.

Rambabu K, Sreenu M, Suresh Kumar RV, Rao TSC. 2011. Incidence Of Udder And Teat Affections In Buffaloes. Tamilnadu J. Veterinary & Animal Sciences, 7(6): 309-311.

S.U. Rathod, P.M. Khodwe, R.D. Raibole and S.H. Vyavahare. 2009. Theloscopy - The Advancement in teat surgery and Diagnosis. Disorder. Veterinary World, Vol.2(1): 34-37.

Saratsis, P.1991. Zur diagnostik von Zitzen- stenosen des Rindes mit Hilfe der Ul- traschalltomographie (Literaturübersicht). Deutsche Tierärztliche Wochenschrift, 98, 441–476.

Scherzer, J. 1992. Ultrasound examination of the bovine teat – influence of teat canal length and other factors on the udder health. Thesis, University of Veterinary Medicine, Vienna, Austria.

Schroeder JW. 2009. Mastitis Control Programs: Bovine Mastitis and Milking Management. 2009;[Online]. Fargo: North Dakota State University Agriculture and University Extension. Available from: http://www.ag.ndsu.edu/pubs/ansci/dairy/as1129w

Seyfried, G. 1992. The sonographic measure- ment of teat structures and the significance for udder health of "Braun-and-Fleckvieh" cows. Thesis, University of Veterinary Medicine Vienna, Austria.

Seykora, A. J. and B. T. McDaniel.1985. Udder and teat morphology related to mastitis re- sistance: A review. Journal of Dairy Sci- ence, 68, 2087–2093.

Sharma S, Singh KB, Oberoi MS, Sood N. 1998. Studies on the occurrence of bovine herpes mammillitis in buffaloes. Buffalo Bulletin, 17:79-81.

Singh J, Singh P, and Amold JP. 1993. The mammary glands. In: Ruminant Surgery (eds. Tayagi RPS and Singh J). CBS Publishers and Distributers, New Delhi, India, Pp: 167 – 174

Singh P, Singh J.and Sharma PD. 2003. Surgical conditions of udder and teats in buffaloes. Intas Polivet, 4(II): 362-365.

Slosarz, P., J. Wójtowski, S. Bielińska, A. Frąckowiak, A. Ludwiczak, J. Krzyżewski, E. Bagnicka and N. Strzalkowska, 2010. Machine induced changes of caprine teats diagnosed by ultrasonography. African Journal of Biotechnology, 9, 8698–8703.

Tiwary R, Hoque M, Kumar B. and Kumar P. 2005. Surgical condition of udder and teats in cows. The Indian Cow.25-27.

Trostle, S. S. and R. T. O'Brien.1998. Ultra- sonography of the bovine mammary gland. Compendium on Continuing Education for the Practicing Veterinarian, 20, 64–71.

Turner, A. J., Morgan, I. R., Sykes W. E. and Nicholls W. A. 1976. Bovine herpes mammillitis of dairy cattle in Victoria. Australian Veterinary Journal, 52: 170-173.

Tyagi, R. P. S. and Singh J. 2012.Ruminant Surgery.11thedn. CBS Publishers and Distributors, New Delhi, pp: 167-174.

Weaver, A. D. 1986. Teat Surgery. Bovine surgery and Lameness, Blackwell Scientific Publications, 141-149.

O'Brein, R. T., K. R. Waller III & J. S. Matheson, 2002. Ultrasonographic appearance of edema caused by injections in the mammary gland attachments of dairy cows. Journal of American Veterinary Medical Association, 221: 408–410.

Transforming Rural Areas through Veterinary Science *Pages 253-258*
Editor: Dipanjali Konwar, Shilpa Sood & Shahid Ahamad
Published by: **ASTRAL INTERNATIONAL PVT. LTD., NEW DELHI**

20 Edible vaccines: A New Ray in Disease Prevention

Dr. Mir Mudasir, Dr. A. K. Pandey, Dr. Nawab Nashiruddullah, Dr. S. A. Khandi, Dr. Utsav Sharma & Dr. Nazam Khan

Introduction

Vaccine is basically an entity which is used to stimulate the production of antibodies and provide immunity against one or several diseases. Vaccines have accomplished near miracles in the fight against infectious disease. Typical vaccines are composed of killed or attenuated disease causing organisms. The administration of vaccines is the cost effective method of combating the spread of diseases. Use of vaccines resulted in the eradication of several diseases like small pox and polio. An international campaign was started in late 1990s with the aim to reduce the annual death toll among the children's which was roughly three million by immunizing all the world's children against six devastating diseases. About 80 percent of infants were immunized under this campaign. Yet these victories mask tragic gaps in delivery. The 20% of infants still missed by the six vaccines-against diphtheria, pertussis (whooping cough), polio, meseales, tetanus and tuberculosis-account for about two million unnecessary deaths each year, especially in the most remote and impoverished parts of the globe. This is due to the limitations on vaccine production, distribution and delivery. It needs to be resolved in order to prevent the spread of infections and epidemics by un-immunized populations in the immunized, safe areas. One hundred percent distribution is desirable, because un-immunized populations in remote areas can spread infections and epidemics in the immunized and safe areas. Immunization through DNA vaccines is an alternative but is an expensive approach, with disappointing immune response. Hence the search for cost-effective, easy-to-store, easy-to-administer, fail-safe and socio-culturally readily acceptable vaccines and their delivery systems is the need of hour.

Edible vaccines are antigenic proteins that are genetically engineered into a consumable crop. The food product from the crop contains protein which is derived from some disease causing pathogens. As the crop is eaten and digested, some of the protein makes its way through the blood stream which is enough to cause an immune response. This immune response would now neutralize the pathogen if encountered in future.

The recent approach for development of novel vaccines stresses the need for edible vaccines that are inexpensive, easily administered and capable of being stored and transported without refrigeration. They comprise alternative and new approach of vaccination. They are cheap, heat stable, require no cold chain maintenance. Like conventional subunit vaccines, edible vaccines are composed of antigenic proteins and are devoid of pathogenic genes. Thus, they have no way of establishing infection, assuring its safety, especially in immunocompromised patients. Conventional subunit vaccines are expensive and technology-intensive, need purification, require refrigeration and produce poor mucosal response. In contrast, edible vaccines would enhance compliance, especially in children, and because of oral administration, would eliminate the need for trained medical personnel. Their production is highly efficient and can be easily scaled up. Edible vaccines are currently being developed for a number of human and animal diseases, including measles, cholera, foot and mouth disease and hepatitis. Development of such kind of vaccination will be highly courageous and fruitful for developing countries to adopt vaccination as the central strategy for preventing some devastating diseases prevailing in such countries.

Concept of Edible Vaccines

The idea of edible vaccines was given by Arntzen in the 1990s. The earliest concept of an edible vaccine was demonstrated from the expression of a surface antigen of the bacterium *Streptococcus mutans* in tobacco which causes dental caries. The preparation of edible vaccines involves the introduction of selected desired genes into plants and inducing these genetically modified plants to manufacture the encoded proteins. This process is known as "transformation" and the altered plants as "transgenic plants". These vaccines are composed of antigenic proteins and devoid of pathogenic genes which make them safer for immunization especially in immunocompromised patients. Traditional subunit vaccines are technology-intensive, require purification, refrigeration and produce poor mucosal response which happens to be big hurdle in the campaigning of world immunization programme. However, edible vaccines proved to eliminate the need of intensive technology and trained personnel for oral administration particularly in children. Moreover, edible vaccines offer numerous advantages like good genetic and heat stability, cheap and do not need cold-chain maintenance. Further, they are easily available and their production can be easily scaled up. For example, hepatitis-B antigen required to vaccinate whole of China annually, could be grown on a 40-acre plot and all babies in the world each year on just 200 acres of land.

Mechanism of Action

In most pathogens the site of predilection is at mucosal surfaces *i,e* urogenital, respiratory and gastrointestinal tracts that makes mucosal immunity as prime line of the defense mechanism. Mucosal immunization largely depends on the oral administration of vaccines which results in the development of mucosal immunity, antibody mediated and cell mediated immune response. The antigens, through the process of bio-encapsulation, are delivered from transgenic plants. The bio-encapsulation, which is provided by the tough outer cell wall, protects them from gastric secretions, and therefore, the antigens are released directly in the intestines. The released antigens are taken up by M cells of the intestinal mucosa overlying payer's patches and gut-associated lymphosid tissue (GALT), passed on to macrophages, local lymphocyte populations and other antigen-presenting cells which in turn generate the serum immunoglobins like IgG, IgE, local IgA and memory cells, that would promptly neutralize the attack by the real infectious agent. Edible vaccines activate both mucosal and systemic immunity after coming in contact with the digestive tract lining. This dual effect would provide first-line defense against pathogens invading through mucosa.

Production of Edible Vaccine

Various methods of production of edible vaccine have been devised but the most commonly used methods are as follows:

1. Desired proteins are expressed in plant virus by genetic engineering. Appropiate plant virus is genetically engineered to express the desired peptides/proteins. The recombinant virus is then inoculated into the plant. These plants containing recombinant viruses are then grown and chimeric viruses are extracted and purified. The resultant plant edible vaccines are utilized for evoking the immune response.
2. Another technique, the gene of interest is integrated with plant vector by transformation. A variety of techniques have been used to introduce transgene into plant cell; these could be grouped into following categories:

a) Agrobacterium Mediated Gene Transfer

The appropriate gene construct is inserted into the T-region of a disarmed Ti plasmid of Agrobacterium. The recombinant DNA is placed into Agrobacterium; a plant pathogen which is co-cultured with the plant cells or tissues to be transformed. The drawback of this method is that it gives low yield and the process is slow. This method worked especially well for dicotelydenous plants like potato, tomato and tobacco. Studies have also proved that the genes are expressed by this method in experimental animals and plants.

b) Biolistic Method

The gene containing DNA coated metal (*e.g.* gold, tungsten) particles are fired at the plant cells using gene gun. Those plant cells that take up the DNA are then allowed to grow in new plants, and are cloned to produce large number of genetically identical crop. This method is quite attractive because DNA can be delivered into cells of plant which makes gene transfer independent of regeneration ability of the species. But the chief limitation is the need for costly device particle gun.

c) Electroporation

Here, there is introduction of DNA into cells by exposing them for brief period to high voltage electrical pulse which is thought to induce transient pores in the plasma lemma. The cell wall presents an effective barrier to DNA. Therefore, it has to be weakened by mild enzymatic treatment so as to allow the entry of DNA into cell cytoplasm.

Advantages of Edible Vaccine

1. Edible vaccines evoke sufficient immune response and do not require adjuvants
2. Edible vaccine can elicit mucosal as well as systemic immunity.
3. Edible vaccines are cost effective in preparation, production and transportation.
4. Edible vaccines do not require skilled persons for administration as they are given orally.
5. Edible vaccines lower the risk of spread of diseases through infected needles.
6. Edible vaccines waive off sophisticated equipments and tools and can be grown easily on rich soils
7. Edible vaccines unlike traditional vaccines are not injectables. Thus, the risk of contamination is meager and the need for sterilized premises and manufacturing area can be avoided.
8. Since the seeds of transgenic plants contain less moisture content and can be easily dried thus offer greater storage opportunities [16].

Veterinary Sciences

The first patented edible vaccine to demonstrate efficacy in animal trials was against the transmissible gastroenteritis virus (TGEV) in pigs and was under planning to be made commercially available [17]. Vaccines against porcine reproductive and respiratory syndrome (PRRS) and other diseases like parvovirus are being investigated. Various transgenic animal feeds are currently undergoing clinical trials in pigs [18].

Future Prospects

Edible vaccines hold central stage of vaccination programme especially in third world countries where transportation cost; poor refrigeration and unavailability of skilled manpower complicate vaccine admintration. These vaccines may lead to a future of safer and more effective immunization and would overcome some of the difficulties associated with traditional vaccines, like costly production, distribution and delivery. Edible vaccine studies demonstrate encouraging progress toward resolving major hurdles in these emerging commercial vaccine technologies. Parasitic infections among domestic animals pose a major challenge in most of the developing countries, especially due to surge of drug resistant strains. However, vaccination seems to be the sole practical strategy in such circumstances. The currently available vaccines are either live or killed vaccines which possess many disadvantages and limited success was achieved using bacterial, yeast, insect and mammalian expression systems. Enhanced use of previously reported and new antigens from transgenic plant is witnessed in recent past which has revolutionized the immunization programme due to their exceptional advantages. Moreover, the regulatory burden for veterinary vaccines is less compared to human vaccines. This led to an incredible investment in the field of transgenic plant vaccines for veterinary purpose. Several plant based vaccine trials have been conducted to combat various significant parasitic diseases like fasciolosis, schistosomosis, poultry coccidiosis, porcine cycticercosis and ascariosis. Besides, passive immunization by oral delivery of antibodies expressed in transgenic plants against poultry coccidiosis is an innovative strategy. These trials may pave way to the development of promising edible veterinary vaccines in the near future.

Conclusion

Edible vaccines holds great potential to combat almost all the problems associated with traditional vaccines and may impose positive effects of vaccines for reaching and to decrease some devastating hazards of parental vaccines. Being cost-effective, easily administrable and storable these vaccines may prove boon to oral immunization particularly in developing countries. Further, due to lack of pathogenic effects these vaccines provide safer way of immunization and reducing the incidence of various diseases like hepatitis and diarrhoea especially in the developing world, which face the problem of storing and administering vaccines. Edible vaccines are specific to provide mucosal activity along with systemic immunity. Thus these vaccines provide a platform for the production of cheap and safe vaccines which might be helpful to combat numerous dreadful diseases in developing world.

References

Arakawa, T., Yu J, Chong, D.K., Hough, J., Engen, P.C. and Langridge, W.H. 1998. A plant based cholera toxin B subunit-insulin fusion protein protects against the development of autoimmune diabetes. Nat Biotechnol. 16; 934-938.

Das, D.K. (2009). Plant Derived Edible Vaccines. Current Trends in Biotechnology and Pharmacy, 3(2): 113-127.

De Aizpura H.J. and Russell-Jones, G.J.(1988). Oral vaccination. Identification of classes of proteins that provoke an immune response upon oral feeding. Journal of Experimental Medicine, 167:440- 451.

Giddings, G., Allison, G., Brooks, D. and Carter, A. 2000. Transgenic plants as factories for biopharmaceuticals. Nat Biotechnol,18:1151-1155.

Krishna, C.V. and Jonnala, U. K. (2006). Edible Vaccines. Sri Ramachandra. Journal of Medicine, 1(1).

Lal, P., Ramachandran, V. G., Goyal, R. and Sharma, R.(2007) Edible vaccines, Current status and future. Indian Journal of Medical Microbiology, 25(2):93-102.

Langridge, W.H.. 2000. Edible vaccines. Science American,283: 66-71.

Ma, J.K., Hiatt, A., Hein, M., Vine, N.D., Wang, F., Stabila. P. et al. 1995.Generation and assembly of secretory antibodies in plants. Science,268:716-719.

Mariotti, D., Faontana, G.S., and Santin. (1989). Genetic transformation of grain legumes: Phaseolus vulgaris L. and P. coccineus. Journal of Genetic Breeding, 43:77-82.

Nochi, T., Takagi, H., Yuki, Y., Yang, L., Masumura, T., Mejima. M, et al. 2007. Rice-based mucosal vaccine as a global strategy for cold-chain- and needle-free vaccination. Proc Natl Acad Sci U S A. 104: 10986-10991.

Pascual, D.W.2007. Vaccines are for dinner. Proc Natl Acad Sci U S A 104: 10757-10758.

Ramsay, A.J., Kent, S.J., Strugnell, R.A., Suhrbier, A., Thomson, S.A. and Ramshaw, I.A. 1999. Genetic vaccination strategies for enhanced cellular, humoral and mucosal immunity. Immunology Review,17: 27-44.

Streatfield S.J., Jilka J.M., Hood E.E., Turner D.D., Bailey M.R., Mayor J.M., et al. 2001. Plant-based vaccines: unique advantages. Vaccine, 19: 2742–2748.

Streatfield, S.J.(2005). Plant based vaccines for animal health vaccines. Rev. Sci. Tech Off Int Epiz, 24 189-199.

Taylor, N.J.and Fauquet, C. M. (2002). Microparticle bombardment as a tool in plant science and agricultural biotechnology. DNA Cell Biology.21:963-977.

Transforming Rural Areas through Veterinary Science *Pages* **259-270**
Editor: Dipanjali Konwar, Shilpa Sood & Shahid Ahamad
Published by: **ASTRAL INTERNATIONAL PVT. LTD., NEW DELHI**

21 Constraints and Strategies for Goat Farming in Hilly and Kandi areas of Jammu

Dr. Surinder K. Gupta & Dr. Suraj Amrutkar

Introduction

Livestock sector is emergent which influence the state economy. The economy of Jammu and Kashmir is still agriculture dependent as wellit is the main occupation of majority of the rural people who earn their livelihood from it. Goat farming is one of the oldest and traditional livestock businesses, which has been established successful since centuries. Goat farm business is intensifying worldwide as the population is growing and non-vegetarian lovers are increasing. There is no religious issue for consumption of chevon as compared to pork or beef. Some people extensively raise goats for meat and some for milk and skin. Rearing of goats is a traditional talent in Jammu and Kashmir people. The tribals viz. *Bakerwals, Gaddies and Changpas*are developed perfect professionalism in sheep and goat rearing. Being the source of their livelihood, they have become the protectors of goats over the centuries. Goats are mainly rearing for meat, milk and fiber (pashmina and mohair), hide and skin. Beside hide and hair; intestine serve as basic raw material for many processing industries of which leather is the most important and accounts for sizeable employment and even export earnings. Goat commonly known as the poor man's cow; and plays a vital role in improving the socio-economic conditions of poor rural masses. This fulfills the requirement of those farmers with marginal grazing lands which due to some reason cannot withstand large animals throughout the milk production cycle. Goat meat from adults is often called chevon. Goat meat is the most commonly consumed red meat in the world.

As per 19th Livestock census(2012), India's livestock sector is one of the largest in the world with a holding of 11.6% of world livestock population which consist of goat (17.93%). The contribution of goat in total livestock population in India is 26.4%.Goat meat comprises 63% of all red meat that is consumed worldwide.

Present Status of Goat in India

Rank of India in goat population is 2nd. The goat population has declined by 3.82% over the previous census and the total goat in the country is 135.17 million in 2012. Goat in China constitutes the 18.19% of the total world goat population.

Total Number of Goat Population State Wise (2012)

Sr. No.	*State*	*Values in thousands*
1	Rajasthan	21666
2	Uttar pradesh	15586
3	Bihar	12154
4	West Bengal	11506
5	Andhra pradesh	9071
6	Maharashtra	8435
7	Tamilnadu	8143
15	Jammu and Kashmir	2018
India		135173

Present Status of Goat of J & K State

The total number of goat in the Jammu and Kashmir state as per 19ths census (2012) is 2.01 million number. There is a 2.44% decline in number of goat population during the inter censuses period (2007-12). The total number of female goat population has decreased from 1.53 million in 2003 to 1.51 million in 2012. The female goat population has decreased by 0.58% over the previous census. The male goat population has also decreased from 0.52 million in 2003 to 0.50 million in 2012. The population of male goat has decreased by 7.58% during the inter censuses period (2007-2012). Rajouri has the major contribution in goat population of 15.16%. The second and third highest contributors are Leh (Ladakh) and Kathua with share of goat population of 11.00 and 10.54%, respectively.

Total Population of Goat in Jammu And Kashmir State in 2003 and 2012

Category	*2007*	*2012*	*% change from 2007 to 2012*
Goat	2068.27	2017.90	-2.44

District Wise Percentage Share of Goat Population

Rajouri	15.16 %	Doda	3.94 %
Leh (Ladakh)	11.00 %	Kishtwar	3.54 %
Kathua	10.54 %	Ramban	2.89 %
Reasi	10.02 %	Baramula	2.69 %
Udhampur	9.55 %	Kupwara	2.35 %
Jammu	8.80 %	Badgam	1.64 %

Punch	4.97 %	Bandipore	1.26 %
Kargil	4.30 %	Anantnag	1.22 %
Samba	4.09 %	Other district	2.00 %

Present Status of India in Meat Production

Total meat production including poultry meat was 5.9 million tonnes in 2012-13. Nearly 45% of the production of meat is contributed by poultry alone.Buffalo, goat, pig, sheep and cattle are contributes 19, 16, 8, 7 and 5% of the total meat products, respectively. Uttar Pradesh produces maximum total meat in India followed by Andhra Pradesh, West Bengal, Maharashtra and Tamilnadu.Maximum meat from buffalo and pig are produced by Uttar Pradesh. Andhra Pradesh produces maximum meat from sheep and poultry.

Nutrient Composition of Different Types of Meat

Nutrients	*Goat*	*Chicken*	*Beef*	*Pork*	*Lamb*
Energy (Kcal)/ 100 gm	122	162	179	180	175
Fats %	2.6	6.3	7.9	8.2	8.1
Saturated fats %	0.79	1.7	3.0	2.9	2.9
Protein %	23	25	25	25	24
Cholesterol (mg)	63.8	76.0	73.1	73.1	78.2

Advantage of Goat Meat Consumption

Goat meat has more nutritional value, greater health benefits; and ideal choice to be considered as compared to the other red meats. Goat meat is a healthy alternative to beef and chicken because of its lower calorie, fat and cholesterol value. It has irreplaceable taste. The amount of saturated fat in goat meat is less than the total amount of unsaturated fats; which improves blood cholesterol level, eases in inflammation and stabilizes heart rhythms. Goat meat reduces the risk of atherosclerosis and coronary heart diseases. Goats are ruminants; and their meat is a good source of Conjugated Linoneic Acid (CLA), a fatty acid that may help to prevent cancer and other inflammatory conditions. Goat meat contains vitamin B complex, which helps to burn fat. Goat meat contains high amounts of lean proteins and low amounts of saturated fat. It helps for controlling weight and reduces the risk of obesity. Mutton contains selenium and choline; which are beneficial in curing off cancer. Goat meat is advantageous for pregnant women because it prevents anemia during pregnancy in both mother and baby by increasing the blood hemoglobin levels in the mother and enhancing blood supply to the baby as it contains high amounts of iron (3 mg iron/100 gm of good meat). If goat meat is included in the diet during pregnancy, it reduces the risk of birth defects in babies, such as neural tube defects etc. Goat meat supports in iron recovery among women during menstruation and provides relief from menstrual pain. Goat meat helps to get healthy skin due to its high content of vitamin B_{12}.Goat meat helps in beating stress and depression due high content of vitamin B_{12}. Goat meat helps to control blood pressure; and prevents kidney diseases &stroke due to high content with potassium and low in sodium.

As goat meat contains niacin; goat meat helps to promote energy metabolism. The protein found in goat meat act as hunger suppressing agents; and keep the stomach full for longer, thus managing weight. Goat meat is rich in calcium, which helps to strengthen the bones and teeth. The meat of goat enhances the production of new cells, thereby delaying ageing. Goat meat helps to maintain thyroid function.

Major Constraints in Goat Farming

- ✰ Heavy losses in goat farming may lead due to lack of knowledge on goat rearing.
- ✰ Larger sizegoat'sfarms of an individual can not tolerate the heavy losses.
- ✰ Poor housing and habitat is primary constraint in failure of commercial goat farms.
  - Need of proper scientific hosing for goats is necessary to run profitable goat farms.
  - Use of latest management equipment to control environment in tropical housing for goats become essential.
- ✰ Unavailability of high genetic potential breeds
  - In spite India is land of genetic diversity even though, here no genetic improvement in goats have been take place since last 60 years.
  - Non descriptive breeding constitutes nearly 80% of the total animals in the field
  - No herd book is maintained to keep standard breed records of goat
  - No registered breeding society is present yet
  - Gap between research scientist and stake holders is large
  - Therefore any entrepreneur who want to run commercial goat farms need to start it from zero.
- ✰ Absence of high productive exotic breed for cross breeding
- ✰ Lack of scientific feeding practices
  - Although feeding standards are available to feed goats at various stages of production but they are grossly ignored and hence farmers and entrepreneurs suffers huge production losses.
  - Properly formulated feed is necessary to keep goat healthy and efficient meat production.
  - Customized feed additive formulations are necessary to run profitable meat goat programme.
- ✰ Health problems
  - Health challenges like PPR, CCPP, Ecto-parasites, Goat pox, Contagious Ecthymia, pregnancy toxemia, strongylosis, FMD, HS and Haemoncosis

- There are some of the major diseases which can be prevented through various precautionary measures but due to carelessness they remain undiagnosed and close the farms.

☆ High kid mortality

- Kids which are main profits of the goat farms are remained ignored.
- 50% and 70% of the total mortality will be occurring in 1st week and 1st month of the kid's life respectively. It means that there would 50% chances that kid die in 1st week.
- Pneumonia and diarrhea are the main causes of the deaths, these are not diseases but managemental problems
- This mortality can be prevented through improve management practices and available medicines administrations
- Extra antioxidant administration to goats in last month of pregnancy improves kids survival rates; provided that kid have sufficient colostrum at birth
- Poor feeding in pregnancy leads to lower birth weight of kids which ultimately leads to low growth rates and poor profits.
- Goat exhaust high amount of energy, water, calcium and electrolyte from the body. These causes calcium and carbohydrate crisis in goats and ultimately lower amount and poor quality of colostrum and subsequent milking.

☆ Poor feeding of goat kids

- Kids are left with goats and no special care is provided to kids.
- It must be keep in mind that in Indian goats are not efficient milk producers and never support the growth potential of kids.
- In such conditions, high energy kid starter and milk replacer are required.
- This milk replacer is needed to give from 7th day after birth upto 10-12 kg weight achievement.
- It is recommended that under proper veterinary consultant's supervision; kids should be weaned on 7th day after birth.
- It should be keep in mind that excess sugar and protein in diet causes Entero- toxemia which causes sudden death of kids.

☆ Goat kids weaning

- Farmers keep kids with the goats which causes management problems in goats.
- Goats with kid will come late into heat and breeding would be delayed.
- Lack of organized market
- Poor marketing channel for goat selling

- Poor and lack of goat transportation facilities
- Unavailability of technical labour
- Improper sanitation facility within the farm
- No specialized feed units
- Lack of properly vaccinated goat stock to start new farm
- Lack of proper scientific information regarding commercial goat farm establishment
- There is lack of extension services
- Many farmers and individuals are unacquainted of available goat farming training programme
- Unavailability of loans and subsidies to start commercial goat farming

Managerial Problems

Profits in goat farming or success rate of goat business is depends on goat kid care and their management.

Newly Born Kid Management

- Never try to cut the navel cord; and let it break naturally used to cut the naval cord
- If you find the naval cord is too long after breaking, you can cut it close to baby goat stomach.
- All the instruments used are sterilized when scissors are used to cut naval cord of baby goat to separate from mother goat.
- To prevent newly born baby goats from any infections and make the cord to dry faster, dip the cord in iodine.
- Provide confortable space for kids to roam around; and ensure the space is dry and warm because wet and cold may cause diseases.
- Should take care of extreme colds
- Goat kids should be exposed to proper ventilation and air flow in the house/shed.
- Keep mother and kids together; and allows the mother goat to clean the baby goat.
- Clean the floor and make it dry after the birth of the kid.
- Provide clean water to the mother goat and monitor the baby goat.
- Goat kids may stop drinking milk either from the mother or bottle. This means that baby goat needs solid feed.
- Goat kids usually start weaning at 4 to 5 weeks of age
- You may introduce pasture or hay to habituate the feeding.
- Provide clean and fresh water along with greens, hay or pasture.

Colostrum Feeding to the Kid

- First milk of the mother goat is called colostrum and this should be fed first time within 1 hour after the birth.
- Ensure the baby goats are fed with the colostrum at least 4 times a day.
- Leave the goat kids with mother for whole day; so that kid may frequent access to try mother milk.
- To prevent any blocks, just pull couple of streams of milk from the mother goat.
- If any cases, goat kids may not drink mother's colostrum after birth; in this case provide bottle feeding with mother goat milk (colostrum) or from any other goat.
- Milking bottle should be sterilized while milk feeding.
- Usually baby goats required 150-160ml of milk during first 3 days after birth. Kids have to be fed with this amount 4 times a day. From 4th day to 10th day, they should be fed with 300 to 325 ml of milk 4 times/day. At 10 to 15 days old, 450-500 ml of milk 3 times/day should be given.

Goat Kids Care

- For safety precaution, you should remove baby goat horn buds.
- Remove of horns should be done at 10 days of age.
- Perform goat kid's vaccination with the help of veterinary doctors.
- Goat requires tetanus and clostridium vaccination around about 4 to 5 weeks of age.
- Carry out de-worming in younger goats in spring and summer.
- Use lice powder to prevent lice and frequently trim the young goat fur.

Shelter Management

- Provide secured and proper shed to the growing goats.
- Always keep the shed floor clean and dry. Make sure that the bedding are dry and warm.
- Keep the goat house with well ventilation and air flow along with good drainage. Keep changing bedding to avoid any wetness on the floor.
- Shelter should protect the young goats from severe climatic conditions such as extreme colds, heats and floods.
- Fence around the shelter; so that young goats cannot jump and this can also provide protection from other predators.

Goat Kids Pasturing

- Don't mix-up the goat kids and adult goats on the same pasture as there is a possibility that goat kids may eat manure in the pasture along with other plants. This may cause goat kids to fall sick very quickly.

- Keep young goats on separate pasture to avoid eating manures. This manure may result in worms and other parasites.
- If find any young goat sick, then isolate that animal
- Never mix-up the young goat with other sick adult goats

Young Goats with Feed

- As goats grow; they should be provided with more supplemental feed along with regular grazing.
- Grains, alfalfa hay, green pasture, maize (corn), barley and oats are best choice of feeding young goats.
- Avoid any poisonous plants in the field.

Nutritional Requirements for Goats

Feeding may be highest expense of any meat goat operation. Goats raised for meat need high quality feed and require an optimum balance of many different nutrients to achieve maximum profit potential. Profitable meat goat production can only be achieved by optimizing the use of high quality forage and browse and the strategic use of expensive concentrate feeds. This can be achieved by developing a year round forage program allowing for as much grazing as possible throughout the year. The goat is not able to digest the cell walls of plants as well as the cow because feed stays in its rumen for a shorter time period. In addition, goats must consume a higher quality diet than cattle because their digestive tract size is smaller with regard to their maintenance energy needs. Relative to their body weight, the amount of feed needed by meat goats is approximately twice. Meat goats require nutrients for body maintenance, growth reproduction, pregnancy and production of products such as meat, milk and hair. The groups of nutrients that are essential in goat nutrition are water, energy, protein, minerals and vitamins.

Daily Nutrient Requirements for Meat Producing Goats

Nutrients	*Young goats*		*Does (50 kg)*				*Bucks (35-55kg)*
	Weanling (15 kg)	*Yearling (30 kg)*	*Pregnant (Early)*	*Pregnant (Late)*	*Lactating (Average milk)*	*Lactating (High milk)*	
Drymatter (kg)	0.91	1.36	2.04	2.04	2.04	2.27	2.27
TDN %	68	65	55	60	60	65	60
Protein %	14	12	10	11	11	14	11
Calcium %	0.6	0.4	0.4	0.4	0.4	0.6	0.4
Phosphorus %	0.3	0.2	0.2	0.2	0.2	0.3	0.2

Breeding Policies for Goat Development

Efforts are being under taken by the Sheep Husbandry Department for development of mutton varieties of goats by introducing improved breeds among the existing goat population of the state, as the native goats exhibit poor growth rate and small quantity of milk due to poor genetic potential.

Local Kashmiri Goat

It is non-descriptive goat, short stature, coloured and weighing 30-40 kg adult stage. It is being found in Hilly tract of Shopian, Kulgam, Trai, Budgam and Kupwara*etc.*

Pashmina/Changra Goat

A sizable portion of goat population of the state *viz.* 3.20 lacs is found in the Leh District of the Ladakh region and major chunk of this goat population comprises of pashmina changra. These goats are reared by changpas, a nomadic race in changthang sub division of Leh, Ladakh situated at an altitude of 12000 to 18000 feet above mean sea level. The area is sandy and mountainous with atmospheric temperature during winter goes down to (-40°C). The goat is hardy, sturdy, small dainty animal with quick moments, capable of surviving in difficult conditions. Animal has short neck and medium sized ears. Horns are narrow towards tips. The entire body is covered with coarse hair with long fibers on the bridges and shoulders with a fine under coat pashmina. Pashmina fiber has a unique position among animal fibers for its fitness, warmth, durability, lightness, softness and ability to absorb dyes and moisture as compared to mohair and wool because of its freeness from inflection. The fiber diamcter of pashnina ranges from 12 to 14 microns.

Angora Goats

Angora goats are reared in Ladakh division and are known for production of Mohair a fine quality fiber which is used by local people in Ladakh for making woolen garments after mixing it with sheep wool.

Alpine Goats

It is an important milch breed with origin in France. The milk yield on an average is 1.5-2.0 kg per day. An adult male weight about 75 kg and female about 62 kg. The breed has introduced in the Valley and Kargir and about 40 % cross have been achieved so far.

Future Policies for Improvement of Goats in the State

Keeping in view, the present scenario of mutton development various mutton breeds of goat are being introduced in the state to bridge the gap between the demand and supply of meat, in addition to increase milk.

Toggenburg

A dual purpose breed has been introduced Jammu division and is still under technical observation for its adaptability vis-à-vis traits of economic importance.

Boer Goats

It isindigenous to South Africa and is a dual purpose and claimed to bear all the attributes which a high yielding improved breed of goat should possess. It is also having adaptability to wide range of climatic conditions. It is said to be very fertile. Addition to it, it produces on average 2 kg milk per day containing 7.9% fat. Boar goats have a birth weight 2.4kg, weaning weight 35 kg and adult weight 115 kg. The breed is likely to be boost meat production in the valley.

Cross-Breeding Programme

Cross breeding of local valley flocks with Alpine is being taken up on a large scale to increase milk production. Similarly a Beetal breed of goats is also introduced in the warmers belts of the valley.

Breeding Policy for Goat Development

Development of goat sector, which remained neglected due to more stress being laid on sheep development, has now been taken up so as to narrow down the gap between demand and supply of meat. The department has accordingly introduced programme for development of goat sector.

Introduction of Beetal Breeds

Under the programme,Beetal bucks are being purchased from progressive breeders of Kathua district and Gurdaspur district of Punjab and from Central Sheep Breeding Farm Hissar (Haryana) and distributed among the breeders of Jammu, Samba, Kathua and Rajouri belt for improvement of their local goats so as to increase the milk production. Dairy Goat Farm, Rajbagh is also maintained a pure Beetal goat breed for breeding purpose.

Conservation of Kagani Goats

Under the progressive belt Kagani bucks are being purchased from progressive goat breeders of Rajouri, Udhampur, Reasi, Jammu and Samba district providing to the breeders having Kagani goats so as to conserve the breed on pure lines and to check inbreeding.

Diseases of Goat

Goat diseases can be prevented by keeping goat healthy which is the first line of defense. You should be known about these goat diseases when buying a goat, so that you can avoid buying a diseased goat. Generally goats are resistant to many diseases. However, when rear more number of animals in one place with insufficiency of pasture facilities; such intensive system of rearing leads to spread of many diseases. This causes reduced production potential and more mortality which in turn causes economic losses to the formers. Hence identification of diseases in goat and its prevention is most important. Health management is more important especially worm load. Hence the kid must be dewormed at first month of age and then in a month upto 6 months of age. Ecto-parasites must be treated carefully because it is not only affect the growth and also affect skin quality.

- ☆ **Bacterial Fiseases:** Anthrax, Haemorrhagic septicemia, Brucellosis, Enterotoxaemia, Pneumonia, Foot rot, and Mastitis etc.
- ☆ **Viral Diseases:** Peste-des-petitis Ruminants (PPR), Foot and mouth disease, Goat pox.

- **Endo-parasitic diseases:** Fluke infection, Tape worm, Round worm and Coccidiosis
- **Ecto-parasitic infestation:** Ticks, Lice etc.

Common Measures for Controlling Disease

- Proper drainage, sprinkling of copper sulphate near water
- Avoid early morning and late evening grazing
- Keep the shed clean and provide clean quality drinking water
- Separate infected animal from healthy one
- Provide proper quarantine measures while purchasing new animals
- Proper disposal of dead animals
- Rotational grazing to control infection

References

Handbook of Animal Husbandry (2011).3rd revised edition, 1233 pp.

Banerjee, G. C. (1998). A text book of Animal Husbandry, 6th edition, 1079 pp.

Sastry, N.S.R. & Thomas, C.K. (2005). Livestock Production Management, 4th revised edition, 642 pp.

Chakrabarti, A. (2011) Text Book of Clinical Veterinary Medicine, 3rd edition, 701 pp.

Verma, D.N. (1999) A text book of Livestock production Management in tropic, 1st edition, 748 pp.

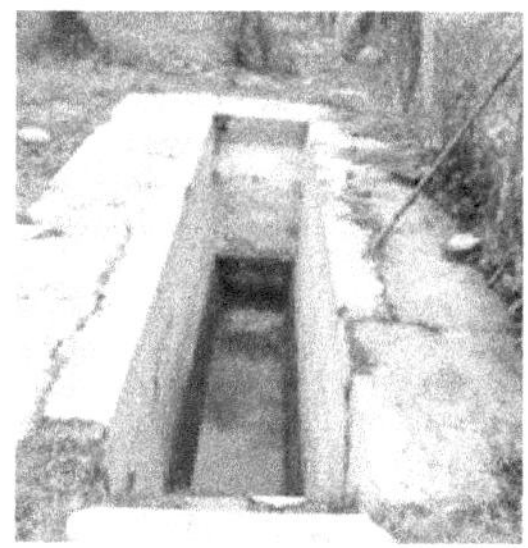

Dipping Bath

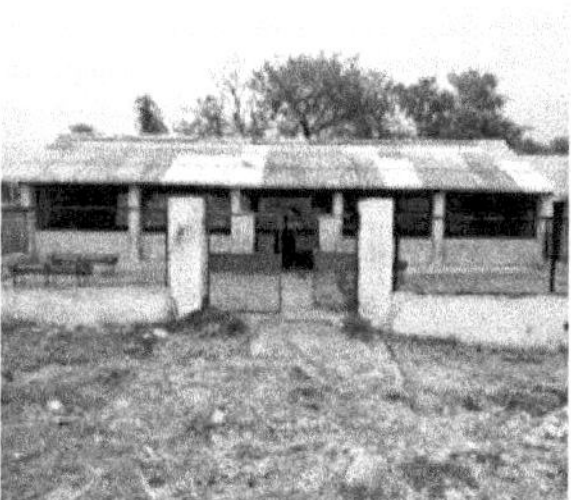

Housing of Goat

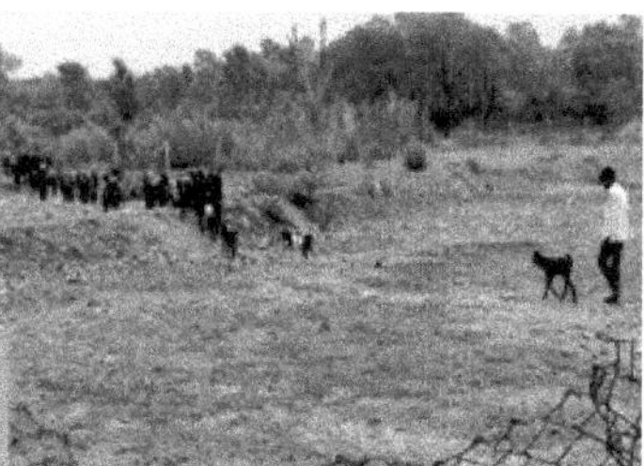

Extensive system of rearing

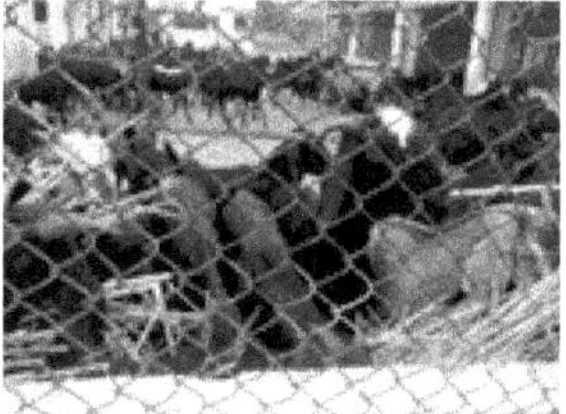

Feeing Fodder

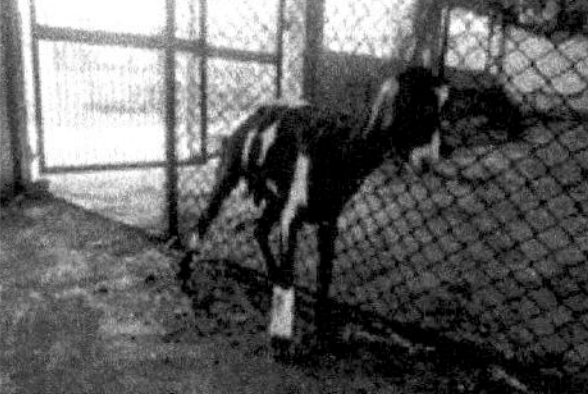

Injured Goat

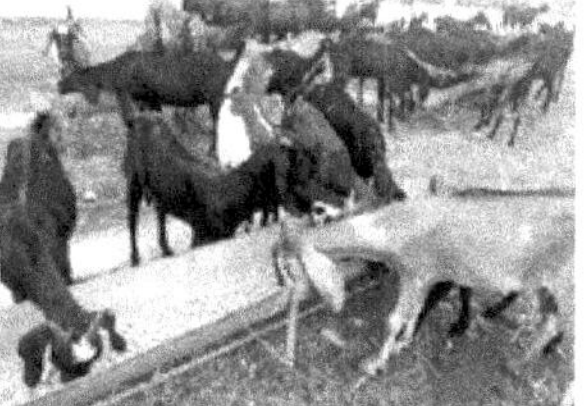

Feeding of Goats

Transforming Rural Areas through Veterinary Science *Pages* **271-284**
Editor: Dipanjali Konwar, Shilpa Sood & Shahid Ahamad
Published by: **ASTRAL INTERNATIONAL PVT. LTD., NEW DELHI**

22 Pig Farming: An Emerging Enterprise in Kandi Areas of Jammu

Dr. Surinder K. Gupta & Dr. Suraj Amrutkar

Introduction

Commercial pig farming in India for meat production is one of the best and profitable business ideas for the Indian people. There are several highly meat producing pig breeds available around the globes. Some of those are very suitable for commercial meat production according to the weather and climate of India. A few years back, pig farming had a bad image in the society, but at present at scenario has changed tremendously and commercial pig farming in India is no more restricted to lower class people. Now peoples are conscious about the economic value of pigs like other domestic livestock animals; andhigher cast, educated people also started commercial pig farming business in a modern and scientific manner.

Pigs convert inedible feeds, forages, certain grain byproducts, meat by products, mill by products, damaged feeds and garbage into valuable nutritious meat. Most of these feeds are either not edible or not palatable to human beings. Pig grows fast and is a prolific breeder, farrowing 10 to 12 piglets at a time. It is capable of producing two litters per year under optimal management conditions. The carcass return is quite high *i.e.* 60-80 percent of live body weight. The farmer can profitably utilize his time and labour in this subsidiary occupation with a small investment on building, equipment, feeding and sound disease control programme. The faeces of pigs are used as a manure to maintain soil fertility. Pig farming is best business for small and landless farmers, uneducated youth, farm women and part time earning for educated youth having agriculture as occupation. Pig population in India is 10.29 million (2012 census) which is decrease by 7.54 % over previous census and it is about 1.3% of its global population (2007 census). National Research Centre PIG is situated at Guwahati, Asaam. China, America, Brazil and West Germany are the world largest pig producing country.

State Wise Pig Population

States	*Values in thousands*
Assam (at 1st rank)	1636
Uttarpradesh	1334
Jharkhand	962
Bihar	650
Chhattisgarh	439
Andhra Pradesh	349
Arunachal Pradesh	356
West Bengal	648
Meghalaya	543

Advantage of Pig Farming

- Most prolific, 6 to12 piglets in every litter
- Fast growing (68 kg in 6-8 months)
- Shortest generation interval
- Pig skin used for light leather goods
- Pig manure contain:- N: 0.70%, P: 0.60% and K: 0.70%
- Pig products such as Pork, Bacon, Ham, Sausages, Lord (pig fat) are increasing in demand

Characteristic of Swine and their Production

- Superior feed conversion ratio (1: 3-3.5)
- Swine store fat rapidly
- Swine are prolific and bring quick return
- A unit of 10 sows and 1 boar will produce about 160 piglets during the first year
- Gilt may be bred between age of about 8 to 9 month farrow when approximately 13 months old and weight about 80 kg in 6 months old
- Enterprise requires moderate investment
- Dressing %: Pig: 65-80, Cattle: 50-60, Sheep & Goat: 45-55
- Pork is most nutritious

Disadvantage

- ☆ Extremely sensitive to unfavorable ration and to careless management
- ☆ Very susceptible to numerous diseases and parasites
- ☆ Sow should have skilled attendants at the time of farrowing

Nutritive Value of Pork

Pork is a high protein food and contains varying amounts of fat. 100 gram pork contain following nutritive value:

Nutrients	*Amounts*
Calories	297
Water	53%
Protein	25.7%
Carbohydrate	0%
Sugar	0%
Fat	20.8%
Saturated	7.72%
Monounsaturated	9.27%
Polyunsaturated	1.87%
Omega-3	0.07%
Omega-6	1.64%

Pork Protein

Like all meat, pork is mostly made up of protein. The protein content of lean cooked pork is around 26% by fresh weight. By dry weight, the protein content of lean pork can be as high as 89%, making it one of the richest dietary sources of protein. It contents all the essential amino acids, necessary for the growth and maintenance of our bodies. In fact, meat is the most complete dietary sources of protein.

Pork Fat

Pork contains varying amounts of fat. The proportion of fat in pork usually ranges from 10-16%, but it can be much higher, depending on the level of trimming and various other sources. The fatty acid composition of pork is slightly different from the meat of ruminants such as beef and lamb. It is low in conjugated linoleic acid (CLA) and is slightly richer in unsaturated fats.

Vitamins and Minerals

Pork is a rich source of many different vitamins and minerals. These are the main vitamins and minerals found in pork. Pork is rich in thiamin, selenium, zinc. Pork may contain useful amounts of many other vitamins and minerals.

Other Meat Compounds

Creatine, Taurine and Glutathione is abundant in pork. Creatine functions as an energy source for muscle. Taurine is an antioxidant amino acid which may be important for heart and muscle function.

Adverse Effects and Individual Concerns

Eating raw or under cooked pork should be avoided altogether especially in developing countries. This is because raw pork may contain several types of parasites that can infects human such as pork tapeworm (Taeniasolium), round worms (Trichinella) and Protozoa (Toxoplasma gondi).

Constraints or Problems

Constraints and problemsarealways there in any kind work, and piggery in Jammu province is not at all exceptional to it.

Feeds

Feed cost constitutes about 70 to 80 percent cost of pork production. Therefore, careful planned feeding programme is important for a successful swine production. It is obvious that pig feeding must be as economical and efficient as possible. Feed plays an important role in successful pig production. The quality of the ration determines the rate of growth of young pigs to great extent. A complete diet for pigs includes protein, carbohydrates, fats, minerals, vitamins and ample good water. The fibre content of pig feed should be in between 5-6%. Garbage, such as kitchen waste and other vegetable waste can be useful feeds, if properly cooked and fed. Poultry farm waste, slaughter house waste, hatchery waste, molasses etc. along with various agro-industrial products can be incorporated in pig rations. Feed is the most important aspects in pork production but this has been sadly neglected in our Jammu province. Pig producers are almost entirely dependent on their own resources of feed. Pigs are mostly reared on kitchen and human waste. Farmers uses waste of shops, *i.e.* waste of military canteen etc.

Good Quality Piglets

Another problems faced by the pig farmers in the lack of easy availability of good quality piglets. Depending on the source of production, piglets may be divided into two categories; *viz.* cross breed and pure breed. The collection of pure breed is better because it is more profitable and suitable for the climatic condition of Jammu province. In reality, due to lack of government breeding farm, farmers have to buy piglets from local market at a high cost. Thus a shortage of piglets is made by the private farms through import from neighboring state like Punjab etc.

Marketing

Middle man plays a significant role in marketing of pigs. The marketing channel for pig enterprise is organized form. The unorganized channel means participation of private traders who have profit making motives.The problems of marketing in Jammu province are numerous and complex. There is a total lack of amenities in providing shelter, water trough and light for the animals.Marketing of animals are also not standardized. There is not provision for maintaining the breeding and production records of animals. The production units are often small and poorly adjusted to the market requirements. The poor and inadequate transportation networks also affect marketing organizations to a great extent. In Jammu and Kashmir, there is no provision for market intelligence services till now. Pork marketing in Jammu province, mostly run by the tribal people is fully unorganized. Due to non-availability of modern slaughter houses, people in this region slaughter the live pigs in the traditional method, which is not conductive for wholesale meat production. Only a few pork selling center have permanent infrastructure and are running smoothly. Many pork selling centers have no permanent structure and run occasionally or once in week in open space. So infestation of meat by flies is a common features usually observed in these pork selling shops.

Financial Problems

Finance has the key role to play for development of piggery. A pig farm should always be equipped with necessary equipments, nutritious food, medicines and chemicals. Pig farmers must be able to bear the labour cost. Hence, the farmers need a good amount of quality production which will yield satisfactory income. In Jammu province, majority of the population live hand to mouth and do not have sufficient money for investment in other financial activities like the pig farming. To get a bank loan, land properties have to be mortgaged. Many farmers are landless. Those who have land property are reluctant mortgage land for fear of losing it in case they are unable to repay bank loan. So most of the farmers, in rural areas go to the lenders, like Mahajan, Dalal and pay higher interest which ultimately minimizes their amount of profit. However, this financial problem can be avoided through implementation of NABARD funded scheme.

Disease Control

Like other domestic animals, pigs are also prone to disease. The common bacterial diseases of pigs are swine plague, swine erysipelas, anthrax and infectious abortions. The diseases of viral origin are swine fever, rinderpest, FMD, viral pneumonia and swine pox. Pigs are also suffered from internal and external parasites. It is obvious that the method of disease control is based on a very high standard of hygiene followed by efficient vaccination programme. Prevention is better than cure and it leads to less chance of incidence of diseases.Successful pig production generally rests on the efficient disease control. Surprisingly, pigs are clean animals by nature and cannot grow in a bad environment. They require good, clean, well ventilated surrounding. Unfortunately most of the farmers neglect diseases and parasites infestation at the early stage which result a serious problems eventually leading to serious losses in the productivity and profitability. It has been proved that adaptation of treatment after outbreak of diseases is more expensive.

Managerial Problems

It consists of all that management problemswhich are facing by farmers while routine operational practices.

The Most Common Breeds Used in India

Large White Yorkshire	Origin : England, Popular English Bacon breed
Middle White Yorkshire	Origin : England, Excellent Pork Breed
Berk shire	Origin : England, Good quality Pork
Other important breeds:	
Landrace	Origin: Denmark, produce Highest quality Bacon
Tamworth	Origin : England, Extremely Good Bacon type
Duroc	Origin : USA, Good meat type
Chester white	Origin : USA
Hereford	Origin : USA

Ghungroo(Desi Breed)

Ghungroo is an indigenous strain of pigs popular among the local people because of high prolificacy and ability to sustain in low input system. This breed/ strain produces high quality pork utilizing agricultural and kitchen wastes. Ghungroo are mostly black coloured with typical "Bull dog" face appearance, with a litter of 6-12 piglets individual weight about 1.0 kg at birth and 7-10 kg at weaning. Both sexes are very much docile and easy to handle. Some of the selected sow has delivered litter size of 17 piglets at birth.

Reproductive Features

- Most gilts reach puberty (age at first estrus): between 6 to 8 months
- Length of oestrus cycle: 21 days (18-24 days)
- Estrous period: 2 to 2½ days
- On the average, ovulation occurs approximately 48 hrs after the onset of estrus
- The interval from the first to last ovulation, at a given estrus varies from 1 hrs in length to perhaps as long as 7 hrs
- Sows are prolific (giving birth to several offspring at one time) animals and the rate of ovulation varies considerably with 10-20 ova being the usual range
- The gestation period of swine averages about 114 days (3 months, 3 weeks and 3 days)
- Domesticated pigs have shorter gestation period than that of wild pigs (124 days)

- Advantage of early weaning from the reproductive point of view is the potential increase in piglets produced per sow per year.
- The boar generally reaches puberty at the age of 8 months

Signs and Detection of Heat

The following are the signs when sows and gilts are showing heat

- ☆ They always assume rigid stance (standing reflex) when pressure is applied in the lower back.
- ☆ The vulva of the pig nearing heat is swollen, red and discharge mucus.
- ☆ Other signs include: loss of appetite, restlessness, alertness, grunting and chomping of the jaws.
- ☆ The grunting and willingness of the sows and gilts to be mounted on is a definitive sign that they are in standing heat.

Flushing of the Sow

- ☆ The increasing of the energy content of sows ration for 6 days or so before the expected time of estrus and for a few days after mating may increase the number of young born.

Preparation for Farrowing

The average gestation period for sows is 114 days. To prepare for farrowing, producers should know when sows are due. However, producers should be ready for delivery prior to the due date because of individual variation in gestation. Newborn pigs have a better survival chance if they arrive in a clean, sanitized farrowing facility. A steam cleaner or high pressure sprayer can be used successfully to clean the furrowing house. A disinfectant can be applied after cleaning. Some producers fumigate, especially those who had a consistent scours problem in a central house. In addition, the sow should be washed with soap and warm water immediately prior to being put into the farrowing pen.

Care and Management of Piglets

The most critical period in the life cycle of a pig is from birth to weaning. On the average, about two piglets per litter are lost during this period. Poor management is the major contributing factor, although the actual cause may be crushing, bleeding from the navel, anemia, starvation or disease. There are many essential tasks to be done shortly after pigs are born. The navelof the day pigs should be disinfected using tincture of iodine.

When piglets are born, they need a warm, dry place to live. New born piglets need temperature of about 90 to 95°F for the first few days and sustained warm temperatures for at least a few weeks. Each week after birth, the ambient temperature can be decreased by 3°F. For bedding, straw or hay works well, with wood chips underneath for absorption. Piglets enjoy chewing and rooting through the hay and burrowing down in the nests they create. Deep bedding will also help maintain warmth. It's best if piglets can get at least some colostrum from the sow. Colostrum helps protect against disease susceptibility and improve growth rates.

Needle Teeth

An examination of the mouth of pigs at birth will show that they have eight small tusks like teeth, two on each side of both upper and lower jaws. These teeth are normal, inclined to flatness, have sharp edges and generally are brown in tinge, at tip. Needle teeth often are the cause of irritation and pain to the sow when pig nurse, especially at first when the udder are tenders. Moreover, the piglets may bite or scratch each other and infection may start and cause serious trouble. Needle teeth has to remove as soon as possible after born.

Anaemia In Piglets

Anaemia is a common iron deficiency disease in piglets. This condition can be prevented and cured by supplying iron either orally or by injection. Oral administration consists of spraying or swabbing the sow's udder with a saturated solution of ferrous sulphate (0.5 kg of ferrous sulphate in 10 litres of hot water). This solution must be applied daily from birth until the piglets start eating creep feed. Intramuscular infection of iron-dextran compounds is the more effective method of preventive anemia.

Hypoglycemia in Neonatal Piglets

Hypoglycemia is a common cause of death in neonatal piglets. Glycogen reserves are soon depleted if piglets become chilled or fail to ingest an adequate amount of milk. Chilling may occurs if the effective temperature in the piglet sleeping area is less than ~95°F during the first week of life. Signs of hypoglycemia include loss of condition, weak vocalization, faltering gait, cold skin and recumbency. These are rapidly followed by paddling, frothing at the mouth, coma and death if intervention does not occur. If chilling occurs, the piglets should be put in a warm environment with a supplemental heat source such as heat lamps. If the piglets are not receiving an adequate amount of milk, cross-fostering or milk supplementation can be beneficial. Porcine milk replacer, bovine colostrum, or evaporated milk diluted equally with water can be used for supplemental nutrition until piglets are able to consume nutrient dense solid food.

Raising Orphan Piglets

The death of a sow after farrowing, mastitis, lactation failure,largerlitter sizeis results in orphan pigs. If another sow has farrowed within a short time previously, the orphan piglets may be transferred to her. This transfer must be made within a few days after farrowing. To ensure acceptance of new pigs, the sow should be separated from her own litter for short time and then the new piglets are brought to her and a disinfectant or other material sprinkled on all the piglets to mask the odors.

Baby Pig Scours

Baby pig scours are major ongoing problems for swine producers. Most common diarrheas are caused by various strains of Escherichia coli, gram-negative bacteria common to the intestinal tract of all mammals. The symptom of E.coli: Induced diarrhea which is watery and yellowish stool. Pigs are most susceptible from 1 to 4 days of age, at 3 weeks of age and at weaning. Although pigs are born with little disease resistance, this resistance increases as they absorb antibodies from their mother's colostrum. It is important that piglets are fed on colostrum soon after birth because pig's ability to absorb antibodies decreases rapidly from birth. Colostrum provides the only natural disease protection; they will have until their own mechanism for antibody production begins to function effectively at 4 to 5 weeks. Disease resistance is lowest at 3 weeks. It is wise to avoid unnecessary stress (castration, vaccination, worming) at this time.In treating common scours, orally administered drugs are usually more effective than injections. A dry, warm, draft-free environment is of primary importance in reducing scours. Sanitation is also very important in reducing the incidence of baby pig scours. Other disease such as transmissible gastroenteritis and swine dysentery may cause more serious diarrhea problems. Contact your local veterinarian if diarrhea persists or does not respond to treatment.

Castration

The male piglets not selected for breeding may be castrated when they are three to four weeks old.

Creep Feeding

Creep feed is that normal feed, given to suckling pigs behind a barrier (or creep) which allows them access to the feed but excludes the sow. In addition to sow's milk, pigs need a creep feed to make maximum gain through weaning. Provide a fresh creep feed at one week of age in a place where pigs can get away from the sow. Creep ration should be high quality, complete mixed feed. Good creep rations can be purchased or mixed on the farm. It has totake particular care to use a high-energy palatable mixture that meets the pig's nutrient needs whilecreep rations are formulated and mixed on the farm. Getting pigs to eat adequate amounts of a creep ration is often a problem. Place the creep feeder in a warm, dry, well-lighted area. Feed small amounts and feed frequently to keep the ration fresh. Sprinkling feed on the floor or placing it in a shallow pan may help pigs start to eat. Pelleted feeds are usually eaten more readily than meal.

Weaning

Normal weaning age of piglets is at 3 to 5 weeks of age. The sow should be separated from the piglets for a few hours each day to prevent stress of weaning and feed is reduced gradually. The piglets should be gradually shifted from 18% protein creep feed to 16 percent grower ration over a period of two weeks. Group of 20 piglets of more or less the same age should be housed in each pen.

Pig Identification for on Farm Management

There are a variety of tracking and identification systems used for managing pigs. For herd management, there are a few ear-marking systems that can be used to identify the individual pigs. Pigs can be permanently identified by notching or tattooing their ears. Number ear tags are also used but are not usually suitable for pigs penned together as the tags can be lost.

Ear Notching

Ear notchingis best done on piglets a few days after farrowing, at the same time as other procedures such as giving an iron supplement. The notches must be carefully done so they can be easily read when the pigs get older. Notches at the base of pig's ear need to be cut deeper than those nearer the tip; otherwise they may grow over in time. If notches are too near the curved base of the ear, they could pass around the curve with age and be overlooked. On the other hand, notches clipped near the tip of the ear should not be too deep otherwise the tip of the ear may droop. This is especially likely to occur if the notches are close together as required in some systems. Shallow notches in this upper section of the ear are easily read. Ear notching should not be done too close to the head along the top of the ear or the ear may droop.

Ear Tattooing

The equipment required is a set of tattoo pliers, three or four sets of 9 mm needle blocks numbers from 0 to 9 and a suitable tattooing ink or paste. Similar systems of identification can be used to ear notching except that numbers rather than positions are tattooed in the ear. Before tattooing, ensure that both the pig's ear and the tattoo blocks are clean. The thinner part of the lower ear is most suitable for tattooing.

Ear Tags

Once gilt and boars have been selected from within the herd or brought into it, they can be identified with easy-to-read numbered plastic tags. There are varying shapes and types of ear tags. Some tags are pre-numbered, others are supplied blank and can be numbered with a special pen.

Electronic Identification

The technology to identify pigs through electronic implants is already developed. The best site seems to be under the skin of the neck at the base of the ear. The system is costly because a large initial outlay is required, as computer, software, data communication and individual transponders are required. Computer-controlled sow feeding stations use electronic identification for feeding purposes. The sows wear a plastic collar, which is embedded with a radio transponder. When the sow enters the feeding stations use electronic identification for feeding purposes. The sows wear a plastic collar, which is embedded with a radio transponder. When the sow enter the feeding station, signal received from the transponder trigger the station's feeding mechanism and the sow received a measured amount of feed.

Pig identification is necessary for accurate performance records. Pigs can be marked with ear notches, ear tattoos or ear tags. Ear notching is the most practical method for commercial farms. Ear tags are useful for re-identifying breeding stock. Electronic identification, if it becomes cheaper may be more widely used in the future.

Housing of Pigs

The house should give adequate protection against direct sunlight and rain. Hogs are sensitive to heat and cold. The floor and wall should be strong to withstand the rooting habits of pigs. Concrete flooring is durable and easy to clean. The walls may be bricks, finished smoothly and doors of strong wooden planks or iron. Feed troughs and water troughs may be placed along the front to facilitate feeding from outside. Pigs thrive well in temperature range of 20-25°C. Provide shade, wallowing tank, cooling devices such as sprinkling of water, washing etc. to maintain thermal comfort. Design should be such that all animals are observable easily from outside and the labour requirement is less. Boars, pregnant and dry sows, gilts and growing pigs are usually kept in open yards with partially sheltered area. Farrowing sows are housed in completely enclosed houses or pens. Simple low costs houses constructed with locally available materials. Uncastrated males and females should not be housed together beyond the age of four months. The walls should have a minimum height of 1.5 m.

Guard Rail

- The guard rail should be raised 8 to 10 inches from the floor and should be 8 to 12 inches from the wall

Floor Space Requirement

Category	*Covered area (m2)*	*Open area (m2)*	*Maximum number of animals per pen*
Boar	6.0-7.5	8.8-12.0	Individual pens
Farrowing pen	7.0-9.0	8.8-12.0	Individual pens
Fattener (3-5 months old)	0.9-1.8	0.9-1.8	30
Fattener (above five months)	1.3-1.8	1.3-1.8	30
Dry sow/gilt	1.8-2.7	1.4-1.8	3-10

Feeds

Urea as Protein Substitute?

- Urea is the compound which used in dairy cattle ration as substitute of natural protein, is **not at all beneficial to pig**
- Thus, the use of **urea in swine ration is completely banned.**

Pre-Starter Ration (Creep Feeding)

The dry pre-starter feeds also known as creep ration or milk replacer are usually offered to the piglets when they are about of 2 kg body weight or 7-10 days old.

This should be continued till piglets are weaned and weight from 6.5 to 8.5 kg body weight. Creep feed should contain about 20% protein, a major portion of which should be animal origin

Starter Ration

The starter ration offered to piglets from day of weaning to about 20 kg body weight. It is almost similar to the pre-starter ration except that the skim milk powder is replaced by either fish meal or meat meal. At some places, where skim milk powder is available at cheaper rate, the pre-starter ration is continued.

Growing–Finishing Ration

After the pigs have a good start and weight about 20 kg, they should be switched from starter to grower diet as by attaining this body weight, it has almost passed a nutritional critical period and after that they will do well on relatively simple ration. The ration contains about 16% protein, having some percentage of animal protein and fibre. When piglets grow about 35 kg body weight, they are offered lighter, bulkier finishing ration for production of lean (bacon) carcasses. These rations contain lower level of animal proteins and energy and during this phase, it is possible to replace larger proportion of cereal grains with grain processing by-products bringing the protein percent upto 13%. The ration in general continued from 35kg till the animals grow upto a body weight of 70 kg, when they are economical for slaughter in India.

Diseases of Pigs

Prevention is always more profitable than treatment, especially for diseases that are difficult to treat.

Mastitis

The inflammation of mammary gland is called mastitis.It occurs in breeding stock.Reduced milk production, loss of appetite and a higher body temperature are symptoms of mastitis in sows. It is caused by a bacterial infection of the mammary glands, where skin discoloration can be seen. Antibiotics, along with anti-inflammatory drugs are effective treatments. Oxytocin may be used to encourage let down of milk and corticosteroids can be prescribed. Hygiene in farrowing housing is important, along with nutrition during late pregnancy to promote immunity. Stress can also be a factor, and it is important to make sure that teats are not being damaged by sow housing facilities. This disease has a significant effect on productivity because of the potential effect of reducing the number of piglets weaned by sows.

Coccidiosis

This disease is very common in suckling piglets and is caused by intracellular parasite coccidia. It causes diarrhea, which can be bloody, often between 10 and 21 days of age and upto 15 weeks of age. Acute cases are treated with fluid therapy and Coccidiostats. Secondary infections can result from damage to the intestinal wall. Hygiene should be improved to the end the cycle of infection; sow feces are a major source, and flies can spread infection. Providing a warm, dry, clean creep area will help to reduce the parasite load and the likelihood of coccidial infection.

Respiratory Diseases

Coughing, sneezing, abdominal breathing, reduced growth rates and potentially mortality are all sign of respiratory diseases. Depending on the cause, antibiotics may be given in feed, water or as an in injectable. Poor ventilation or environmental conditions can exacerbate respiratory conditions.

Swine Dysentery

Animal with this disease suffer from diarrhea, with or without the presence of blood. It is caused by the bacteria *Brachyspirahyodsenteriae.*Growth rates of post weaning pigs are reduced, and in some casessudden death occurs. Antibiotics are used to treat the disease, either in feed, water or as an injectable. Reducing stocking density can be an effective way of reducing infection pressure and stress in the herd. As well as improving hygiene levels, rodent control is a high majority; rodents are a vector for this disease.

Exudative Dermatitis (Greasy Pig)

The symptoms of this disease are skin lesions, caused by an infection of the bacteria staphylococcus hyicus. In severe cases, mortality can occur, as the bacteria damage the liver and kidneys. Lesions first present as dark areas of skin, which spread and become flaky with a greasy feel. Antibiotics are used to treat the infection, along with skin protectants, autogenously vaccine have also been used with success. Improving hygiene in piglet housing is key to preventing this condition, along with teat dipping of sows pre and post farrowing.

Conclusion

Pork is the world's most popular type of meat. It is a rich source of high quality protein, as well as various vitamins and minerals. For this reason, it may promote muscle growth and maintenance and improve workout performance. The pig husbandry is still solely depends on small scale production system. The production system is traditional with zero to minimum input involvement and low remunerative. Considering the demand of pork in the region, immense opportunities prevail in improvement of productivity through adopting scientific intervention in routine management and health care services. Entrepreneurship development in major sectors like feed formulations and supply, establishing pig breeding unit, artificial insemination facilities, mobile vaccination services, pork processing and use of pork products could make the enterprises a profitable one and generate employment opportunities for farmers and youth engaged in this sector.

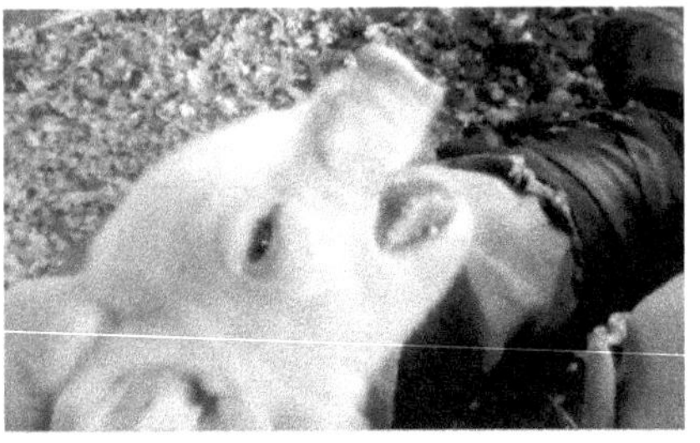

Drinking Milk

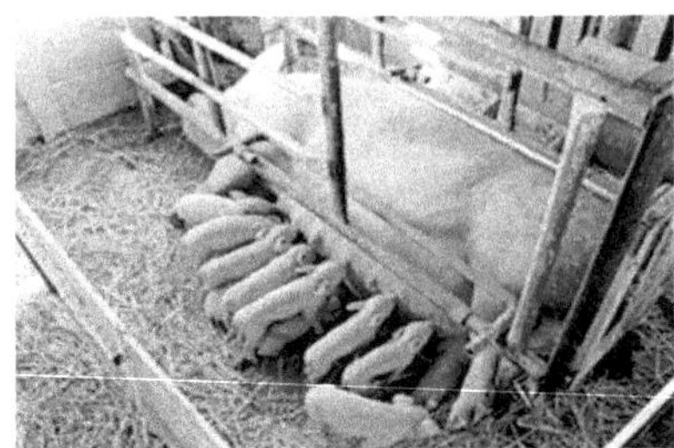

Cultural Feed of Pig

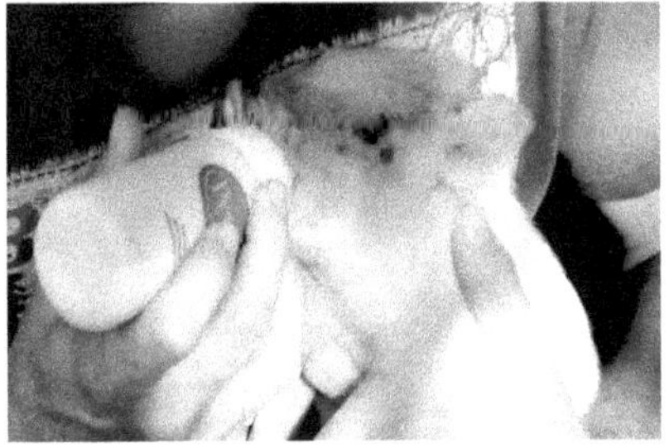

Ear Tagging in Pig

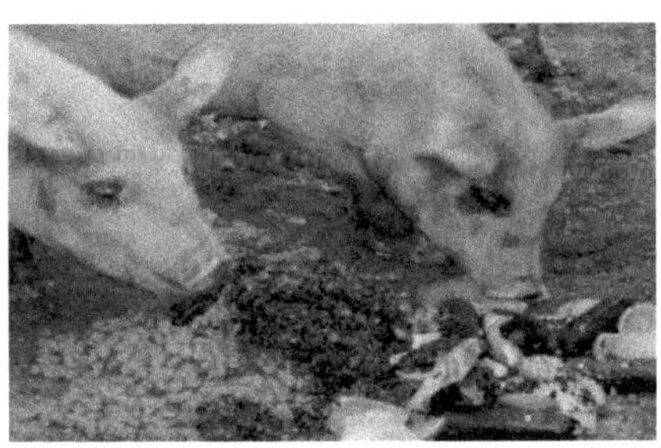

Ear Notch in Pig

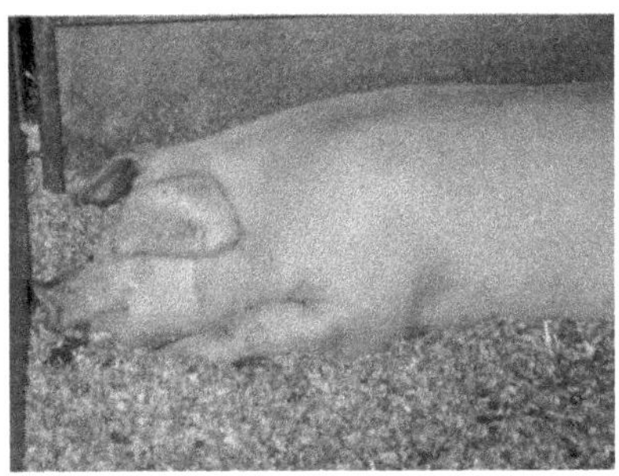

Needle Teeth

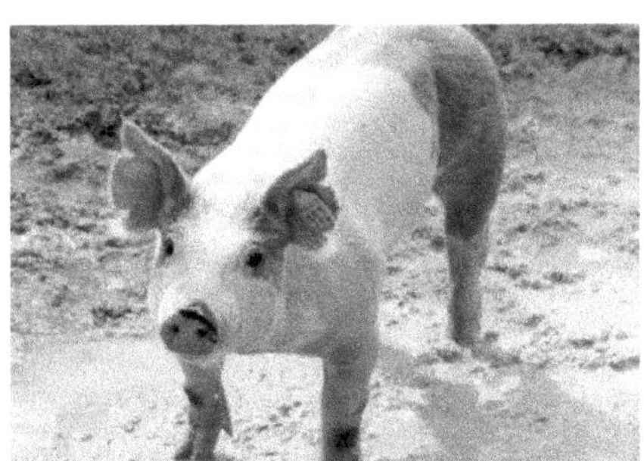

Farrowing Pen

Transforming Rural Areas through Veterinary Science *Pages* **285-308**
Editor: Dipanjali Konwar, Shilpa Sood & Shahid Ahamad
Published by: **ASTRAL INTERNATIONAL PVT. LTD., NEW DELHI**

23 Improvement in Dairy Production and Productivity: Role and Future Perspective of Livestock Management

Dr. Biswajit Brahma & Dr. Rakhshan Jeelani

Dairy farming is a class of agriculture for long-term production of milk, which is processed for eventual sale of a dairy product. The rising demand for fresh and packaged dairy products and ethnic dairy specialties is broadening the base of India's modern dairy sector, which accounts for almost 17% of India's expenditure on food. The Indian dairy market was valued at USD 5.4 billion, in the year 2010, which raised to USD 11.8 billion in the year 2015. By the year 2020 the dairy industry market in India is expected to be valued at USD 22.5 billion based on the projections and past trends. Affluent farmers are seeking to establish dairying units on a commercial level, with a big herd size of 30-50 animals and modern machinery. These large commercial farms are required to cope with a growing population, higher incomes, increasing health consciousness, and the consequent explosion in demand for pouch milk and value added products across the country. Thus, farmers will have to shift towards adopting modern dairy farming techniques in order to increase their production. India ranks first among the world's milk producing Nations since 1998 and has the largest bovine population in the World. Milk production in India during the period 1950-51 to 2017-18, has increased from 17 million tonnes to 176.4 million tonnes as compared to 165.4 million tonnes during 2016-17 recording a growth of 6.65%. FAO reported 1.46% increase in world milk Production from 800.2 million tonnes in 2016 to 811.9 (Estim) million tonnes in 2017. The per capita availability of milk in the country which was 130 gram per day during 1950-51 has increased to 374 gram per day in 2017-18 as against the world estimated average consumption of

294 grams per day during 2017. Most of the milk is produced by animals reared by small, marginal farmers and landless labours. Of the total milk production in India, about 48% milk is either consumed at the producer level or sold to non-producers in the rural area. The balance 52% of the milk is marketable surplus available for sale to consumers in urban areas. Out of marketable surplus it is estimated that about 40% of the milk sold is handled by the organized sector (20% each by Cooperative & Private Dairies) and the remaining 60% by the unorganized sector. According to a UN report released **(27 May 2015, Rome)** The number of hungry people in the world has dropped to 795 million – 216 million fewer than in 1990-92, or around one person out of every nine. But because of increase in population world's 70% of the population will be in hunger in 50 years from now (2060) according to the estimation by Food and Agriculture Organisation of the United Nations (FAO). The world human consumption for the animal protein was 29 g per capita daily (or 10 kg per capita consumption). However, there is an increasing trend towards per capita demand for animal source foods and it is occurring primarily in developing countries (80% of world population). India is the world's largest producer and consumer of dairy. The dairy industry in India was worth INR 5,000 billion in 2016. India is also globally the largest milk producing country since 1997. In India, the co-operatives and private dairies have access to only 20% of the milk produced. Approximately, 34% of the milk is sold in the unorganized market while 46% is consumed locally. This is in comparison to most of the developed nations where almost 90% of the surplus milk is passes through the organized sector. The Indian ice cream industry is one of the fastest growing segments of the dairy or food processing industry. Currently the ice cream market in India is estimated to be over INR 4,000 crores, and is growing at a rate of 15-20% year-on-year. It is projected that by 2019, the market will reach a value of approximately INR 6,198 crores. Growing population, changing lifestyles, expanding urbanization and accelerated climate changes are creating new challenges in Bovine breeding systems. In the past, the challenge was to ample feed, but now it is to provide essential nutrients to promote health especially reproductive health; and in the future, the challenge would be to provide optimal nutrients based on an animal's genetic profile and productivity. Fortunately, along with challenges, the developments in science are creating new avenues for tackling the challenges.

Livestock Sector in J&K: A Brief Overview

Dairy sector has emerged as one of the key components of poverty lessening, rural growth and nutritional security policies. In J&K, the dependence over livestock is far more due to topographical challenges that make other activities difficult and unsatisfactory. Agriculture and allied sectors contribute about 38 per cent to the state gross domestic product of which 11 per cent is contributed by the livestock. The economy of Jammu and Kashmir is still agriculture dependent with main occupation of majority of the rural people who earn their livelihood from it. The contribution of Agriculture and livestock to total GSDP has increased from 5.04%% in 2007-08 to 18.52% in 2013- 14. Integrated Sample Survey (2011-12) revealed that total livestock population of Jammu region had demonstrated an increase of 8.40% over the year 2009-10 and reached to 78.908 lakhs from 72.79 lakhs. Kashmir region also witnessed an increase of 4.63% as livestock population had reached to 74.994 lakhs from 71.67 lakhs. However, in Ladakh region livestock population slipped by 1.44% from 6.60 lakhs to 6.505 lakhs during the same period. J&K state witnessed 30% increase in its contribution towards national milk production. Approximately 95.38 thousand metric tonnes (TMT) of liquid milk have been imported through Lakhanpur inter-state border terminal, up to February in 2014-15, from 76.61 TMT in 2013-14 and 72.16 TMT in 2012-13. The total milk production by the state in 2011-12 from total milch animal population of 1228 thousand animals (703 thousand crossbred cows of age above 2.5 yrs, 524 thousand indigenous cows of age above 3 yrs and 417 thousand buffalo females of over 3 yrs age) was 1614 thousand tonnes. The dairying marketing channels in Jammu and Kashmir is largely under-developed. Jammu and Kashmir Milk Producers Cooperative Limited (JKMPCL) is the oldest organization with two milk plants, one each at Srinagar and Jammu, and is the state level federation of 186 and 130 dairy cooperative societies, respectively. The pasteurization capacity of these two plants is 30000 litres / day (LPD) each and presently, 10000 -12000 LPD and 7000–8000 LPD are sold from Srinagar and Jammu, respectively. Khyber Agro farms Pvt. Ltd is the biggest milk plant of Jammu and Kashmir functioning in the Kashmir Valley with pasteurization capacity of 1 lakh LPD. Presently, it sells 50000–60000 LPD, of which 60 per cent is procured from the neighbouring state of Punjab and 40 per cent from the local network of vendors / wholesalers, etc. Milk distribution system in J&K has been quite exploitative and traditional with the organized sector handling only 1.70 and 5.0 per cent of the total liquid milk production and marketed surplus. The situation is alarming in the state and to reverse these trends, it is essential that an integrated dairy development project is planned and implemented to boost milk production, to provide a regular and remunerative market to the milk producers and capture a major share of urban milk markets with regular supply of quality milk.

As per the Integrated Sample Survey Report (ISS), 2011-12, total estimated meat production of State was worked out to be 322.781 Lakh Kg consisting of 80.79% of (260.762 Lakh Kg) Red Meat and 19.21% (62.019 Lakh Kg) of White Meat. As per the latest Integrated Sample Survey Report (ISS), 2010-11, total estimated meat production of State was worked out to be 308.986 Lakh Kg. As per estimated results of ISS survey 2011-12, the meat availability was worked out to be 2.701 Kg per person per year against 2.650 Kg for 2010-11.Meat production registered a growth from 308.986 Lakh Kg to 322.781 Lakh Kg in the year 2011-12 over the previous year resulting into 4.47% growth. Average wool yield per annum is 26.218 Kg for cross-breed sheep and 17.495 Kg for local-breed sheep. During the year 2011-12 the total wool production estimated for the State was 75.295 Lakh Kg which consisted of 61.586 Lakh Kg (81.79%) from Crossbreed Sheep and 13.709 Lakh Kg (18.20%) of Local-breed Sheep. During the year 2010-11, the total wool production estimated for the state was 73.819 Lakh Kg.

Animal diseases continue to be a major constraint in livestock productivity and agriculture development. Rinderpest has been eliminated in the state, whereas Anthrax, Black Quarter, Hemorrhagic septicemia, Foot and mouth disease and helminthic infections have been controlled substantially. However, ectoparasitic infestation and protozoan infections are still a major issue hampering livestock health status in animals. One of the major reason for low production in dairy sector is Jammu and Kashmir's diversified climate e.g. cold desert in Ladakh region and temperate climate in Kashmir region and humid sub-tropical climate in Jammu region. Small size of land holding is another hurdle for limited milk production in the state as state does not produce enough fodder because of lack of modern technologies in small and marginal farmers. Area specific dairy mineral mixture should be given to the dairy farmers to fulfill the diet of dairy animals. The dairying marketing channels in Jammu and Kashmir is largely under-developed. Lack of a regular outlet of milk has made the producers extremely dependent on the milk vendors/ shops, who exploit them by not paying remunerative prices, thereby discouraging the producers to increase their milk production. The situation is alarming in the state and to reverse these trends, it is essential that an integrated dairy development project is planned and implemented to boost milk production, to provide a regular and remunerative market to the milk producers and capture a major share of urban milk markets with regular supply of quality milk, which is otherwise being captured rapidly by the neighboring state of Punjab. The population of sheep has stagnated except a marginal increase between 2003 and 2007. The wool production has declined to around 40 million kg, of which fine wool is only 10%. The major bottlenecks in improving sheep and goat production are lack of pastures and fodder shrubs and trees in the area where the sheep and goat thrive The higher stocking rates, excessive grazing pressure, change in plant composition of grazing areas and reduced biomass availability have rendered migratory system of rearing difficult to sustain. Excessive parasitic load in migratory flock, higher energy spent while covering greater distance during migration along with other factors lead to body weight loss resulting into poor remunerative price realization by migratory Sheppard community.

Main Challenges and Problems of the Dairy Industry

Shortage of Feed and Fodder

There is an excessive number of unproductive animals which compete with productive dairy animals in the utilization of available feeds and fodder. The grazing area is being reduced markedly every year due to industrial development resulting in shortage of supply of feeds and fodder to the total requirement. Ever increasing gap between demand and supply in feeds and fodder limits performance of dairy animals. Moreover, provision of poor quality of forage to dairy cattle restricts animal production system. The low capability of purchasing feeds and fodder by the small and marginal farmers and agricultural labourers engaged in dairy development result in inadequate feeding. Non-supplementation of mineral mixture results in mineral deficiency diseases. High-cost Feeding reduces the profits of the dairy industry.

Breeding System

Late maturity, in most of the Indian cattle breeds, is a common problem. There is no effective detection of heat symptoms during oestrus cycle by the cattle owners.

The calving interval is on the increase resulting in a reduction in efficiency of animal performance. Diseases causing abortion leads to economic loss to the industry. Mineral, hormone and vitamin deficiencies lead to fertility problems.

Education and Training

A vigorous education and training programmes on good dairy practices could result in the production of safe dairy products, but to succeed they have to be participative in nature. In this regard, education and training of all the employees is essential so that they understand what they are doing and develop a sense of ownership. However developing and implementing such programs in the dairy sector requires a strong commitment from the management, which at times, is a stumbling block.

Health

Veterinary health care centres are located in far off places. The ratio between cattle population and veterinary institution is wider, resulting in inadequate health services to animals. No regular and periodical vaccination schedule is followed, regular deworming programme is not done as per schedule, resulting in heavy mortality in calves, especially in buffalo. No adequate immunity is established against various cattle diseases.

Animal and Product Hygiene

Many cattle owners do not provide proper shelter to their cattles leaving them exposed to extreme climatic conditions. Unsanitary conditions of cattle shed and milking yards, leads to mastitis. Unhygienic milk production leads to a reduction in storing quality and spoilage of milk and other products.

Less Emphasis on Indigenous Breeds

The native cattle is more resistant to diseases and environmental conditions, but very less attention is given to indigenous cattle and their breeding programmes. More emphasis is given to cross breds which are not adapted to the local climatic conditions.

Marketing and Pricing

Dairy farmers are not getting remunerative price for milk supply. Due to the adoption of extensive crossbreeding programme with Holstein Friesian breed, the fat content of crossbreed cow's milk is on the declining condition and low price is offered as the milk price is estimated on the basis of fat and solid nonfat milk content. There is also a poor perception of the farmers, due to lack of marketing facilities and extension services, towards commercial dairy enterprise as an alternative to other occupation.

Welfare Problems

Despite the relaxing image of outdoor farming, several industry practices negatively affect dairy cows. To meet production demands, dairy cows are subject to a continuous cycle of impregnation, induced calving and milking.

Tail-docking and horn removal are routinely performed without pain relief. Lameness is another major animal welfare problem, often the result of environmental pressures, such as tracks, herd size and handling. The average lifespan of a dairy cow is six to seven years, whereas generally cows can live for 20 to 25 years.

One of the most controversial issues is young "bobby" calves. A bobby calf is a newborn calf, less than 30 days old, who has been purposely separated from their mother. Immediately after separation, cow and calf call out and search for each other. Most bobby calves are slaughtered within the first week of their life. Handling and transport pose added problems for young calves who have not developed herding behaviours, are vulnerable to stress, and are forced to go without their mother's milk. Each year, 450,000 bobby calves are slaughtered.

The Environmental Impact

The effect of thermal stress on livestock is multidimensional, affecting metabolism, production, product quality, health and reproduction negatively (Babinszky *et al.*, 2011). The feed intake of animal is reduced and as a result the energy is used for maintenance purpose of the animal and nothing is left for the production purpose. In India, an estimated loss of 1.8 million tonnes of milk annually, is attributed to heat stress amounting to a fiscal loss of approximately Rs. 2661 crore (Upadhayay, 2010).

High Perishability of Dairy Products

In India, ice cream industry is mostly regional and there is a multitude of brands focusing on only one or two districts or in some case only one state. There are very few national brands and the major reason behind slow growth of the smaller players is the high perishability of ice cream products.

Unavailability of Records

As per 19th Livestock census, there are 88 million In-Milk animals whose records are unavailable on an annual basis even. Records of those in breeding stage, their productivity, treatment and vaccination are also not properly maintained by State Animal Husbandry Departments. This is because the system for maintaining records on the above aspects has not yet evolved in complete shape due to lack of prioritisation. Impediments like lack of animal identification and traceability, inability to meet sanitary and phyto sanitary conditions also need to be addressed in this connection.

A Brief History of Dairy Development Programmes in India

Government of India has made efforts for strengthening infrastructure for production of quality milk, procurement, processing and marketing of milk and milk products through following Dairy Development Schemes in the recent pasts.

Military Dairy Farms

The earliest attempts at dairy development can be traced back to British rule, when the Defense Department established military dairy farms to ensure the supply of milk and butter to the colonial army.The first of these farms was set up in Allahabad in 1913 and subsequent facilities were established at Bangalore, Ootacamund and Karnal. These farms were well maintained and even in early stages, high quality milch animals were raised. But it failed to supply milk to urban consumers and it catered to only the needs of the military personnel.

The Royal Commission on Agriculture

The first attempt to conceive a set of policies for livestock development in India was the Royal Commission on Agriculture (1928). Following the report of the Royal Commission on Agriculture, interest in promoting development of animal husbandry gradually came to focus on ways to increase milk production and to improve the quality of milch cattle. However, in the pre-independence period attempts to improve the quality of the bovine population in the country were limited in scale and geographical coverage.

Key Village Scheme

Key Village Scheme (KVS) was the most important component of the animal husbandry development programmes during the first three Five Year Plans. Initially, its main focus was on increasing the supply of breeding bulls in the country by setting up bull breeding farms in the major cattle tracts. Gradually the KVS was transformed into a more comprehensive programme for general cattle development intended to improve the productivity of cattle by giving simultaneous attention to better feeding, improved breeding, effective disease control measures, scientific management practices and organized marketing facilities. Towards the end of the second plan nearly 600 KVS centres were functioning in the country covering an estimated 6 million cows and she-buffaloes, that is, about 10 per cent of the total stock. However in the absence of stable and remunerative market for milk, production remained more or less stagnant. During the two decades between 1951 and 1970 milk production grew by barely 1 per cent annually while percapita milk availability declined by an equal ratio.

Intensive Cattle Development Project

The perceived failure of the KVS to make significant impact and the shortage of milk in the rapidly growing urban areas led to the formulation of the Intensive Cattle Development Project (ICDP). Its primary purpose was to increase the production of milk to feed public sector dairy plants in the Hinterlands of the main urban centres. Consequently they placed great emphasis on cross-breeding in indigenous cows with exotic dairy breeds and tended to be concentrated in milk shed areas of large cities and towns. Animal health and breed improvement remained common elements in the project. The scheme envisaged provision of all necessary inputs and services simultaneously to milk producers. The ICDP is, thus, distinguished from KVS by the shift of attention to the cross-breeding component and closer link up with dairying and urban milk supply programmes. By 1960, 62 centers were functioning in the country under the ICDP. In areas where ICDP existed, the KVS was merged into the ICDP. In areas where ICDP did not exist, KVS was continued in the original form.

Establishment of Cattle Colonies and Milk Schemes

During 1960s various state governments tried out different strategies to develop dairying, including establishing dairies run by their own departments, setting up cattle colonies in Bombay, Calcutta and Madras. These government projects had extreme difficulties in organizing rural milk procurement and running milk schemes economically, yet none concentrated on creating an organized system for procurement of milk, which was left to contractors and middlemen. Milk's perishable nature and relative scarcity gave the milk vendors leverage, which they used to considerable advantage. This left government -run dairy plants to use large quantities of relatively cheap, commercially imported milk powder, which resulted in a decline in domestic milk production.

AMUL and the Evolution of the Anand Model

AMUL formed the basis for the Anand pattern of dairying, referring to its origin in Anand District, in the state of Gujarat. Under the Anand pattern structure individual farmers are joined in village level dairy co-operative societies which are joined to form district level unions which, in turn, are joined in state level marketing federations. In each state the Anand Pattern has the following features:

a. Decentralised milk production by the small milk producers

b. Milk procurement by the village level dairy co-operative societies.

c. Centralized milk processing by the district-level unions.

d. Marketing of milk and milk products by the state level federation.

The primary milk producers democratically govern this entire federal co-operative structure to ensure that higher-tier organizations serve the purpose of the lower levels and that the gains at all levels go back to the milk producers in significant measure. The core feature of the Anand pattern model is farmer control of the three stages following production, that is, procurement, processing and marketing of milk and milk products.

Emphasis on Cross-Breeding Strategy

The Board of Agriculture and Animal Husbandry Wing of the Government of India, in 1958, and the expert committee appointed to evaluate the KVS, in 1959, have recommended a shift of policy to the cross-breeding of indigeneous non-descript cattle with exotic stock for rapid increase in milk production. Though the Third Five Year Plan referred to the need to evolve better dual-purpose breed for increasing the work capacity and milk production potential of the Indian cattle, its programmes gave high priority to cross-breeding for increased milk production. Such a shift of policy was the need of the time to meet the increasing demand of milk in the urban and sub-urban centres of the country.

National Dairy Development Board (NDDB)

It was constituted by the Ministry of Agriculture and Irrigation, under the Societies Registration Act, in 1965. Its headquarters were established at Anand.

During its initial stages NDDB was assisted financially by the Government of India, the Danish Government and by AMUL. In 1969, NDDB formulated an integrated dairy development programme under Dr. Varghese Kurien, its founding Chairman. It was accepted by Government of India in 1970 and it functioned as a corner stone for the Operation Flood I.

Indian Dairy Corporation (IDC)

In 1970 the Government of India established a public sector company, the Indian Dairy Corporation (IDC). It functioned as a finance and promotion link for the Phase I programme of NDDB. The IDC was given responsibility for receiving the project's donated commodities, testing their quality, their storage and transfer to user dairies and receiving the dairie's payments.

Dairying in Period of Operation Flood (1970-1996)

Government of India launched a massive dairy development programme popularly known as Operation Flood (OF) from 1970 to 1996. The programme was initially started with the help of the World Food Programme (WFP) and later continued with diary commodity assistance from the European Economic Community (EEC) and a soft loan / credit from the World Bank. The OF programme established milk producers' cooperatives in villages and made modern technology available to them. The broad objectives were to increase milk production ("a flood of milk") , augment rural incomes and transfer to milk producers the profits of milk marketing that were hitherto enjoyed by well-to-do middlemen. This kind of innovative effort has greatly increased milk production and ushered in a "White Revolution", making India the world's largest milk producer.

Implementation of Operation Flood

The programme was implemented in three phases:

Operation Flood I [1970-1981]

Operation Flood II [1981-1985]

Operation Flood III [1987-1996]

Operation Flood I [1970-1981]: Started in 1970, it envisaged certain specific targets:

a. The organization of one crore farmers into 30,000 village cooperatives in virtually all the states of India.

b. Establishing a national bufferstock of skim milk powder and butter oil.

c. The evolution of a national milk grid covering all parts of India and connecting all the major consumption and production centres.

d. dTo help the State Dairy Co-operative Federations to set up processing facilities and to develop the National Milk Herd of one crore improved buffaloes and dairy cattle.

e. To increase the daily per capita consumption of milk from 107 grams in 1970 to 144 grams in 1985.

During its first phase, the project aimed at linking India's 18 best milksheds with the milk markets of the four metropolitan cities of Delhi, Mumbai, Calcutta and Madras. The programme visualized organizing dairy cooperatives at the village level, creating the physical and institutional infrastructure for milk procurement, processing and marketing services at the union level and establishing dairies in Indias major metropolitan centres.

Operation Flood II [1981-1985]

The second phase of the programme was implemented between 1981 and 1985. It was an extension and intensification of the first phase to cover more cities and districts in India. Both in terms of the financial outlay involved [Rs. 4800 million] and of the geographical coverage (160 districts) it was one of the biggest dairy development projects ever undertaken in India by the National Dairy Development Board. The main objectives of the project are:

a. to build up the infrastructure for the development of a growing and self-reliant dairy industry consisting of 10 million rural families of milk producers and a national milch herd of about 14 million crossbred cows and she-buffaloes by middle 1980s;

b. to link up the rural supply sources and urban demand centres (with a population of 150 million) through the establishment of approximate marketing arrangements; and

c. to increase per capita consumption of milk in the national diet.

With Operation Flood II, a self-sustaining system of 43,000 village co-operatives covering 4.25 million milk producers had become a reality. Phase II mainly emphasized to build infrastructure for technical input services and management services. Phase II built on the foundations established by Phase I.

Operation Flood III (1987-1996)

The third phase of the Operation Flood (1987-1996) enabled dairy co-operatives to expand and strengthen the infrastructure required to procure and market increasing volumes of milk. Phase III consolidated India's dairy co-operative movement by adding 69,600 new dairy co-operative societies and thereby covering 90 lakhs milk producer members. These co-operatives form part of the National Milk Grid which today links the milk producers with consumers in more than 799 towns and cities, bridging the gap between the seasonal and regional variation in the availability of milk while at the same time ensuring a remunerative price to the producers and supplying quality milk and milk products to the consumers. For the five years ending March, 2003, the average milk procurement by dairy co-operatives grew at 7.3 per cent whereas the marketing of milk by co-operatives grew at 3.2 per cent. Phase III gave increased emphasis to research and development in animal health and animal nutrition. Innovations like vaccine for Theileriosis, bypass protein feed and urea-molasses mineral blocks, all contributed to the enhanced productivity of milch animals.

Introduction of Milk and Milk Products Order

The Government introduced the Milk and Milk Products Order (MMPO) in 1992 under the essential commodities act of 1955 to regulate the production of milk and dairy products. The order required permission from State/Central registration authorities to set up units handling more than 10,000 litres of milk per day or milk solids upto 500 tons per annum, depending on the capacity of the plant. The order included sanitary and hygienic regulations to ensure product quality. However, concerns were raised about these government controls and licencing requirements for restricting large Indian and multinational firms from making significant investments in this sector. The government, therefore, amended the MMPO in March, 2002, and restrictions on setting up milk processing and milk product manufacturing plants were removed and the concept of milkshed was abolished. This amendment is expected to facilitate the entry of large companies, which would definitely increase competition in the domestic markets.

Uruguay Round Agreement on Agriculture

The second major development in Indian dairy sector policy came when India signed the Uruguay Round Agreement on Agriculture (URAA) in 1994 and became a member of the World Trade Organization (WTO), which made India open up its dairy sector to world markets. The import and export of dairy products were delicenced and decanalized and trade in dairy products was allowed freely with certain inspection requirements. The first major step was taken in 1994-95, when the import of skim milk powder and butter oil were decanlized. Restrictions on the remaining products were removed in April 2002. Now India has bound its import tariffs for dairy products at low levels according to the Uruguay Round decisions.

Strengthening Co-Operative Business

Perspective 2010 aims to recruit, train and motivate increasing number of women to work for co-operatives, to achieve significant improvements in dairy husbandry, as they primarily shoulder animal husbandry related responsibilities in rural India. It visualizes the consolidation and growth in milk and milk product marketing, promoting better equity for regional co-operative brands and developing qualified and skilled manpower. It also aims to persuade the State and Central Governments to remove the shackles on cooperative laws so that co-operatives can compete on equal terms with other forms of enterprise. Expanding the market is a major target of perspective 2010. It offers financial and technical help to milk unions and federations in areas such as sales promotion, consumer education, infrastructure development etc. As part of sales promotion it recommends standardization of artwork, colour, logo and retail outlet design across regional co-operative brands with a view to promote better recall by consumers under a common mnemonic umbrella. Another target is increasing women membership in dairy co-operatives to 50 per cent and improving women participation in the governance of dairy co-operatives at all levels.

Production Enhancement

Perspective 2010 stresses to improve the production potential of indigenous breeds of cattle such as Sahiwal, Gir, Rathi and Kankrej and breeds of buffalo such as Murrah, Mehsana and Jaffarbadi through appropriate selection programme. It gives proper direction to crossbreeding technology to increase production in such a way that crossing of non-descript cattle with Holestein Friesian in areas with adequate feed and fodder and with Jersey in resource poor areas. As a step to increase production and availability of fodder, it appeals to unions, NGOs and co-operatives to put common property area under improved pasture and fodder tree. It promotes first aid coverage through village level societies and disease Free Zones in the country.

Quality Assurance Programmes

As part of increasing quality it facilitates improvement of hygiene, sanitation, food safety and operating efficiency in the dairy plants and sensitize dairy personnel to product quality aspects as per international standards. It promotes encouragement of quality incentives supported by educational programmes for dairy co-operative society staff, transporters and farmer producers. Quality is assured through facilitating dairy co-operatives in ISO 9000-2000 (Quality Management Systems), ISO HACCP (Safety Management Systems) certification and maintain the required plant conditions under the accreditation on a sustainable basis.

Information and Development Research

'Perspective 2010' plans to link large Co-operatives, Unions, Federations and NDDB in a national network that collects and disseminates information to all. It ensures the availability of analytical information for policy planning and implementation. The integrated dairy industry information service facilitates decision making at various levels in co-operative institutions with the help of an extensive on-line computer network that analyses relevant data obtained from Dairy Co-operative Societies, District Milk Producers' Union, State Milk Marketing Federations, NDDB and research institutions.

Perspective 2010 also proposes the need of a National Database that generates data on milk supply (producer, animal and village data) data on milk and milk product demand (consumer and urban data) performance data (societies, unions and federations) and secondary data (domestic and international).

Role of Modern Management

Management of Diary

The scheme for diary, farming should include information on land, livestock markets, availability of water, feeds, fodders, veterinary aid, breeding facilities, marketing aspects, training facilities, experience of the farmer and the type of assistance available from State Government, dairy society/union/federation.

(A) Technical Feasibility – This Would Briefly Include

1. Nearness of the selected area to veterinary, breeding and milk collection centre and the financing bank's branch.
2. Availability of good quality animals in nearby livestock market.
3. Availability of training facilities.
4. Availability of good grazing ground/lands.
5. Green/dry fodder, concentrate feed, medicines etc.
6. Availability of veterinary aid/breeding centres and milk marketing facilities near the scheme area.

(B) Economic Viability – This Would Briefly Include

1. Cost of for feeds and fodders, veterinary aid, breeding of animals, insurance, labour and other overheads.
2. Output costs i.e. sale price of milk, manure, gunny hags, male/female calves, other miscellaneous items etc.

Modern and well established scientific principles, practices and skills should be used to obtain maximum economic benefits from dairy farming.

Reducing Preweaning Mortality

A nutritional intervention for decreasing mortality in young livestock would include the use of colostrum for neonates. Colostrum contains high levels of energy and nutritionally important proteins, and neonates depend on the early infusion of nutrients to maintain body temperature because their energy stores are low at birth.

Improving Grass Forage

Many forage-fed animals in the tropics grow slowly and produce small amounts of milk because their diets are inadequate in protein, energy, and micronutrients. The types of forage available to the animals are mainly the C4 grasses (so named for the metabolic pathway used to fix carbon dioxide). The C4 grasses that predominate in the tropics are less digestible than temperate C3 grasses and have low energy and protein content. Until recently, there was little work on characterization of forage traits that need improvement, and temperate forage still receives far more attention than that grown in the tropics (Spangenberg, 2005; Smith et al., 2007). In general, tropical forage plants have received little attention from plant breeders with a few notable exceptions: alfalfa, which is grown in some tropical highlands; *Brachiaria* spp.; *Pennisetum purpureum* (elephant or Napier grass); and *Panicum maximum* (Guinea, colonial, or Tanganyika grass (Jank et al., 2005). The collections of germplasm of tropical forage are poorly funded, and loss of current accessions is threatened. The collections include diverse accessions that may be important sources of disease resistance, increase in digestibility, or increase in biomass production. For example, the most recent outbreak of a smut (*Ustilago kamerunensis*) is affecting Napier grass. In much of eastern and southern Africa, farmers rely heavily on Napier grass because it produces copious amounts of reasonably high-quality forage. The smut has the potential to affect the small-holder dairy industry seriously and has already reduced forage yields in much of the Kenyan highlands (Farrell et al., 2002; Mwendia et al., 2007). Research to understand smut biology and to develop resistant strains of Napier grass is important for the rapidly growing dairy industry in the Kenyan highlands. A better understanding of plant chemistry and lignin synthesis could help plant breeding programs to improve the nutritional value of forage because the lignin cross-linkages affect whether plants are easily digested (Spangenberg, 2005). There may be advantages in attaching work on this problem to the burgeoning international interest in biofuels, such as switchgrass. There is a common interest in understanding how lignin cross-linkages can be broken down, whether in the context of biofuels or with respect to the processes occurring in forage digestion by ruminants.

Improving Legume Forage

In temperate areas, legumes, especially alfalfa and clover, are high protein, highly digestible forage that permit cows to sustain milk production as high as 20 kg/day on forage alone. In the tropics, however, many promising legume species contain high concentrations of anti-nutritional factors (such as proanthocyanidins, hydrolyzable tannins, alkaloids, and terpenoids) that confer disease resistance on the plants. Condensed tannins have both beneficial and deleterious effects on domestic animals (Mueller-Harvey, 2006). The adverse effects of consuming high-tannin forage include lower feed intake, lower protein and dry matter digestibility, inhibition of microbial and mammalian enzymes, reduced live weight gain and milk yield, and systemic effects that are due to absorption of phenolics and are sometimes offset by lower urinary nitrogen loss, greater parasite resistance, and improved efficiency of nutrient use (Mueller-Harvey, 2006). The apparently contradictory research results are due largely to the heterogeneity of tannin structures and to variation in the quantities ingested. Achieving the goal of developing disease resistant legumes that provide animals with needed nutrients requires research on tannin chemistry linked to legume breeding programs. Progress has been made in understanding some aspects of tannin synthesis, but the polymerization process that affects tannin chemistry and anti-nutritive effects remains poorly understood (Xie and Dixon, 2005).

Evolving Technologies

Improving Animal Germplasm

Since the beginning of domestication of animals, substantial progress has been made in improving their characteristics as food and fiber producers by selectively mating individual animals that had advantageous traits (phenotypes). The importance of phenotypic information is sometimes lost in this age of genomics, and it is astonishing to recognize that animal breeders could triple average milk yield of dairy cattle in 50 years without knowing a single gene involved or having any genome sequence information to guide them. They simply needed to know the milk production traits of members of the dairy cattle family and select the right mates to breed.

Although it is possible to practice breeding of that type on a farm or village scale, small-herd owners in SSA and SA are likely to have difficulty in systematically improving the genetic potential of their livestock by using only locally available germplasm. Nor can small-holders apply modern quantitative breeding practices on the basis of the knowledge of genotypic associations with specific traits; information systems to collect phenotypic and genotypic data from populations of the desired species or breeds systematically have not been put into place.

The use of quantitative phenotypic methods to improve breeding requires collecting data on a large number of animals in a family that exhibit wide variation in the traits of interest. That kind of effort typically takes place in breeding centers, where resource populations of animals can be developed over a decade or two and individual phenotypes can be collected and recorded to make it possible to identify genetically superior animals (Meuwissen and Goddard, 2000, 2001). Infrastructure is needed to distribute the germplasm to farmers through artificial insemination and embryo transfer techniques. In industrialized countries, that approach has been used over the last 50 years to develop animals with superior genetics, and it is the model used in developing countries, often successfully. However, the scientific community is now in a position to bypass many of the heavily resource-dependent approaches used in the industrialized world. Emerging technologies offer potentially practical approaches for more rapidly discovering superior livestock genetics and delivering them to subsistence farmers in SSA and SA.

Leapfrogging Selective Breeding with Molecular Sampling: DNA-Derived Pedigrees

The buffalo is a primary source of milk protein and is used for draught and as a supplementary source of meat in parts of Asia.Ten major breeds exist in India, some having been selected and maintained for each of the three functions, which are essential to the farm economy. National programs to improve milk and meat production have been initiated and are being termed the "white" and "red" revolutions, respectively, in keeping with the name of the Green Revolution.

Genetic improvement for production traits and disease resistance in buffalo does not benefit from the availability of the powerful genomic tools recently generated for domestic cattle in the United States, for two mainreasons: the areas of the world where buffalo are economically important lack the financial resources for genomic research, and the application of genomic research to identify genetically meritorious individual animals can be applied only within families of animals. There is no such information on *Bubalus bubalis*, the Asian water buffalo, or on any farm animals (such as goats and hair sheep) raised by subsistence farmers in SSA and SA, so the use of well-established quantitative genetic tools is precluded. However, it may be possible to construct an equivalent dataset from the bottom up with the aid of molecular genetic tools. To implement that approach, a reference genome of the breed of interest would need to be generated with DNA sequencing, and DNA samples and phenotypic data would have to be collected from several thousand animals in geographic regions that have common environmental stresses. Single nucleotide polymorphisms (SNPs) would be generated from the DNA samples by sequencing regions of the genome that have proved to be informative in related species. The database of tag SNPs generated from the sequencing data would be aligned with the reference sequence to build family pedigrees. With pedigrees in hand, traditional quantitative tools could be applied to identify animals of superior genetic merit. The approach requires several lines of research. An inexpensive field kit for preserving DNA in tissue samples (ear snips, buccal swabs, or the equivalent) that does not require refrigeration would have to be developed, as would an effective questionnaire for gathering trait phenotypes. Whole genome sequencing (6X coverage) of *Bubalis Bubalis*, the African buffalo (*Syncerus caffer*), *Bos indicus* cattle, sheep, and at least a few representative milk- and meat-producing breeds of goats and sheep should be included in the sequencing project. Finally, substantial investment in developing informatics algorithms for what is essentially reverse engineering of pedigrees from SNP data would be needed. With today's sequencing capability, it might take 2 years to generate a reference genome sequence for a species. It might take a year each to develop a DNA tissue-sample preservation kit and a phenotype questionnaire, 3 to 5 years to collect DNA samples and phenotypic data, and a year to build pedigrees and test the hypothesis that animals of high genetic merit can be identified with this approach. All the steps except the last can be conducted in parallel, the overall timeframe of the project to reach proof of concept would be 6 to 10 years. If the project were successful, its impact would be large. DNA-enabled approaches to building a pedigree would leapfrog existing approaches by eliminating the decades of breeding needed to create resource populations, the usual starting point of contemporary genetic-genomic analyses. The substantial costs of housing and feeding such a population would be eliminated. Most important, it would provide a tool to identify genetically superior animals without having to develop the enormous infrastructure currently used in the developed world.

Genetic Engineering

For the first 8 to 10 millennia since animal domestication began, selective breeding has been the method by which desirable phenotypes were enriched in a population. The dramatic diversity generated in dog breeds and improvement in the efficiency of producing dairy cattle are just two examples of the power of selective breeding (Weller, 1994; Pennisi, 2007). However, the approach has limitations, of which the largest is the inability to introduce a trait if genetic information on the trait does not exist in the species of interest. For example, endowing swine with the ability to synthesize lysine *de novo*, which would eliminate the need to supplement feed with what is now an essential amino acid, is impossible because the biochemical pathway does not exist in any breed of swine. The pathway does exist in bacteria and yeast, but that is of no use to the animal breeder. Furthermore, selective breeding lacks precision. There are many examples of selecting for one important economic trait at the expense of another, such as sacrificing the reproductive performance of dairy cattle for increased milk production (Wicks and Leaver, 2004). But, as previously described, the most serious constraint in applying modern tools of genetic selection is the time needed to build resource populations and harvest the phenotypic information needed to populate the genetic algorithms for each breed of interest. In 1981, a new method for altering the genetic makeup of mammalian offspring led to the ability to place genes from one species (transgenes) into the genome of another (Gordon and Ruddle, 1981). Transgenes can encode completely novel natural or synthetic information, modulate the level of gene expression, or switch transcription on or off conditionally or permanently (Niemann and Kues, 2007). In the last 2 decades, genetically engineered cattle, chickens, goats, pigs, rabbits, and sheep have been produced (Hammer et al., 1985; Salter *et al.*, 1987; Bondioli et al., 1991; Ebert et al., 1991; Krimpenfort *et al.*, 1991). Transgenic livestock applications have been diverse and range from projects focused on animal well (Wall *et al.*, 2005) to drug manufacturing (Edmunds *et al.*, 1998). Transgenic animal technology has now advanced to the point where specific genetic information can be introduced precisely into any desired location of the genome (Richt *et al.*, 2007). In theory, the technology provides a vast array of new ways to address challenges in animal agriculture.

Engineering Animals for Disease Resistance

Transgenic technology can be used in many ways to reduce susceptibility to disease in animals. It can be directed at a specific pathogen or a wide variety of pathogens, depending on the protein encoded by the transgene. There are dozens of examples of successful application of genetic engineering to protect mice, and many are expected to be predictive of outcomes of transgenic livestock experiments. However, to date there is only one example of genetic engineering that has protected a livestock species from disease (Wall *et al.*, 2005). In general, a transgenic strategy for disease resistance involves identifying an anti-pathogenic protein to be expressed in the animal and determining in which tissue and at what developmental stage expression should occur. The transgenic protein should cause no harm to the animal itself or to the consumer that eats it. If possible, the transgene product should avoid interfering with endogenous homeostatic feedback loops. The recombinant protein produced should be benign to the environment. Finally, a plan should be devised to prevent the target pathogen from developing resistance to the transgene product.

RNA Interference

RNA interference (RNAi), is an evolutionarily conserved mechanism of plants and animals that processes microRNA (miRNA) and destroys double-stranded RNA, targeting, in a sequence-specific manner, both messenger RNA and retroviral genomes (Hannon, 2002; McCaffrey *et al.*, 2002). Theoretically, it should be possible to target any virus with this mechanism. Retroviruses, with their RNA genomes, are an obvious potential target but DNA viruses could be targeted if their provirus encodes a unique mRNA that could serve as a target. The RNAi approach to targeting HIV-1 infection has been demonstrated in cell-culture studies (Anderson and Akkina, 2005). And RNAi approaches have been devised to inhibit viral evolution of resistance (Anderson *et al.*,2007). The idea of using RNAi as a viral therapeutic is not new but has not been fully explored, possibly because of a number of potential hurdles (Silva *et al.*, 2002) and because the focus has been on using the technology in basic research (Hannon and Rossi, 2004; Silva *et al.*, 2005). But it is clear that targeting gene expression can be achieved with this approach in mammals (Kunath et al., 2003; Dann et al., 2006), and RNAi has recently been shown to work against influenza virus in mice (Zhou *et al.*, 2007).

Germ Cell Distribution

No matter how the genetics of indigenous farm animals are improved, there needs to be a means of distributing the improved genetics to farmers. Whether by quantitative genetics (selective breeding) or transgenic technology, the germplasm of the lineage progenitors will be produced at a hightechnology center that resembles a modern-day artificial insemination (AI) stud farm. A distribution system must be in place to allow farmers access to the superior genetic material; the lack of a distribution system seriously constrains the improvement of the genetic potential of subsistence farmers' livestock. Since the 1950s, genetic improvement of the livestock herds in industrialized nations has been achieved primarily by distributing gametes (spermatozoa) from outstanding sires and more recently by distributing embryos from meritorious females (Hasler, 1992; Foote, 1998; Thibier, 2005). As currently practiced, AI and embryo transfer (ET) require a ready supply of inexpensive liquid nitrogen. Liquid nitrogen must be available during the initial gamete- or embryo-freezing process and thereafter as a storage medium. On-farm storage dewars require replenishment (commonly every 4 to 6 weeks) that depends on use and environmental temperature. Furthermore, the use of preserved spermatozoa or embryos requires a specific knowledge of female reproductive physiology and highly skilled and practiced people to transfer the gametes or embryos into the recipient females. Even in developed countries, AI and ET are practiced mainly in intensively managed livestock operations, such as medium to large dairy, swine, and poultry farms. Less intensively managed enterprises, such as beef-cow and -calf operations or small farms, do not use these reproductive strategies, primarily because of the cost of estrous cycle management, the lack of availability of skilled AI technicians, and the low return on investment. Attempts have been made to eliminate the dependence on liquid nitrogen for preservation of gametes. At first, freeze-dried spermatozoa were not very successful (Norman *et al.*, 1958; Foote *et al.*, 1962; Wakayama and Yanagimachi, 1998). Recent refinements in freeze-drying protocols have resulted in live-born mice from spermatozoa stored for over a year at 4°C (Bhowmick et al., 2002; Ward et al., 2003; McGinnis et al., 2005). Such freeze-dried spermatozoa are not viable in the traditional sense, but viable offspring can be produced by injection of their nuclei into an oocyte (intracytoplasmic sperm injection, ICSI). Storage at –20°C or –80°C improves the success rate of ICSI over storage at 4°C (Li *et al.*, 2007). Most recent attempts to adapt this technology to a non-rodent species have been unsuccessful (Meyers, 2006; Nakai *et al.*, 2007). Modern cryobiology may eventually develop room-temperature storage methods that will preserve the genome of gametes. But it is also likely that any such technique will require some highly sophisticated method, such as ICSI, to introduce the stored genetics into a living organism. Such an approach would be impractical for production of breeding stock.

Spermatogonial Stem Cell Transplantation

The use of an emerging technology called spermatogonial stem cell (SSC) transplantation may be able to overcome the infrastructure and technical skill deficiencies that will inhibit subsistence farmers from taking of meritorious germplasm when it is available. SSC transplantation (also known as male germ-cell transplantation or germline stem cell transplantation) involves transplanting self-renewing male germ-cell stem cells from one male to another. The recipient male becomes the mechanism for spreading the genetics through a herd. In the early 1990s, it was demonstrated that the stem cells that give rise to spermatozoa in a male mouse could colonize the testes of another mouse, and the recipient mouse could sire offspring with the donor-derived spermatozoa (Brinster and Avarbock, 1994; Brinster and Zimmermann, 1994). The SSCs can also be frozen and stored at –196°C and, on thawing, be used to colonize a recipient's testes after transplantation (Avarbock *et al.*, 1996). The technique also works in rats (Ryu *et al.*, 2007), and it has been shown that it can be used to restore fertility in two mouse models of infertility (Ogawa *et al.*, 2000). Most relevant here are reports that demonstrate the potential of applying the technology to livestock. SSCs isolated from immature pig testes have been transplanted (Honaramooz *et al.*, 2002), and the transplanted spermatogonia remained in the seminiferous tubules of the recipients for at least a month; somewhat surprisingly, not only did SSCs colonize the seminiferous tubules and generate spermatozoa capable of siring offspring, but this was possible in recipients unrelated to the host. Several studies also demonstrated the feasibility of the approach in goats (Honaramooz *et al.*, 2003; Honaramooz *et al.*, 2007). One attempt has been made to demonstrate its efficacy in cattle: testicular cells were isolated from *Bos taurus* bull calves and transferred, after fluorescent staining, into *Bos indicus* prepubertal recipient calves (Herrid *et al.*, 2006); *Bos taurus* fluorescently labeled cells were found in the testes of recipients up to 6 months after transfer. It is envisioned that once this technology has been refined and adapted to local breeds, SSCs harvested from males with superior genetic merit will be distributed to males of average genetic merit but good libido. The recipient males, harboring the "good genetics," could then be distributed to farmers. Alternatively, because the transplantation procedure can be performed in the field, the SSCs from genetically superior males could be frozen, transported to farms (or villages), and transplanted into farmers' (villages') own breeding males by someone skilled in the surgical procedure. The main constraint limiting the technology is the acquisition of enough SSCs. It is possible on rare occasions to harvest enough SSCs from a donor to distribute to four recipients (Ina Dobrinski, University of Pennsylvania, presentation to the committee, October 15, 2007). Protocols are needed for multiplying SSCs in culture so that dozens, if not hundreds, of males can be serviced by a single genetically superior donor. In addition to a propagation system, there is a need for more efficient SSC-enrichment methods. Finally, methods to improve the ability of the newly acquired SSCs to dominate the testes of the recipient will need to be devised. The current literature on this new procedure is not vast, but there are enough examples to suggest that SSC transplantation should be applicable in a wide array of species. It will be necessary to confirm that SSC transplantation can be implemented in the breeds and species of interest in SSA and SA and, if so, that it can be optimized for each species.

Improving Animal Health

Improving the health of animals can have a substantial impact on the livelihood of farmers, especially subsistence farmers that rely on animals for labor, food, and additional income. Some of the ways to improve animal health discussed below include fortification of neonatal passive immunity, development of animal vaccines for diseases affecting SSA and SA, and use of animal disease surveillance. Not explored by the committee are the development of novel drugs and drug delivery strategies for animal disease infections in SSA and SA, two areas in which innovations have been lacking.

Neonatal Passive Immunity

In Kenya, calf mortality after weaning ranges from 6 to 70 percent, depending on health and nutritional management (Homewood et al., 2006; Lanyasunya *et al.*, 2006). Almost all the primary causes of high preweaning mortality-including failure to ensure that the young receive colostrums within 6 hours of birth, respiratory diseases, diarrhea, and inadequacy of maternal milk production can be substantially reduced with currently available, low-cost management interventions. These include giving young animals the same salt- and sugar-based rehydration solutions made with clean water as are given to children who have diarrhea. The application of existing knowledge to raising calves, lambs, and kids could reduce mortality to below 9 percent, a commonly accepted target, and improve animal productivity and profitability. Technologies are used to enhance colostrum quality by vaccinating pregnant dams. Also, the preparation and preservation (freeze-drying) of serum antibody extracts are used as artificial colostrums substitutes. There are some truly nutritional interventions to prevent preweaning mortality, such as enhancing the nutrition of the lactating dam and providing nutritional supplements to the diets of lactating animals. The issue of access to veterinary services by the poor in SSA and SA is critical. The delivery of appropriate medicines and information on livestock health has been compromised by privatization of veterinary services in many countries. Now only those able to pay have access to veterinary services, so livestock productivity is low and the risk of outbreaks of zoonotic and other diseases is high. Very simple interventions in providing education, medicines, and vaccines could have a major impact in protecting the health and productivity of animal populations in SSA and SA. Reversing the situation would make meeting the projected increased demand for meat products more feasible without large increases in the number of breeding females.

Animal Vaccine Development

Disease is a major constraint on livestock productivity in developing Countries. Infact, when the committee asked several experts what could have a major effect on improving the life of poor farmers, they noted that effective vaccines already exist to prevent globally endemic disease, such as brucellosis,leptospirosis, and bovine virus diarrhea (Hans Draayer and Raja Krishnan, Pfizer Animal Health, presentation to committee, September 24, 2007). However, some factors that affect the use of current vaccines in SSA and SA include strain variations, costs of vaccines, and the need to have an effective cold-chain for transportation, marketing, distribution, and delivery to the animals in the field. Technologies to develop thermostable vaccines, such as the development of a thermostable attenuated vaccine for Newcastle disease in chickens in Australia and Malaysia, can compensate for the lack of a cold-chain. A focus on infections for which vaccines exist and on others that cause respiratory and intestinal diseases in young, preweaned animals could reduce mortality and improve productivity. The other two categories of opportunity identified by experts the committee consulted were zoonotic diseases, particularly those associated with foodborne illness, and endemic infections peculiar to SSA and SA (Guy Palmer, Washington State University, and Roy Curtiss, Arizona State University, presentation to committee, September 24, 2007). SSA and SA are home to the most severe vector-borne diseases, including trypanosomiasis, babesiosis, and theileriosis (the last two of which are parasitic diseases spread by ticks). Diseases, such as trypanosomiasis, have been the subject of vaccine investigations for many years and have thwarted vaccine effectiveness because of the great variability of surface proteins of the parasite, which the organism is able to "switch" under the pressure of the host immune system. The greatest challenge for these vaccines is the discovery of antigens that will result in a protective immune response in the host. Such a discovery will be assisted by the complete genome sequences that have been completed for all six major vector-borne pathogens in the last 2 years, including *Anaplasma marginale, Babesia bovis, Ehrlichia ruminantium, Theileria parva, T. annulata,* and *Trypanosoma bruci*. For example, it is known that immunity to East Coast fever, caused by the tick-borne parasite *T. parva*, can be created by inoculating a host with sporozoites of the parasite in conjunction with long-acting oxytetracycline. However, until the *T. parva* genome was available, the antigens involved in the immune response were unknown. Using gene prediction methods, investigators were able to identify candidate genes in the genome that were associated with a secretion signal on the basis of the idea that secreted proteins would be the first to become associated with the host major histocompatibility complex apparatus. Screening of the protein products of those genes narrowed the search to the ones involved in establishing immunity and paved the way to future vaccine development (Graham *et al.*, 2006). Zoonotic diseases were suggested as targets for disease control because of their implications for limiting the spread of diseases to humans and back to animals. Effective vaccines exist for some of the diseases, including brucellosis, salmonellosis, and listeriosis; but problems related to supply, cost, and delivery mechanisms slow their widespread use.

DNA Vaccines

DNA vaccination stimulates the immune response by introducing into the host naked DNA that codes for antigens of a pathogen. The protein synthesis machinery of the host cell expresses the antigen and stimulates a response by the host's immune system. In theory, DNA vaccines can be manufactured far more easily and less expensively than vaccines composed of inactivated pathogens, protein subunits, or recombinant proteins. Other potential advantages include stability, resistance to extreme temperatures, efficacy as an oral vaccine, and the ability to introduce multiple antigens (Mwangi *et al.*, 2007). However, substantial development is needed before DNA vaccines become an alternative to conventional methods. Most of the experimental DNA vaccines have not shown as great protective immunity as conventional vaccines, but new technologies, such as the coating of colloidal gold with DNA, that are in development could improve effectiveness. If future research can deliver a DNA vaccine that offers protective immunization, this approach would add flexibility to the custom designing of vaccines for regional needs. For instance, it is easier to change the sequence of an antigenic protein or to add heterologous epitopes. The protective immunity of the expressed protein can be easily evaluated after the DNA is injected into a model animal, such as the mouse. This simple, elegant method could quickly allow researchers to learn about the effectiveness of candidate antigens. The final goal of effective DNA vaccines is considered to be far in the future because of the many unresolved problems,but the potential high payoff will continue to draw investment.

Animal Disease Surveillance

It is pointless to develop and deliver drugs and vaccines without knowing which syndromes are present in a region, because protecting an animal against one pathogen only to have it succumb to another will not reduce the burden of disease on a small-holder farmer. Developing a database of such information will require field research, trained technicians, and diagnostics. The relatively new World Animal Health Information Database managed by the World Organization for Animal Health (OIE) is a significant database that tracks disease prevalence in all regions of the world. In cooperation with the Food and Agriculture Organization of the United Nations (FAO), the OIE is investigating disease rumors that surface on ProMED or other non-scientific sources of information; these early warning systems serve as good alert systems for emerging disease outbreaks. The use of satellite-based remote sensing technologies could be useful as early warning systems for the emergence of serious infectious diseases, particularly those that are transmitted by arthropods. The FAO's Emergency Prevention System (EMPRES) for Transboundary Animal and Plant Pests and Diseases program currently uses remote sensing technologies to determine the Normalized Difference Vegetation Index (NDVI), and the use of such data has led to the successful advanced prediction of Rift Valley fever outbreaks (FAO, 2008). Similar technologies have been used for the advanced notification of blooms of desert locus and of outbreaks of Venezuelan Equine Encephalomyelitis (FAO, 2008). Inexpensive diagnostic tests, like that developed for rinderpest (Yilma, 1989; Ismall et al., 1994), are needed for disease detection and vaccination campaigns. Other similar rapid pen-side tests for the recognition of infectious diseases have been developed and are in use, such as the field diagnosis of human and avian influenza outbreaks. Increasing in greater numbers are the development, validation, and deployment of rapid RT-PCR technologies for accurate diagnosis of a variety of diseases affecting SSA and SA. These tests require only a nasal swab as a sample and are not sensitive to the effect of higher temperatures in the transportation to diagnostic laboratories. Furthermore, emerging technologies, such as biosensors are promising because of their sensitivity, speed, portability, and ease of use and could be developed for a variety of surveillance efforts and especially useful in resource-constrained countries in SSA and SA. Moreover, if farmers have tools to detect the presence of disease, they are more likely to seek out a drug or vaccine. Farmers' confidence in medical treatment and vaccination depends on their seeing a benefit, which they will not if a problem is not solved by a drug or vaccine that targets a single pathogen.

Conclusions

The sustainability prospects for livestock farming remain depressing unless the main stream perceptions about the problems are not changed. The development strategies are essential for formulating farmer responsive plans, giving due consideration to the nature of marginality, fragility, diversity and niches of each area. It will help to ameliorate the impact of the marginalization of livestock farmers and in achieving social equity by building on the comparative advantages of key land resources.

Transforming Rural Areas through Veterinary Science *Pages* ***309-322***
Editor: Dipanjali Konwar, Shilpa Sood & Shahid Ahamad
Published by: **ASTRAL INTERNATIONAL PVT. LTD., NEW DELHI**

24 Constraints and Strategies for Mutton & Wool Production in Hilly and Kandi areas of Jammu & Kashmir

Dr. Surinder K.Gupta & Dr. Suraj Amrutkar

Introduction

Sheep farming is the traditional business and occupation of the people of Jammu & Kashmir state. Sheep is a domestic animal from the ancient time. Sheep farming means, rearing of sheep commercially for the purpose of meat, milk and wool production. Although sheep farming is not a good decision for commercial milk production but sheep are suitable for meat and wool production. Commercial sheep farming business is very profitable and get investment back within a short period. Sheep meat from adults is often called mutton. Sheep meat is the most commonly consumed red meat in the world. Livestock sector is emerging sector which influence the state economy. The economy of Jammu and Kashmir is still agriculture dependent and is the main occupation of majority of the rural people who earn their livelihood from it.

Present Status of Sheep in India

As per 19th Livestock census (2012), livestock sector of India's is one of the largest in the world with a holding of 11.6% of world livestock population which consist sheep (7.14%) population. The contribution of sheep in total livestock population in India is 12.71%. India has 3rd rank in sheep population. The total population of sheep in our country is 65.06 million numbers in 2012 which declined by about 9.07% over the 2007 census.

State Wise Sheep Population of India (2012 Census)

Sr. No.	*State*	*Values in thousands*
1	Andhra Pradesh	26396
2	Karnataka	9584
3	Rajasthan	9080
4	Tamilnadu	4787
5	Jammu and Kashmir	3389
6	Maharashtra	2580
7	India	65069

Present Status of Sheep in J & K State

The total sheep population in the Jammu and Kashmir state is 3.38 million numbers. There is 17.87% decrease in number of sheep during the inter censuses period (2007-12). The number of indigenous sheep has decreased from 1.40 million in 2003 to 2.31 million in 2012. The percent changes in number of exotic/crossbred and indigenous sheep are (-5.6%) and (-35.86%), respectively during the inter censuses period (2007-2012). The district of Rajouri has the highest contributors in sheep population with 12.67% in Jammu & Kashmir state. The second and third highest contributors are Kathua and Udhampur with share of sheep population of 9.04% and 7.74%, respectively.

Jammu & Kashmir State Population of Sheep: (Values in Thousands)

Category	*2003*	*2012*	*Percent change from 2007 to 2012*
Exotic/crossbred			
Male	659.00	700.09	717.96
Female	1343.00	1752.69	1597.51
Total Exotic cross bred	2002.00	2452.78	2315.46
Indigenous			
Male	463.00	501.01	319.69
Female 946.00		1173.37	754.33
Total indigenous	1408.00	1674.37	1074.02
Total Sheep	3411.00	4127.15	3389.49

District-Wise Share of Sheep Population

District	*Population %*	*District*	*Population %*
Rajouri	12.67	Ramban	3.55
Kathua	9.04	Punch	3.53
Udhampur	7.74	Kupwara	3.18
Doda	7.29	Kulgam	3.17

District	*Population %*	*District*	*Population %*
Reasi	6.61	Pulwama	2.94
Baramula	5.31	Shupiyan	2.48
Kishtwar	5.24	Leh (Ladakh)	2.40
Badgam	5.23	Jammu	2.32
Anantnag	4.39	Ganderbal	1.65
Kargil	4.39	Srinagar	1.52
Bandipore	4.08	Samba	1.27

Total Population of Sheep in Jammu And Kashmir State in 2003 and 2012

Category	*2007*	*2012*	*% change from 2007 to 2012*
Sheep	4127.15	3389.49	-17.89

Present Status of India in Meat Production

Total meat production including poultry meat was 5.9 million tonnes in 2012-13. Nearly 45% of the production of meat is contributed by poultry alone. Buffalo, goat, pig, sheep and cattle contributes 19, 16, 8, 7 and 5 % of the total meat products, respectively. Uttar Pradesh produces maximum total meat in India followed by Andhra Pradesh, West Bengal, Maharashtra and Tamilnadu. Maximum meat from buffalo and pig are produced by Uttar Pradesh. Andhra Pradesh produces maximum meat from sheep and poultry.

Advantage of Sheep Farming

Sheep are raised mainly for their wool, milk, skin and manure production. Sheep meat is very tasty, nutritious and popular to all types of people throughout the world. Sheep farming business can be a great source of income for eradicating poverty from the barren, desert, semi-arid and mountainous areas. It is also a reliable income source for the people who are engaged with animal farming business.

- No need to have a huge capital for starting a sheep farm
- No need to make an expensive house for sheep
- Require less labour than any other livestock farming business.
- Sheep give birth of kids frequently, so the size of herd will be large within a shorter period.
- Sheep eat different kinds of plants, compared to other kind of livestock animals.
- Sheep can use for cleaning unwanted plants from your garden or field.
- Sheep hardly destroy trees than goats.
- Sheep can survive by consuming low quality grass and turn the feed into meat and wool.
- Sheep products such as wool, meat and milk are used for different purposes.

- ☆ They are very hardy animal, and can adopt themselves with almost all types of environment.
- ☆ Sheep require less space for living; even sheep can rise with other livestock animals.
- ☆ By proper care and management, commercial sheep farming business can be a great source of earning and employment.
- ☆ Unemployed educated young can also a make a good income and employment source through raising sheep commercially.

Problems of Sheep Farming

You can't run any business without any problem; and sheep farming is not an exception in case of sheep farming business. You might face some common problems, such as protecting the sheep from predators, shelter management, protection from the cold weather, and diseases etc. Among those problems, predators and diseases are harming the sheep so much. So make a suitable fence for protecting the sheep from predators. Diseases are also great threat for the sheep. So vaccinate them timely to stay free from various types of diseases.

- ☆ **Problems Relating to Grazing Lands:** The shortage of grazing lands was a pressing problem. Grazing land is gradually shrinking in area of the state. It is due to illegal encroachment of common land by the private parties.
- ☆ **Problems in Marketing of Sheep:** As the rearers are illiterates and ignorant of prices, they were exploited by the middlemen. It was found that nearly all the rearers faced this problem, and had to sell their sheep at unremunerated prices. The buyers had a dominants way in the price fixation, as a result of which the sheep rearers could not obtain better returns.
- ☆ **Seasonal Diseases:** Sheep are exposed to seasonal diseases. There are number of diseases which expose the sheep. One of the most deadly disease affect sheep is "blue tongue disease".
- ☆ **Unusual Rates of Interest Charged by Money Lenders:** In some cases, shepherds borrowed funds from local money lenders at high rate of interest. This is often worked out to be non-economical for the shepherds. At time on demand the money lenders, the borrowed shepherds had to sell away their flocks at low rates to clear of their loans.
- ☆ **Reluctance on the Part of the Bankers in Meeting the Financial Needs of the Sheep Rearers:** Since, the shepherds are illiterates; they are not familiar with the bank transactions. A majority of shepherds did not find access to banks loans.
- ☆ **Thieves' Threat:** Since, flocks have been rested in the open place, thieves find it is easy to steal in the nights.
- ☆ **Absence of Wool Cording Unit:** Most of the places wool cording unit is absent.

- **Superstitious Beliefs:** High rate of illiteracy has been noticed among the shepherds. They are found to be more gullible and superstitious in their outlook.
- **Lack of Awareness About Diseases by the Shepherds:** The veterinary services are found to be inadequate, and staff of the veterinary department could not meet shepherds by way conducting awareness camps to sensitize the shepherds about the probable diseases that would often affect the sheep. Ignorance on a part of shepherds suffered high losses on account of death of entire flocks.
- **Lack of Government Assistance:** Adequate veterinary services have not been made available. It is often reported that the veterinary hospitals most of the times, did not have sufficient medicines.
- **Acute Water Scarcity:** Water is not found in the tanks in summer. Shepherds face acute water scarcity in summer. Hence shepherds tend their sheep to the neighboring district where canal flows.
- **Attack by Wild Animals:** Wild animals such as wolves and dogs attacked on the sheep flock because the flock of sheep is always found grazing, and under resting in the open area.
- **Road And Train Accident:** On either side of railway tract, goat quality fodder available. The rearers tend their flock for grazing purpose on either side of the railway tract. So road and train accident is common.
- **Extent of Adoption of Management Practices:** The practices of recommended management practices in any enterprise will help in increasing the present income levels.

Farm Location

Selecting a suitable location for starting a sheep farm is very important. Consider the essential facilities for raising sheep, while selecting the place.

- A good clean and fresh water source
- Availability of adequate amount of greens
- Good medications
- Suitable transportation
- Proper marketing

Purchase Quality Breeds

Always try to purchase quality breeds from famous farms or breeders. There are numerous sheep breeds available around the world. But all of those breeds are not suitable for farming in all areas. Some breeds are suitable for commercial meat production and some breeds are suitable for wool production. Choose suitable breeds according to desired production purpose. You can also consider your local breeds.

Housing

- ☆ Usually an adult sheep requires about 20 sq.ft. floor space.
- ☆ Keep the roof at least 6 feet high from the floor
- ☆ Make good ventilation system
- ☆ Always try to keep the house clean and dry
- ☆ Ensure flow of sufficient air and light inside the house
- ☆ Make a proper drainage system inside the house.

Floor Space Requirement for Indian Condition

Age groups	*Covered space (sq.m.)*	*Open space (sq.m.)*
Up to 3 months	0.2-0.25	0.4-0.5
3 months to 6 months	0.5-0.75	1.0-1.5
6 months to 12 months	0.75-1.0	1.5-2.0
Adult animals	1.5	3.0
Male, pregnant or lactating ewe	1.5-2.0	3.0-4.0

Feeding and Watering Space Requirement

Type of animal	*Space per animal (cm)*	*Width of manger/ water trough (cm)*	*Depth of manger/ water trough (cm)*	*Height of inner wall of manger /water trough (cm)*
Sheep	40-50	50	30	35
Lamb	30-35	50	20	25

Feeding

Good feeding is must for proper growth and maximum production. High quality feed also helps to keep the animal healthy, productive and disease free. So always try to feed your goat's high quality and nutritious food. Usually all types of grasses, plants and corns are favorite food of sheep. In accordance with providing high quality and nutritious foods always provide your sheep adequate amount of clean and fresh water according to their demand.

Reproductive Characteristics of Ewes

Characteristics	*Average*	*Range*
Age at puberty	5 to 12 months	
Length of estrus cycle (Days)	17	13-19
Duration of estrus (Hrs)	30	18-48
Timing of ovulation	20-30 Hrs after start of estrus	
Gestation (Days)	146-147	138-149

Reproductive Parameters of Sheep

- Breeding age: 6 - 8 months
- Comes heat after lambing: 21 days after
- Length of pregnancy: 147 days (ranges between 144 to 152 days)
- Male female ratio = 1: 20
- Estrus period is repeated every 16-17 days on average in ewes
- The estrus period lasts for about 24-36 hrs in ewes

Estrus Sign of Sheep

- Redden of the vulva and discharge from vulva
- Tail wagging
- Mounting on other animals
- Seeking male
- Frequent bleating
- Push her back
- Standing for mating (standing reflex)

Preparation of Female and Male for Breeding

Flushing

Flushing is feeding of extra concentrate to ewes prior to onset of breeding season, normally 3 or 4 weeks before breeding. This increases the ovulation rate of ewes, so that the number of twins and triplets increase. Flushing can be done by supplementing 250 gm of concentrate daily or 500 gm of good quality legume hay per head per day. Flushing increases the lambing rate by 10-20%.

Eyeing

To prevent wool blindness in some breed, the excess wool around the eye should be clipped away regularly. This process is referred to as eyeing.

Crutching

Removal of wool around the perennial region and base of the tail of the ewe is known as crutching.

Ringing

Before breeding season start, the wools should be completely removed from all over the body of the ram. He should be at least clipped from the neck and from the belly particularly at the region of the penis. This process is referred as ringing. This process makes it easier for the ram to have proper mating.

Care of Pregnant Animals

The pregnant ewes should not be handled frequently. The ewes in advanced stage of pregnancy should be separated from the flock and effective care should be taken in their feeding. Extra feed during the later part of pregnancy (3-4 weeks before parturition) will be beneficial for the condition of the pre-parturient ewes which will help in improving milk production of ewes and birth weight and growth of lambs. Inadequate and poor nutrition in pregnant animals may result in pregnancy toxaemia, abortion and premature birth of weak lambs. Ewes in advance stage of pregnancy should be kept in a separate lambing shed, 4-6 days before parturition and maximum comfort like soft clean bedding and individual lambing pen should be provided. The pregnant ewes should be protected from cold weather condition.

Care During Lambing

After lambing, the ewe naturally licks the lamb. Allow to lick the lambs, which helps in early drying, sensitizing and stimulating the lamb and thereby attracts the new born with motherly instinct towards udder. If ewes are not do, so better remove the membranous attachment from over the face, nostril, eyes, mouth as well as body parts. Apply tincture iodine on the navel after cutting the navel cord 1" below with a new sterilized blade. Do not leave the navel cord in hanging position; it may attract the crows in open causing bleeding injury the navel. Allow the lambs to suckle the mother within 20 minutes of birth so that the lambs get vitamins-A rich colostrum and immunoglobulin essential for the lambs. Give the ewe warm cereal meal to drink. In case of heavy milker, if not sucked by the lamb; she should be milked out soon to extent of relieving her udder pressure. The first 1 to 2 hrs after birth is the vital period for establishment of bond between the new born and the mother. Hence, the ewe should be kept in a calm place without disturbance from stray dogs and other animals.

Sheep Breeds of Jammu and Kashmir:

Favorable agro-climatic conditions and other natural endowments including rich alpine pastures made the sheep and goat rearing as the core activity of rural masses of the Jammu and Kashmir state from the times immemorial to play a vital role in the socio-economic upliftment of the weaker sections of the society viz. Chopans, Gujjars, Gaddies, Changpas and Bakerwals. However, at that time, the economic returns from sheep and goat rearing were non-significant due to low productivity of the available genetic materials. As the developmental activities related to sheep and goat were carried out in the state under the auspices of Animal Husbandry Department, no concrete sheep development programme could be under taken except some cross breeding experiments/trials till 1962, when sheep breeding and developmental department was carved out of Animal Husbandry Department for look after of sheep husbandry sector. The newly formed department of sheep Husbandry right from its inception laid maximum emphasis on cross-breeding programme which resulted in substantial progress in production of wool and mutton.

Breeds Maintained

Besides various fine wool breeds like Australian merino, Russian merino, Russian stevropol; the department has introduced some dual purpose breeds of sheep like Correidale and Polldorset in areas like Sonawari, Shopian and Kulgam to quickly enhance the production of mutton. The Correidale breed has adapted well to the local environment and proved quite popular among the breeders. However, the details of breeds maintained at various farms are given as under:

Farm	*Breed maintained*
Sheep Breeding Farm, Dachigam	Kashmir Merino
Sheep Breeding Farm, Goabal	Kashmir Merino
Sheep Breeding Farm, Kralpathri	Corriedale and Kashmir Merino
Sheep Breeding Farm, Zawoora	Corriedale
Sheep Breeding Farm, Kewa	Corriedale and Polldorset
Sheep Breeding Farm, Daksum	Australlian & Russain Merino crosses

Some of the breeds found in Jammu and Kashmir are given below:

Gurezi

- ☆ **Habitat:** Gurez Tehsil of Kashmir
- ☆ **Wool Yield:** 1250-1500 kg/annum
- ☆ **Wool Quality:** Medium fine about 6 inches long and lacking kemps.
- ☆ **Characteristic:** Gurezi sheep is the biggest among the Kashmir breeds. Animals are coarse woolen dairy animals, usually white and polled. Majority of sheep are hornless. However, recently some animals even with more than two horns (poly-ceros conditions) were observed. These sheep have short ears and wool in predominantly white. However, a number of coloured sheep are also maintained for getting wools of natural shades of grey, black and brown. The animals graze rich grasses at 8000 feet in summer but are stall fed in winter.

Gaddi

- ☆ **Habitat:** Kistwar and Baderwah Tehsils of Jammu and Kulu
- ☆ **Wool Yield:** 0.817 kg/annum
- ☆ **Wool Quality:** Medium fine with average fiber dia-meter 34.90 μ and staple length 10.10 cm. The wool in good sheep is lustrous and under coat is used for manufacture of Kulu shawls and blankets
- ☆ **Characteristic:** Gaddies are hills tribes who are traditional sheep breeders raising this breeds. These sheep are small in size but have sturdy legs with short tails and ears. They live on scrubs forest during winter and in summer they migrate to poddar and other neighboring ranges. The fleece is generally white with brown coloured hair on the face. The rams are horned and ewes hornless.

Kashmir Valley

- **Habitat:** Kashmir Valley at attitude of 5000-6000 ft.
- **Wool Yield:** 0.860 kg per annum
- **Wool Quality:** Admixture of coarse and medium fine with fiber diameter and staple length varying from 28-34 µ and 8-10cm, respectively.
- **Characteristic:** Animals are smaller in size with predominantly coloured fleece yielding an admixture of medium fine and coarse wool. These animals have short tails with males having small horns.

Karnahi

- **Habitat:** Karnah Tehsil at an attitude of 1200-4600 meters.
- **Wool Yield:** 1000-1250 kg/annum
- **Wool Quality:** Medium fine wool having average fiber diameter of 29.70 µ and staple length of 9.36 cm.
- **Characteristic:** The animals are robust, having long face and prominent nose. Rams have big curved horns. The fleece is relatively fine though shorter than that of Guresi, breed of sheep.

Bakerwali

- **Habitat:** Migratory sheep reared by the nomadic tribe called Bakerwals. Their movements include high ranges of Pirpanchal mountains, Kashmir Valley and other low lying Hills of Jammu and Kashmir. Being migratory, these sheep live in open throughout the year.
- **Wool Yield:** 1600 kg/annum
- **Wool Quality:** Coarse wool is 6 inches long
- **Characteristic:** These sheep are hardy and sturdy and are excellent climber in-spite of its big bulk. The males are generally horned and ewes hornless. Some flocks are fat tailed. Ears are generally long, broad and dropping. These sheep grow coloured wool, which is used locally for manufactures of coarse Lohis (small blankets).

Changthangi

- **Habitat:** Changthang sub-division of Leh District
- **Wool Yield:** 1.5 kg/annum
- **Wool Quality:** Coarse and long wool
- **Characteristic:** Animals are big sized, usually coloured, coarse woolen. Sheep are used as a transport animal in the mountains.

Poonchi

- **Habitat:** Poonch and surrounding places situated at high elevation in the state
- **Wool Yield:** 1.6 kg/annum
- **Wool Quality:** Medium fine with average fiber diameter 32μ
- **Characteristic:** Animals are long sized, mostly hornless with short tail but thick at the base. Ears are generally short and colour is predominantly white. These sheep are best for wool production and are raised on rich summer pastures and are stall fed during winter on stored grasses and fodders.

Diseases of Sheep

Viral Diseases

- Blue Tongue disease
- Foot and Mouth disease
- Peste-des-petits-ruminants (PPR)
- Sheep pox

Bacterial Diseases

- Black legs
- Enterotoxemia
- Johne's disease
- Listeriosis

Fungal Diseases

- Facial eczema

Protozoal diseases

- Babesia species
- Trypanosoma species
- Toxoplasma gondii
- Eimeria species

Helminths

Flat Worms

- Fasciola species
- Schostosoma bovis
- Dicrocoelium dendriticum

Tape Worms

- Echinococcus granulosus
- Taenia ovis
- Taenia hydatigena
- Moniezia species

Round Worms

- Trichuris ovis
- Haemonchus contortus
- Dictyocaulus filoria
- Oesophagostomum species
- Cooperia species

Blue Tongue Disease

Blue tongue disease is a contagious, insect-borne, viral disease of ruminants, mainly sheep and less frequently cattle, goat and buffaloes. It is caused by the Blue Tongue virus (BTV). The virus is transmitted by the midge culicoides imicola, culicoides variipennis and other culicoides. The virus belongs to family: Reoviridae and Genus: Orbivirus.

Signs: Major signs are high fever, excessive salivation, swelling of the face and tongue and cyanosis of the tongue. Swelling of the lips and tongue this sign is confined to a minority of the animals. Nasal signs may be prominent, with nasal discharge and stertorous respiration. Some animals also develop foot lesion beginning with coronitis, with consequent lameness. In sheep, this can lead to knee walking. Not all animals develop signs, but all those that do lose condition rapidly and the sickest die within a week. For affected animals which do not die. Recovery is very slow, lasting several months. The incubation period is 5-20 days and all signs usually develop within a month. The mortality rate is normally low, but it is high in susceptible breed of sheep.

Control & Prevention: The main prevention for blue tongue disease is vaccination.

Conclusion

Sheep farming is a traditional Livestock farming business. Before starting a sheep farm, choose proper breeds because maximum profits mostly depend on selecting high quality and healthy sheep breeds. If possible visit some farms practically in your areas and gather experience and finally do it.

References

Handbook of Animal Husbandry (2011). 3rd revised edition, 1233 pp.

Banerjee, G. C. (1998). A text book of Animal Husbandry, 6th edition, 1079 pp.

Sastry, N.S.R. & Thomas, C.K. (2005). Livestock Production Management, 4th revised edition, 642 pp.

Chakrabarti, A. (2011) Text Book of Clinical Veterinary Medicine, 3rd edition, 701 pp.

Verma, D.N. (1999) A text book of Livestock production Management in tropic, 1st edition, 748 pp.

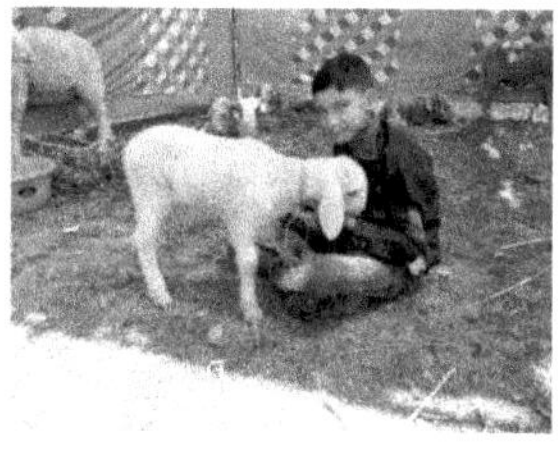
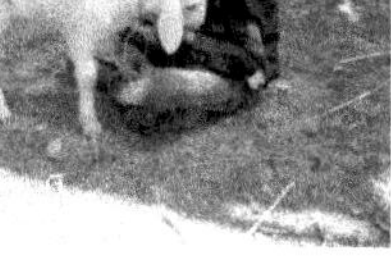

Lamb

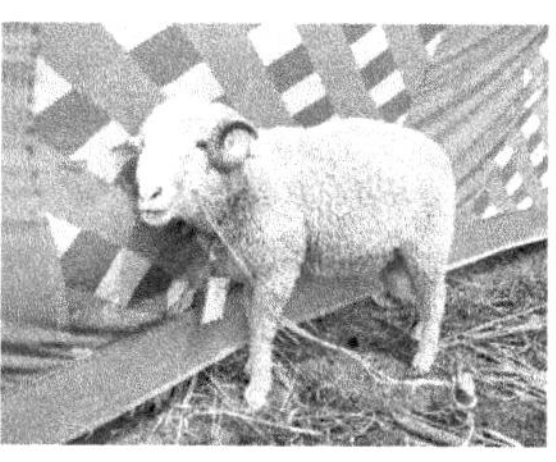
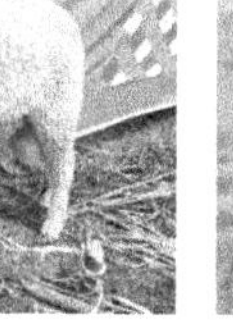

½ Breed RAMBOULLET
Male Adult

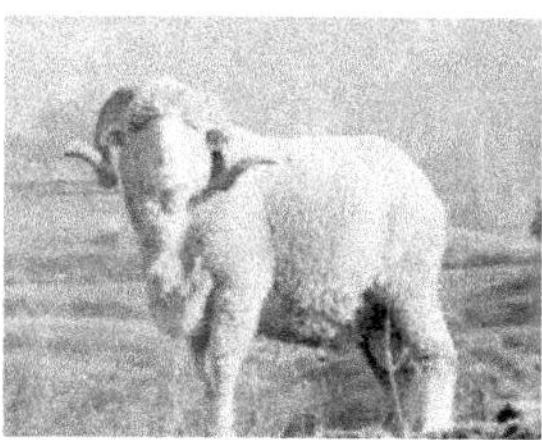

Kashmir Merino

Transforming Rural Areas through Veterinary Science *Pages 323-330*
Editor: Dipanjali Konwar, Shilpa Sood & Shahid Ahamad
Published by: **ASTRAL INTERNATIONAL PVT. LTD., NEW DELHI**

25 Yak: Largest Animal of Cold Desert of Ladakh Region

Dr. Surinder K. Gupta & Dr. Suraj Amrutkar

Introduction

The domestic yak (*Bos grunniens*) is a long haired domesticated bovine found throughout the Himalayan region of the Indian subcontinent as well as in the Tibetan plateau, Mongolia and Russia. Theyareoriginated from the wild yaks. Yaks are belonging to the genus *Bos* and are therefore related to cattle. The yak is the only bovine species (ruminant) whichresides in the high hills of the Himalayas even at altitudes of 6000 meters above the mean sea level. The normal living range of yak is at 3000 to 4500 meters height from the mean sea level which are tree less uplands. Similar to domestic cattle and goat, chromosomes number of yak is 60. Zoological name of yak is *Poephagus grunniens* or *Bos grunniens*.

Ladakh is a region in the Indian state of Jammu & Kashmir that currently extends from the Siachen Glacier in the Karakoram Range to the main great Himalayas to the south, inhabited by people of Indo-Aryan and Tibetan descent. It is one of the most sparsely populated regions in Jammu and Kashmir and its culture is history is closely related to that of Tibet. The Ladakh is renowned for its remote mountain beauty and culture. Yak is the dominant livestock species that support livelihood. Yak is a main source of livelihood for the high altitude residents in Ladakh.

Distribution

The distribution of Yak is majorly found in Northern Ladakh, the plateau of Tibet and part of the Kansu province in China. Within India, yak mostly found in Changechenmo valley in Ladakh and spiti valleys of Himachal Pradesh, and also in North Eastern states, particularly in Arunachal Pradesh, Sikkim and Nagaland. Small number of yaks is also found in Garhwal district of Uttar Pradesh. It is native in Tibet country as well as surrounding countries in Central Asia. The yak is also found in Pakistan, NorthernAfghanisthan, Bhutan, Mongolia and in China.

Zoological Classification

The Yak is belongs to the Phylum: Chordata (Vertebrates), Class: Mammalia (milk giving), order: Artiodactyla (even toed hoofed animals), Family: Bovidae.

Yak Population Status

Yak population in India is 77000 number.

State Wise Population of India

States	*Population*
Jammu and Kashmir	54000
Arunachal Pradesh	14000
Sikkim	4000
Himachal Pradesh	3000
West Bengal	1000
Total (India)	77000

Population Status of Jammu & Kashmir

Category	*2003*	*2007*	*2012*	*% change from 2007-12*
Male Yak	15	28.71	24.0	-16.41
Female Yak	32	33.20	30.09	-9.37
Total Yak	47	61.91	54.49	-11.98

Research Station

The Indian Government established a research center for Yak husbandry under ICAR, National Research Centre on Yak, in 1989. NRC Yak is located at Dirang, Arunachal Pradesh and maintains a yak farm in the Nyukmadung areas at an altitude of 2750 m above sea level. Scientist of this stationare conducting various surveys and the study on feeding, breeding management and disease control aspects of yak at hilly regions in India to improve its productivity and utility.

Yaks Sports

Yak racing is a form of entertainment at traditional festivals and is considered an important fragment of Tibet culture. More recently, sport involving domesticated yaks, such as *Yak skiing* or *Yak polo* are being marketed as tourist attractions in Central Asian countries.

Domestic Yak

The yak had been domesticated thousands years B.C. by the Tibetans. The domestic yaks are considerably smaller than its wild ancestor. Domestic yaks has brown, yellow, reddish-grey and piebald colour. The wild yaks are black and pure white in colour. Domestic yaks coat are resemble with the wild ones. The horns are weaker; even hornless animals are not too rare, at a ratio of 1:100. Now the domestic yaks have a much wider distribution than the wild yaks. Domestic yaks make frequent grunting sounds in dissimilarity to the wild yak. Domestic yak is also called *"grunting ox"*. Both wild and the domestic yaks have the most surefooted mountain animals.They can proceed without stumbling along the worst mountain paths, with a wall of rock on one side and a void on the other side but without ever falling. Yaks from centuries past been domesticated at the Himalayas by interbreeding with domestic cattle.Two kinds of hybrids are known which *i.e.* horned (ZO) and hornless (Zum). Yaks are also interbreeding with several other members of the genus Bos, such as Bison, Banting, Gajal, Zebu and European cattle. Interbreeding with buffaloes is not possible in case of yak.The resultant male offspring of all crossbreeds with yaks are always sterile. More than 90% yaks found in Mongolia are hornless. Like other bovines, yak love to stand or wallow in running water (the icy streams which spring from the snow of the glacier).

Wild Yaks

Yak's sense of smell is excellent, although its eye sight is only ordinary. In general, they are resident of the coldest, widest and most desolate mountains, where both arctic and desert conditions prevail. In fact wild yak's survival is one of continuous struggle against the adverse forces of its environment. It is one of the animals in the world which live at higher level. In summer time, yaks are living at elevations ranging from 4270 to 6100 metre and even in winter they do not descent much below this level.The colour of a wild yak is a uniform blackish brown with a little whitish muzzle but in the domestic yaks usually have patches of white on the chest and tail. Usually they live in small herds, except during the spring when the newly sprouting grass attracts large groupings. In high altitudes where neither man nor wolf go, yaks usually achieve the record age of about 25 years when they finally die of old age.The wild bull's horns are much more massive than those of domestic yaks.

Physical Characteristic

Yak is a heavily built animal with a bulky frame, sturdy legs rounded cloven hooves and extremely dense, long fur that hangs down lower than the belly.Male yak weight is 350-580 kg and female yak weight is 225-255kg. Male yak is comparatively heavier than female yak. Wild yaks are heavier as compared to domestic yak, bulls reaching weight upto 1000 kg. Depending upon the breed of domestic yak, males are 115-138cm high at withers while female yak are 105-117cm high at the withers. Both sexes have long shaggy hair with a dense wooly undercoat over the chest, flanks and thighs to protect them from the cold. Especially in bulls, this may form a long "skirt", which can reach the ground. The tail is long and horse like rather than tufted like cattle or bison.Domesticated yaks have a varied range of coat colours with some individuals being white, grey, brown, roan or piebald. The udder in female and scrotum in males are small and hairy as safeguard against the cold. Female yak has four teats.Yak is grunting animal unlike cattle and are not known to produce the characteristic bovine lowing (moving) sound which inspired the scientific name of the domestic yak variant, *Bos grunniens* (grunting bull).

The wild yak is massively built animal which has drooping head, high humped shoulders, a straight back, and a short sturdy limbs. The dewlap is absent. The yak has 14 pairs of ribs instead of 13 in all other bulls. The withers are formed by an extended spinal process of the vertebra, and since the 7th cervical vertebra is much higher, the line gently slopes to the crops. The skull is bulky, broad and well-proportionate because of the considerable length of the frontal and nasal bone. The horns are beautifully curved. The size of the base is 50 cm apart. In female, the horns are much weaker and more irregularly shaped. The coat on the top of the head, wither and back is rather short but densely matted, while on the shoulders and sides of rump it longer like a mane. The head hair is curly. The yak has a thin muzzle, small & dilatable nostrils, enlarged nasal cavity which is highly coiled, large thoracic cavity and well developed lungs. These features help the animal in having better oxygen carrying capacity and mechanical economy in movements on the hills.

Physiology

Yak physiology is well adapted to high altitude. Yak has larger lungs and heart than cattle found at lower altitude. Yak has greater capacity for transporting oxygen through their blood due to persistence of foetal hemoglobin throughout life.On the other hand, yaks have trouble thriving at lower altitudes, and are prone to suffering from heat exhaustion above about 15°C (59°F). Additional adaptations to the cold include a thick layer of subcutaneous fat, and an almost complete lack of functional sweat glands. As compared to domestic cattle, the rumen of yaks is unusually large, relative to the omasum. It allows them to consume greater quantities of low quality food at a time, and to ferment it longer so as to extract more nutrients. Yak consume the equivalent of 1% of their body weight daily but cattle require about 3% to maintain body condition.

Odour

Yak and their manure have little to no detectable odour when maintained in pastures or paddocks with adequate access to forage and water. Yak's wool is naturally odour resistant.

Reproduction

Yaks mate in summer typically between July and September. In the rest of the year, many bulls wonder in small bachelor groups away from the large herds, but, as the rut approaches, they become aggressive and regularly flight among each other to establish dominance. In addition to non-violent threat displays, yak also start bellowing and scraping the ground with their horns, repeatedly charging at each other with heads lowered or sparring with their horns. Like Bison, but unlike cattle, males wallow in dry soil during the rut; often while scent marking with urine or dung. Female enter estrus upto four times a year, and females are receptive only for a few hours in each cycle. Gestation period of yak is about 257 - 270 days, so that the young yakis born between May and June, and results in the birth of a single calf. The cow finds a separate location to give birth, but the calf is able to walk within about 10 minutes of birth and the pair soon rejoins the herd. Female of both the wild and domestic forms typically gives birth only once every other year; although more frequent births are possible if the food supply is good.Calves are weaned approximate at one year and become independent shortly thereafter. Wild calves are initially brown in colour and only later develop the darker adult hair. Females generally give birth for the first time at 3 to 4 years of age and reach their peak reproductive fitness at around six years. Yaks may live for more than 20 years in domestication or captivity, although it is likely that this may be somewhat shorter in the wild.

The mating (rutting) season begins in September and lasts for one whole month. The old bulls like to live singly or in small groups of 3 to 5 except for mating season when they join the cows for some weeks and have bitter rival fights among themselves during which each animal tries to push his horn into the opponents flank. However, the wounds heal quickly in the sterile air at these altitudes. Only during the mating season,wild yaks make strange grunting sounds. The rest of the time,it is not a common. Cows give birthto their calves during April to June after a gestation period of 9 months when the new-grown grass ensures a good feed supply. Calving takes place only during second year because the young are dependent on them for the year. The yak is considered to be fully grown only at 6 to 8 years old. In case of domestic yak, the oestrus is irregular, cows in contrast to wild form calves every year in April or May.

Inbreeding can be minimizes by exchanging bulls among different herds. Reproductive efficiency can be improved by nutritional supplementation during winter. Early weaning or restricted suckling may shorten the duration of postpartum cyclicity; however, it is impractical due to reduced growth rates and increased winter mortality of early weaned calves. A single treatment with either GnRH, or PGF_{2alfa} successfully inducedestrus in yak cows that calved in previous years (with or without calf), did not calves in the current year, however, it has little effect in cows, nursing a calf born in the current year.

Hybrid yak

In Nepal, Tibet and Mongolia, domestic cattle are cross bred with yaks. They gives rise to the infertile male also called as *Dzo*, as well as fertile female also called as *Dzomo or Zhom* which may be cross again with cattle. Crosses between yaks and domestic cattle (*Bosprimigenius Taurus*) have been recorded in Chinese literature for at least 2000 years. Successful crosses have also been recorded between Yak and American Bison and Gaur, generally with similar results to those produced with domestic cattle.

Relationship with Humans

Domesticated yaks have been kept for thousands of years primarily for their milk, fibre and meat. Their dried droppings are an important fuel. Yaks transport goods across mountain passes for local farmers and traders as well as for climbing and trekking expeditions. They are also used to draw ploughs. Yaks milk is often processes to a cheese called *Chhurpi* in Tibetan and Nepali languages. Butter made of yak's milk is an ingredient of the butter tea that Tibetans consume in large quantities and is also used in lamps and made into butter sculptures used in religious festivities.

Composition of Yak Milk

Nutrients		*Quantity*
Fat		10.90 %
Water	81.85%	
Protein		4.06%
Total solids		19.25%
Ash		0.98%
pH		6.6 (Slightly acidic)

Composition of Yak Meat

Nutrients	*Quantity*
Fat	7%
Water	68%
Protein	20%
Ash	5.1%
Calcium	1.28 %
Phosphorus	1.08%

Utility

The utilities of yak are summarized below:

- Since domestic yak requires little food and is insensitive to cold temperature, it is the best suited domestic animal in Asia at elevations above 2000 metres.
- Without yak, travel and trade in lonely trans-Himalayas regions would be extremely difficult. It easily carries loads of 150 kg over the steepest mountain paths.
- The milk production is somewhat lower with averages about 500 litres/ per year, but the milk has a high nutritious value with a fat content of 7 to 11 percent. The composition varies from area to area, and also on the quantity and quality of feed. In Tibet, a milk powder is prepared (besides butter and cheese) by a special process of coagulation.
- Occasionally, the yak is slaughtered at old age for meat particularly in many parts of hilly tracts. The meat tastes good but is highly rich is in fat content. The meat fiber is finer than those of beef and resembles mutton fibers.
- The yak annually produces 300-600gm of down hair and 1000-2000gm of coarse hair. The down hair is similar to pashmina which is used for making garments. The coarse hair is used for preparing bags, ropes, carpets and tents.
- The yak's manure is often the only fuel in the highlands of Tibet where there are no trees or bushes.

- Yak bullocks (castrated) are used for ploughing and threshing grains. Crosses between yak and zebu also give milk & better meat and are excellent work animals for carrying loads at moderate altitudes. The cross-bred males are always sterile.

Feeding

Very little is well-known about the feeding of yaks. They are livingon small herds, except during the spring when the newly sprouting grass attracts large assemblages. In summer, their food contains mainly of wiry tuffs of grass and small shrubs which clothe the barren plateau. They also eat much of the salt encrusted earth.Winter is a time of great hardship, when many die of starvation and exposure. When grazing at extreme heights, melting snow is their usual liquid nourishment. When grass is extremely scarce, and cattle and horses cannot survive for long, the yaks are capable of existing by eating up broken and wilted blades of last year's grass which have been blown by the wind and particularly embedded in the soil. In such areas, yak may spend upto 8 hours a day licking up dead grass, and thus remain alive and keep on working. For this purpose, yaks travel in single file, each animal carefully places its feet in the imprints left by the hoofs of the one preceding it.

In India during June, the yak herdsmen moves their herds to pastures situated 4000-5000 meter above the mean sea level, after making a journey of 3 to 4 days from their villages. At this height, the herdsmen live in temporary huts, bearing high winds and occasional snowing. The average temperature during this period is 4-5°C. The yaks are allowed to graze from morning to evening, and milked once in a day. Cash sale is rare, and most transaction is done through barter system. With the onset of winter in October, the herdsmen come down to their villages along with their yaks. The winter pastures of the middle altitudes are very poor both in quantity and nutritive values. Even in summer pasture lands are almost devoid of legumes and are profusely infested with weeds resulting suboptimal production among yaks. Yaks grazing in snow covered Himalayan Mountains. They are most commonly found in alpine meadows with a relatively thick carpet of grasses and sedges.

Diseases of Yak

Yak and cattle often share the same habitat, especially during the winter season. It is not surprising that many of the diseases observed in cattle are also reported in yak.

- **Bacterial Diseases:** Anthrax, Botulism, Brucellosis, Chlamydia infection, Leptospirosis, Lymphadenitis, Mastitis, Pasteurellosis, Salmonellosis, Tetanus, Tuberculosis, Black quarter, Coxiellaburneti infection, Kerato-conjunctivitis and Camphylo-bacteriosis.
- **Viral Diseases:** FMD, Infectious Bovine Rhinotracheitis, Rinderpest and Viral diarrhea/Mucosal disease
- **Parasitic Disease:**
    - ***Ecto-Parasites:*** Ticks, Fleas, Lice and Mites

- *Protozoa:*Babesiosis

☆ *Endoparasites:*Gid disease (Coenurosis), Liver fluke and Round worms

☆ **Miscellaneous Conditions:**Contagious skin disease, Contaminated water and Mineral and trace elements deficiency

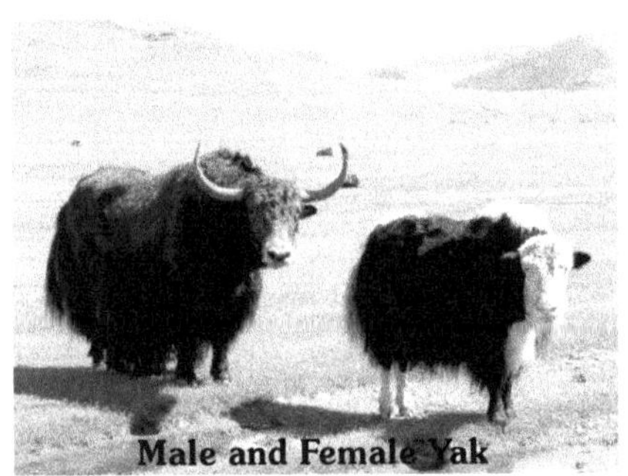
Male and Female Yak

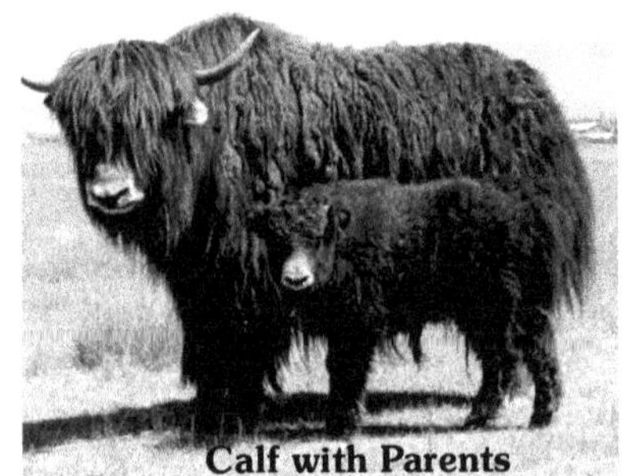
Calf with Parents

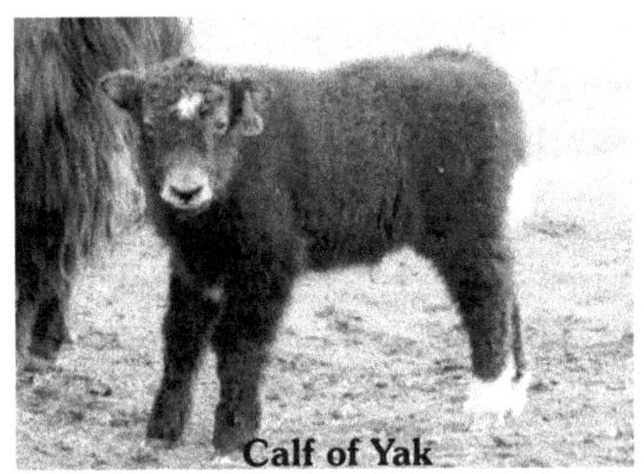
Calf of Yak

Transforming Rural Areas through Veterinary Science *Pages* **331-336**
Editor: Dipanjali Konwar, Shilpa Sood & Shahid Ahamad
Published by: **ASTRAL INTERNATIONAL PVT. LTD., NEW DELHI**

26 Strategies to Check Mastitis in Dairy Cow

Dr. Surinder K. Gupta & Dr. Suraj Amrutkar

Introduction

Bovine mastitis is the persistent, inflammatory reaction of the udder tissue due to physical trauma or infections microorganisms. Mastitis is a potentially fatal mammary gland infection. Mastitis is the most common diseases in dairy cattle in India and worldwide. It is the most costly disease to the dairy industry because it affects the whole economics of dairy farmers.

Prevention and control of mastitis requires regularity in sanitizing the cow barn facilities, proper milking procedure and segregation of infected animals. Mastitis takes place when white blood cells (leukocytes) are released into the mammary gland, usually in response to bacteria invading the teat canal or occasionally by trauma on the udder. Milk secreting tissue and various ducts throughout the mammary gland are damaged due to toxins released by the bacteria,and it results in reduced milk yield and quality. Meanwhile the quality and quantity of the milk is influenced by mastitis. It is considered to be one of the most important causes of economic losses in the dairy industry worldwide. Somatic cells are the part of the natural defense mechanism which includes lymphocytes, macrophages, polymorpho nuclear cells and some epithelial cells. Somatic cells count can be measured by California Mastitis Test. It is a simple, easy and low cost screening test for subclinical mastitis at dairy farms.

Mastitis in cows is the inflammation of the cow's udder tissue. This disease is a major endemic disease of dairy cattle but can also affect all other lactating mammals. When bacteria get entry into the udder through the teat canal, they find nutrients in the udder and multiply rapidly.Their metabolic byproducts cause poisoning of the udder tissues which results into an inflammation.This inflammation is due to the cow's auto immune response to the toxic metabolites released by the bacteria. Mastitis can also occur due to chemical, mechanical or thermal wound to the cow's udder. The bacterial byproducts released in the udder tissue can damage the milk secreting tissues and ducts through-out the udder. In some situation, the damage is permanent and the udder losses its functionality. Acute cases can lead to fatalities whereas cows that recover will be incapacitated for the rest of their lactation lives.

Identification

This disease can be recognized by abnormalities in the udder such as swelling, heat, redness, hardness or pain (if it is clinical). Other symptoms of mastitis may be abnormalities in milk such as a watery appearance, flakes or clots. When infected with sub-clinical mastitis, a cow does not display any visible signs of infection or abnormalities in milk or on the udder.

Mastitis is an inflammation of the mammary gland caused by bacteria that enter the udder through the teat end. *Mastitis is nearly always caused by bacteria that invade the udder through the teat end and multiply there. Mastitis can be either clinical or sub-clinical.*

Clinical mastitis is mastitis in which an abnormality of the udder or abnormal secretion is observed. Clinical mastitis can be mild, moderate or severe. Cows with mild clinical mastitis typically have abnormalities in the milk such as clots and flakes with little or no swelling of the gland or systemic illness. Cows with severe clinical mastitis typically have a sudden onset of udder inflammation, abnormal milk, and systemic sign such as fever, increased heart rate, dehydration, weakness and depression.

Sub-clinical mastitis is a form of mastitis in which the udder condition is normal as well the milk appears normal. *However, micro-organisms can usually be cultured from the milk and inflammatory changes in the milk can be detected by measuring the somatic cell count.*

Status of Mastitis

Due to mastitis in cows causes severe wastage of milk, and undesirable milk quality. It is major challenging trait while selecting breed for breeding development as well as during nutritional management, control of internal parasitic diseases in dairy development of tropics.

Subclinical mastitis was found more in India, varying from 10-50% in cows and 5-20% in buffaloes than clinical mastitis (1-10%). Some cattle breeds are highly susceptible for mastitis disease. The incidence was highest in pure bred Holsteins and Jerseys and lowest in local cattle and buffaloes.

Monsoon season was more prone to sub-clinical mastitis than summer or winter. Incidence increases with higher lactation number and animals in 4th-5th month of lactation were found more susceptible (59.49%), and hind quarter were found more affected (56.52%) than fore quarters (43.47%). The factors like herd size, agro climatic conditions of the region, variations in socio-cultural practices, milk marketing, literacy level of the animal owner, system of feeding and management were found important affecting the incidence of subclinical mastitis.

Etiology

Disease causing bacteria are called pathogens. The most common mastitis pathogens are found in the udder tissues, spreading from cow-to-cow (contagious pathogens) or in the herds surroundings (environmental pathogens), such as bedding materials, manure and soil.

Contagious pathogens that cause mastitis tend to live on the cow's udder and teat skin and transfer from affected cow (or quarter) to unaffected cow (or quarter) during milking. They adhere easily to the skin, colonizing the teat end and then grow into the teat canal, where infection occurs, because of this, post milking teat disinfection and dry cow therapy play in important role in controlling contagious mastitis. Farms with high levels of contagious mastitis often have high Somatic Cell Counts.

Environmental mastitis pathogens present in the housing and bedding can transfer during milking or between milking, when the cows is loafing, eating or lying down. The pathogens can enter the teat canal by force during milking, for example, when liner slippage occurs. These environmental pathogens do not generally possess the same ability as contagious pathogens to adhere to and colonise in the teat; dry cow therapy has little value in their control as these type of infections do not carry from one lactation to the next.

Most common bacteria known to cause mastitis are *Pseudomaonas aeruginosa, Streptococcus agalactiae, Streptococcus uberis, Staphylocossus aureus, Staphylocossus epidermidis, Brucella melitensis, Corynebacterium bovis, Mycoplasma bovis, Escherichia* coli, *Websiella pneumonia, Klebsiella oxytoca, enterobact eraerogenes, Pastuerella species, Proteus species etc.*

Transmission

Mastitis is most frequently transmitted by repetitive contact with the milking machine and through contaminated hands and materials. Another route of transmission is via oral-to-udder among calves.

Effects on Milk Composition

Mastitis can cause a decline in potassium and increase in lactoferrin in milk. It also results in decreased casein which is the major protein in milk. As most calcium in milk is linked with casein, the disruption of casein synthesis contributes to lowered calcium in milk. The milk protein continues to deterioration during processing and storage. Milk from mastitis cows also has a higher somatic cell count. The higher somatic cells count leads to the lower the milk quality.

Losses of Farmers Due to Mastitis

Mastitis cow milk has to throw away by the farmers because the milk may contaminate by medication for being unfit for consumption. The cows will produce less milk during the illness. A permanent udder tissue injury will negatively affect the milk yield. The farmers have to spend extra labor for the management of the sick/mastitis cows. Medication and veterinary services for treating the sick cows is very high. Sick cow has a lesser productive lifespan due to the injured udders. Cross contaminations in the farm can lead to loss of the entire herd due to premature culling. Dairy cows have many predisposing factors to mastitis infections such as the risk of contamination from milking equipments, hygiene of the milking equipment handlers and cleanliness of the cleaning water.

Detection of Mastitis

Visualization and Palpation of the Udder

In clinical mastitis, the udder may turn hard, red and hot to the touch. Palpation of the udder may be painful to the cow. These symptoms arise from the changes in vascularity and blood flow of the gland when inflamed.

Vasculization of the Milk

Gross changes in the milk may be observed at the time of milking such as the presence of flakes, clots or serous milk. This is the most common means of detection of clinical mastitis. Stripping the first few squirts of milk from each quarter into a strip cup at the beginning of milking is a preferred method of detecting flakes or clots in the milk.

California Mastitis Test

The California Mastitis Test (CMT) is a simple cow-side indicator of the somatic cell count of milk. It operates by disrupting the cell membrane of any cells present in the milk sample, allowing the DNA in those cells to react with the reagent, forming a gel. It provides a useful technique for detecting subclinical cases for mastitis. The reaction between Sodium hydroxide and milk resulted in the thickening of mastitis milk. The utility of this reaction in a field test was limited because the reaction was sometimes difficult to observe and would eventually occur even in normal milk.

A four well plastic paddle is used, one well for each quarter of the cow to be tested. Foremilk is discarded, and then a little milk drawn into each well. An equal volume of test reagent is added, and gently agitated. The reaction is scored on a scale of 0 (mixture remains unchanged) to 3 (almost solid gel forms), with a score 2 or 3 being considered a positive result. A special reagent for the test is marketed under the name "CMT-test" but domestic detergents are frequently used instead, being cheaper and more readily available.

Modified California Mastitis Test (MCMT) is more sensitive (96.16%) and specific (98.02%) test.

Treatment

Treatment is possible with long-lasting antibiotics. The antimicrobial susceptibility test revealed that most of the bacterial strains (gram positive, gram negative and mixed) isolated from sub-clinical mastitis milk samples, which were highly sensitive to Enrofloxacin (53.91%), Least sensitive to Oxytetracycline (17.39%) &Ampicillin (7.83%); and resistant to Streptomycin. *The therapy with Enrofloxacin and Nimesulide was found more effective (92.30%) in treating sub-clinical mastitis cows.* Treatment of the disease may also carry out by penicillin injection with sulphur drug.

Control Measures to Check Mastitis

Mastitis control program can reduce economical loss and increase herd efficacy and milk hygiene. Epidemiological data including mastitis prevalence, mastitis causing organisms, predisposing factors and response to treatment are necessary for the establishment of a mastitis control programme. Following are the some measures given to control mastitis:

Environmental

- ✩ Animals should always be housed in a clean, dry environment
- ✩ Keep cow clear of manure, mud, pools of water and high moisture areas
- ✩ Keep the calving area as clean as possible for both cows and calf
- ✩ Keep the standard same for dry and lactating cows

Bedding

- ✩ Regularly clean out the old bedding, and add new bedding
- ✩ Refresh bedding and more often in warm & wet weather
- ✩ Choose bedding wisely such as inorganic materials like sand which helps bacteria at a minimum level because it is low in nutrient and moisture

Udder Cleanliness

- ✩ Always pre-and-post dip at milking
- ✩ Use a germicidal dip to keep germs at a minimum, and which helps to prevent the spread of contagious organisms
- ✩ Try to keep udders as clean and dirt free as possible

Dry Cow Therapy

- ✩ Complete on all four quarters of dairy cows at dry off to control environmental streptococci

Milking Procedures

- ✩ Have a standard operating procedures for your milking routine-outline pre-and-post dipping, length of time dip is on, the percentage of the teat that should be covered with dip, what to do with wet or unclean udders, *etc.*

Other Control to Prevent Environmental Mastitis Cows Cases

Maintain your milking machine to prevent liner slips and teat end conditions that can increase the rate of mastitis cows. Ensure cow's ration has enough vitamin-E and Selenium. Consider a vaccination programme against Coliform bacteria.

Practices such as good nutrition, proper milking hygiene, and the culling of chronically infected cow can helps to prevent mastitis. Ensure that cow has clean dry bedding which decreases the risk as well as transmission of infection. Dairy workers should wear rubber gloves while milking; and machines should be cleaned regularly to decrease the incidence of transmission of infection.

A good milking routine should be dynamic. This usually consists of applying a pre-milking teat dip or spray such as iodine spray, and wiping teats dry prior to milking. The milking machine may use for milking. After milking, the teats can be cleaned again to remove any growth medium for bacteria. A post milking products such as *iodine-propylene glycol dip*may be used as a disinfectant which work as a barrier between the open teats and the bacteria in the air. Mastitis can occur after milking because the teat holes are open up to 15 minutes, in this period infection may get entry if the animal site in a dirty place with feces and urine.

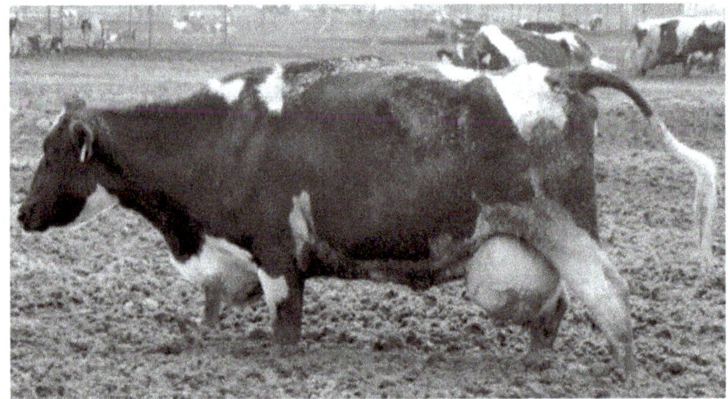

Clinical Mastitis in Cow

Index

A

B

C

D

E

F

G

H

I

O

P

Q

R

S

T

U

V

W

Y

Z